Color Atlas of
Cosmetic
Dermatology

Color Atlas of
Cosmetic Dermatology
Second Edition

Zeina Tannous, MD
Chief, Mohs/Dermatologic Surgery, Boston VA Medical Center
Massachusetts General Hospital, Dermatology Laser & Cosmetic Center
Affiliate Faculty, Wellman Center for Photomedicine
Faculty Director for Dermatopathology, Department of Dermatology, Harvard Medical School
Assistant Professor in Dermatology, Harvard Medical School
Boston, Massachusetts

Mathew M. Avram, MD, JD
Director
Massachusetts General Hospital, Dermatology Laser & Cosmetic Center
Faculty Director for Procedural Dermatology Training, Department of Dermatology, Harvard Medical School
Affiliate Faculty, Wellman Center for Photomedicine
Boston, Massachusetts

Sandy Tsao, MD
Director of Procedural Dermatology
Harvard Medical School
Massachusetts General Hospital, Dermatology Laser & Cosmetic Center
Boston, Massachusetts

Marc R. Avram, MD
Clinical Professor of Dermatology
Weill Cornell Medical School
Private Practice—905 Fifth Avenue
New York, New York

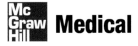

New York   Chicago   San Francisco   Lisbon   London   Madrid
Mexico City   Milan   New Delhi   San Juan   Seoul   Singapore   Sydney   Toronto

Color Atlas of Cosmetic Dermatology, Second Edition

1 2 3 4 5 6 7 8 9 0   CTP/CTP   15 14 13 12 11

ISBN 978-0-07-163503-5
MHID 0-07-163503-3

Notice

Medicine is an ever-changing science. As new research and clinical experience broaden
our knowledge, changes in treatment and drug therapy are required. The authors and the
publisher of this work have checked with sources believed to be reliable in their efforts to
provide information that is complete and generally in accord with the standards accepted
at the time of publication. However, in view of the possibility of human error or changes
in medical sciences, neither the authors nor the publisher nor any other party who has
been involved in the preparation or publication of this work warrants that the information
contained herein is in every respect accurate or complete, and they disclaim all responsi-
bility for any errors or omissions or for the results obtained from use of the information
contained in this work. Readers are encouraged to confirm the information contained
herein with other sources. For example and in particular, readers are advised to check the
product information sheet included in the package of each drug they plan to administer to
be certain that the information contained in this work is accurate and that changes have
not been made in the recommended dose or in the contraindications for administration.
This recommendation is of particular importance in connection with new or infrequently
used drugs.

This book was set in TradeGothic by Aptara, Inc.
The editors were Anne M. Sydor and Cindy Yoo.
The production supervisor was Sherri Souffrance.
Project management was provided by Saima Ghaffar, Aptara, Inc.
Design adapted from original by Alan Barnett; the cover was designed by Pehrsson Design.
Cover image of woman having a neurotoxin injection (c) Image Source/Corbis.
China Translation & Printing, Ltd., was printer and binder.

Library of Congress Cataloging-in-Publication Data

Color atlas of cosmetic dermatology. – 2nd ed. / Zeina Tannous ... [et al.].
p. ; cm.
  Cosmetic dermatology
  Rev. ed. of: Color atlas of cosmetic dermatology / Marc R. Avram ... [et al.]. c2007.
  Includes bibliographical references and index.
  ISBN-13: 978-0-07-163503-5 (hardcover)
  ISBN-10: 0-07-163503-3 (hardcover)
  1. Skin–Care and hygiene–Atlases. 2. Skin–Diseases–Treatment–Atlases. 3. Surgery,
Plastic–Atlases. 4. Dermatology–Atlases. I. Tannous, Zeina. II. Title: Cosmetic dermatology.
  [DNLM: 1. Cosmetic Techniques–Atlases. 2. Skin Diseases–therapy–Atlases. WR 17]
  RL87.C65 2011
  616.50022'3–dc22
                          2010041090

DEDICATION

I would like to dedicate this book to the memory of my beloved father,
who always gave me his ultimate love and support.

Zeina Tannous, MD

I would like to dedicate this book to my wonderful parents, Morrell and
Maria Avram. You have provided me unconditional love and endless
support since the day I was born. I love you.

Mathew M. Avram, MD, JD

To my husband, Hensin. You are my strength and inspiration. Your love, wisdom and
encouragement help me realize anything is possible. You are a wonderful husband,
father and best friend. I will love you always. To my sons, Sebastian and Hunter. Your
unconditional love, enthusiasm and sense of adventure help me remember what is truly
important. You brighten my days and fill my life with happiness and love.

Sandy Tsao, MD

This book is dedicated to my wife Robin and my two sons Robert and Jacob.
I thank them for the love and support that they give me every day.

Marc R. Avram, MD

CONTENTS

Preface ix

SECTION ONE: PHOTOAGING

Chapter 1: **Analysis of the Aging Face and Non-Facial Regions** 2

Chapter 2: **Topical Treatment Options** 7

Chapter 3: **Soft Tissue Augmentation** 14

Chapter 4: **Botulinum Toxin** 21

Chapter 5: **Chemical Peels** 29

Chapter 6: **Nonablative Laser Resurfacing** 39

Chapter 7: **Ablative Laser Resurfacing** 43

Chapter 8: **Nonablative Fractional Laser Resurfacing** 52

Chapter 9: **Ablative Fractional Laser Resurfacing** 57

Chapter 10: **Tissue Tightening** 62

Chapter 11: **Dermatochalasis** 64

Chapter 12: **Poikiloderma of Civatte** 67

SECTION TWO: DISORDERS OF SEBACEOUS GLANDS

Chapter 13: **Acne Vulgaris** 72

Chapter 14: **Rosacea** 76

Chapter 15: **Sebaceous Hyperplasia** 81

SECTION THREE: DISORDERS OF ECCRINE GLANDS

Chapter 16: **Hyperhidrosis** 86

SECTION FOUR: DISORDERS OF HAIR FOLLICLES

Chapter 17: **Hirsutism** 92

Chapter 18: **Pseudofolliculitis** 99

Chapter 19: **Male Pattern Hair Loss** 103

Chapter 20: **Female Pattern Hair Loss** 126

Chapter 21: **Low Level Light Therapy (LLLT) and Hair Loss** 133

SECTION FIVE: DISORDERS OF PIGMENTATION

Chapter 22: **Café Au Lait Macule** 136

Chapter 23: **Ephelides** 139

Chapter 24: **Lentigines** 144

Chapter 25: **Melasma** 149

Chapter 26: **Nevus of Ota** 154

Chapter 27: **Postinflammatory hyperpigmentation** 158

Chapter 28: **Vitiligo** 163

SECTION SIX: VASCULAR ALTERATIONS

Chapter 29: **Angiokeratoma** 168

Chapter 30: **Cherry and Spider Angiomas** 170

Chapter 31: **Granuloma Faciale** 174

Chapter 32: **Infantile Hemangioma** 177

Chapter 33: **Keratosis Pilaris Atrophicans** 181

Chapter 34: **Port-wine Stains** 183

Chapter 35: **Pyogenic Granuloma** 188

Chapter 36: **Facial Telangiectasias** 192

Chapter 37: **Lower Extremity Telangiectasias, Reticular and Varicose Veins** 198

Chapter 38: **Venous Lakes** 203

Chapter 39: **Warts** 206

SECTION SEVEN: BENIGN GROWTHS

Chapter 40: **Angiofibroma** 212

Chapter 41: **Becker's Nevus** 216

Chapter 42: **Epidermal Inclusion Cyst** 219

Chapter 43: **Epidermal Nevus** 222

Chapter 44: **Lipoma** 226

Chapter 45: **Milium** 229

Chapter 46: **Neurofibroma** 231

Chapter 47: **Seborrheic Keratosis** 234

Chapter 48: **Syringoma** 238

Chapter 49: **Dermatosis Papulosa Nigra** 241

Chapter 50: **Xanthelasma** 243

SECTION EIGHT: CUTANEOUS CARCINOMAS

Chapter 51: **Actinic Keratosis** 248

Chapter 52: **Basal Cell Carcinoma** 252

Chapter 53: **Squamous Cell Carcinoma** 256

SECTION NINE: INFLAMMATORY DISORDERS

Chapter 54: **Lichen Planus** 262

Chapter 55: **Morphea** 265

Chapter 56: **Psoriasis** 267

SECTION TEN: ADIPOSE TISSUE ALTERATIONS

Chapter 57: **Gynecomastia** 272

Chapter 58: **Cellulite** 276

Chapter 59: **HIV Lipodystrophy/Facial Lipoatrophy** 280

Chapter 60: **Striae Distensae** 285

SECTION ELEVEN: WOUND HEALING ALTERATIONS

Chapter 61: **Hypertrophic Scars, Keloids, and Acne Scars** 290

SECTION TWELVE EXOGENOUS CUTANEOUS ALTERATIONS

Chapter 62: **Ear Piercing** 298

Chapter 63: **Tattoo Removal** 300

Chapter 64: **Torn Earlobe** 308

Index 311

PREFACE

There has been a revolution in the treatment of medical and cosmetic disorders of the skin. In large part, this is due to the availability of procedures and technologies that produce clear, cosmetic benefit with few side effects and little downtime. With the advent of lasers and light sources over the past 20 years, cosmetic improvement is a matter of quick, relatively painless procedures. Non-laser treatments such as soft tissue fillers, botulinum toxin injections, sclerotherapy, hair transplantation and others have also dramatically expanded the scope of this field. These procedures coincide with the busy lifestyle of many patients who seek an improvement in appearance that does not interfere with their professional, social or personal obligations.

These procedures, however, are not without potential side effects or complications. Physicians who perform these treatments in the absence of training or education are certain to encounter poor results, complications and irate patients. Because patients are pursuing elective treatments for cosmetic benefit, any worsening of appearance will understandably anger patients who under-go these procedures. The decision as to when *not* to treat a patient is perhaps the most important in this field.

With this in mind, *Color Atlas of Cosmetic Dermatology, Second Edition* seeks to provide a succinct yet broad overview of cosmetic therapy. There are a plethora illustrations and graphs to elucidate consultation, management, treatment and side effects of numerous cosmetic procedures. Its practical format is geared to the busy practitioner or trainee who seeks a quick, comprehensive reference for approaching the cosmetic patient. It also emphasizes pitfalls of treatment in order to educate the reader as to potential problems with certain treatments. It serves as an invaluable resource to both the experienced and novice.

Zeina Tannous, MD
Mathew M. Avram, MD, JD
Sandy Tsao, MD
Marc R. Avram, MD

ACKNOWLEDGMENTS

We would like to thank two people who provided significant help in the production of this textbook, Dr. Rox Anderson and Dr. Gary Lask. In addition, we would like to thank the office staff at the Massachusetts General Hospital Dermatology Laser & Cosmetic Center and the office staff of Dr. Marc Avram for their hard work and dedication in obtaining high-quality photographs.

Finally, we would like to thank the professional staff at McGraw-Hill for their great help and devotion in producing this book. Thank you for pushing us to strive for the best possible Atlas.

SECTION ONE

Photoaging

CHAPTER 1 | Analysis of the Aging Face and Non-Facial Regions

The face is the focal point of human beauty. Although various factors influence facial beauty, the aging process is the most common aspect prompting non-surgical and/or surgical intervention. Aging is a dynamic and continual process. Different cultural, ethnic, and gender norms (Table 1.1) of beauty exist; however, there are certain features which globally transcend these differences to determine what is perceptually pleasing. Heredity and environmental factors (eg, sun exposure, wind, trauma) are the main determinants of aging. In addition, cigarette smoking and estrogen loss can accelerate the aging process. As one ages, changes can be observed in all facial and non-facial anatomical compartments, including the skin, subcutaneous fat, muscle, and bony structure. Use of a systematic approach in the analysis of facial and non-facial aging will allow for the selection of appropriate, safe, and effective therapies.

TABLE 1.1 ▪ Facial Age-Related Contour Changes
Malar crescent
Cheek depression
Nasolabial fold formation
Prejowl sulcus
Platysmal bands
Jowl formation

ANATOMIC CONSIDERATIONS

Successful rejuvenation of the face and non-facial regions requires a thorough understanding of age-related contour changes (underlying soft tissue aging) and textural changes (skin aging) (Tables 1.1 and 1.2).

TABLE 1.2 ▪ Age-Related Textural Changes
Superficial and deep rhytides
Pigmentary disturbances
Telangiectasia formation
Loss of skin elasticity
Actinic keratoses

A youthful face can be divided into three facial zones: upper, middle, and lower zones, as well as the upper neck.

The upper face includes the forehead, temple, and periorbital region. Aging results in flattening of the brow arch, eyelid skin redundancy, pseudo fat herniation, and formation of dynamic rhytides at the lateral canthus. Horizontal forehead skin creases develop secondary to sustained contraction of the frontalis muscle in a subconscious attempt to elevate the sagging brows. A rim sulcus deformity develops between the cheek and the eyelid with upper cheek

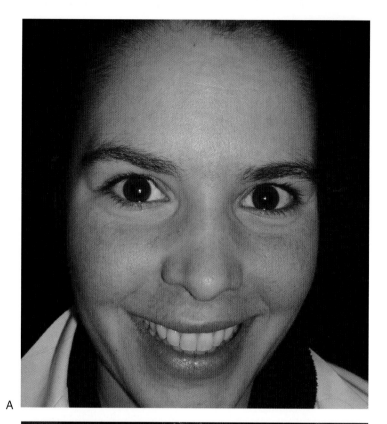
A

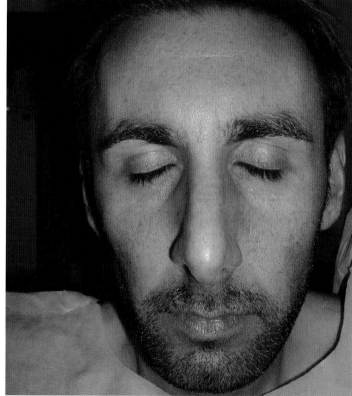
B

Figure 1.1 A&B *Glogau type 1 photoaging. Minimal signs of aging present*

thinning. This sulcus is exacerbated by a preexisting tear trough deformity. Orbicularis oculi muscle ptosis can create a malar fullness, referred to as a malar crescent.

The midface includes the cheekbones that form a smooth continuous convexity from the eyelid to the lip. The melolabial fold represents a flat, smooth junction between the lower cheek and the upper lip. The aging face results in a downward migration of the malar soft tissue, accentuating skeletonization of the orbital rim. Central cheek fat ptosis creates a fullness lateral to the melolabial fold, referred to as nasolabial folds.

The lower face possesses a well-defined mandibular border and a well-defined cervicomental angle. With aging, platysmal muscle ptosis and cheek fat ptosis along the mandible produce "jowls" overlying the jawline. Soft tissue atrophy anterior to the jowls creates a "prejowl sulcus" which accentuates the skeletonized appearance. Platysmal ptosis of the upper neck blunts the cervico-mental angle, creating platysmal bands or a "turkey neck" deformity.

Facial textural changes include superficial and deep rhytides, pigmentary disturbances, telangiectasia formation, loss of skin elasticity, and actinic keratoses.

PREOPERATIVE EVALUATION

An individualized treatment plan designed to minimize surgical risk is essential. The goal is a youthful and natural postoperative result. A strategy should be formulated for each of the three facial zones as well as each individual non-facial region, as each anatomic region requires a specific management which influences the remaining anatomic regions.

A systematic evaluation should include the degree of textural changes, rhytid formation, pigmentary changes, loss of subcutaneous fat, changes in facial musculature, cartilaginous and bony structures, and elasticity loss.

■ Glogau Photoaging Classification— Wrinkle Scale

The Glogau Photoaging Classification has been devised which broadly defines the changes that may be seen at different ages with cumulative sun exposure.

Type 1—"no wrinkles" (Fig. 1.1)

- Early photoaging
  - Mild pigmentary change
  - No keratoses
  - Minimal wrinkles
- Patient age: twenties or thirties
- Minimal or no makeup use

Type 2—"wrinkles in motion" (Fig. 1.2)

- Early to moderate photoaging
  - Early senile lentigines visible

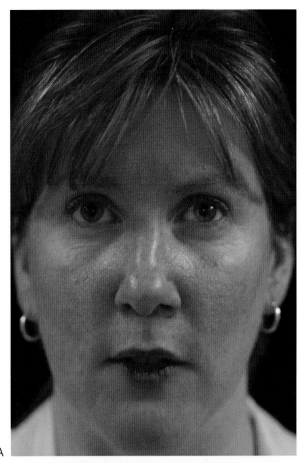

A

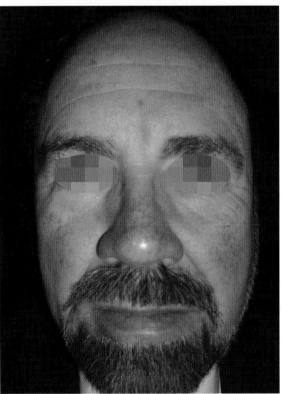

B

Figure 1.2 A&B *Glogau type 2 photoaging. Fine lines barely visible. Minimal pigmentary changes noted*

– Keratoses palpable but not visible

– Parallel smile lines beginning to appear

• Patient age: late thirties or forties

• Usually wears some foundation

Type 3—"wrinkles at rest" (Fig. 1.3)

• Advanced photoaging

– Obvious dyschromia, telangiectasia

– Visible keratoses

– Wrinkles even when not moving

• Patient age: fifties or older

• Always wears heavy foundation

Type 4—"only wrinkles" (Fig. 1.4)

• Severe photoaging

– Yellow-gray [A3] color of skin

– Prior skin malignancies

– Wrinkled throughout, no normal skin

• Patient age: sixties or seventies

• Cannot wear makeup—"cakes and cracks"

■ Pigmentary Changes

A vital aspect of the patient evaluation is the determination of the patient's skin response to erythema-producing doses of ultraviolet light. Fitzpatrick's classification of skin types provides a strong indication of the potential for post-inflammatory hyperpigmentation and hypopigmentation and potential for dyschromia upon epidermal and/or papillary dermal injury (Table 1.3).

TABLE 1.3 ■ Fitzpatrick's Classification of Skin Types

Skin type	Color	Reaction to sun
I	Very white or freckled	Always burns
II	White	Usually burns
III	White to olive	Sometimes burns
IV	Brown	Rarely burns
V	Dark brown	Very rarely burns
VI	Black	Never burns

A patient's treatment response can be determined by assessing both the degree of photodamage present and the pigmentary skin type. A procedural risk—benefit ratio will differ, depending on the patient's individual findings (Figs. 1.5 and 1.6). In general, patients with Fitzpatrick skin types I–III can tolerate more epidermal and dermal injury with minimal risk of residual dyschromia. Patients with Fitzpatrick skin types IV–V have a high risk of residual dyschromia with increased skin injury that may preclude the use of many treatment modalities.

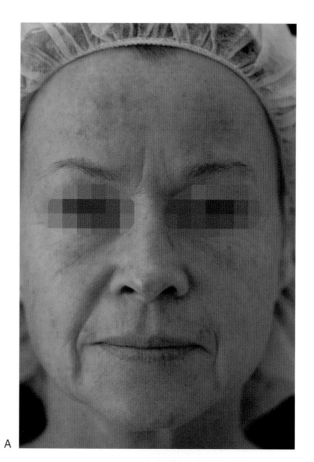

A

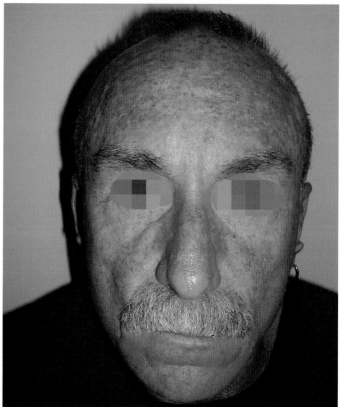

B

Figure 1.3 A&B *Glogau type 3 photoaging. Dyspigmentation and wrinkles are evident*

■ Subcutaneous Fat Atrophy

Aging results in a significant degree of loss or redistribution of subcutaneous fat, especially of the forehead, temporal fossae, perioral area, chin, and premalar areas. This leads to a skeletonized appearance. Restoration of volume loss results in the reshaping of the face for a fuller, rounder appearance.

■ Facial Musculature Changes

Aging also results in muscular atrophy, contributing to volume loss. As well, dynamic rhytides, which are muscular in origin, often create an angry, tired, or aged appearance. Selective chemical denervation provides marked relaxation of these lines.

■ Changes in Cartilage, Bony Structures, and Underlying Supportive Structures

Aging results in sagging and loss of resiliency. Redraping, repositioning, and judicious removal of skin and soft tissue assist in the restoration of a youthful appearance.

Once a systemic approach has been followed, the four Rs of facial rejuvenation—relax, refill, redrape, and resurface—can be applied solely or in combination to help restore a more youthful appearance.

BIBLIOGRAPHY

Chung JH, Eun HC. Angiogenesis in skin aging and photoaging. *J Dermatol.* 2007;34(9):593-600.

Davis RE. Facelift and ancillary facial cosmetic surgery procedures. In: Nouri K, Leal-Nouri S, eds. *Techniques in Dermatologic Surgery.* London: Mosby; 2003, pp. 333-344.

Fitzpatrick T. The validity and practicality of sun-reactive skin types I through VI. *Arch Dermatol.* 1998;124:869-871.

Glogau R. Aesthetic and anatomic analysis of the aging skin. *Semin Cutan Med Surg.* 1996;15(3):134-138.

Montagna W, Carlisle K, Kirchner S. *Epidermal and Dermal Histological Markers of Photodamaged Human Facial Skin.* Shelton, CT: Richardson-Vicks; 1988.

Paes EC, Teepen HJ, Koop WA, et al. Perioral wrinkles: Histologic differences between men and women. *Aesthet Surg J.* 2009;29(6):467-472.

Shaw RB Jr, Katzel EB, Koltz PF, et al. Aging of the mandible and its aesthetic implications. *Plast Reconst Surg.* 2010;125(91):332-342.

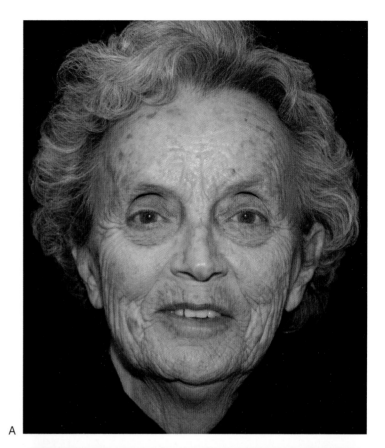

A

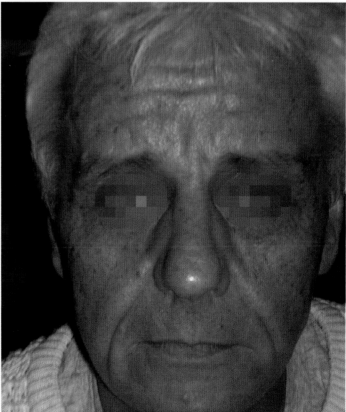

B

Figure 1.4 A&B *Glogau type 4 photoaging. Extensive wrinkles and prominent dyspigmentation*

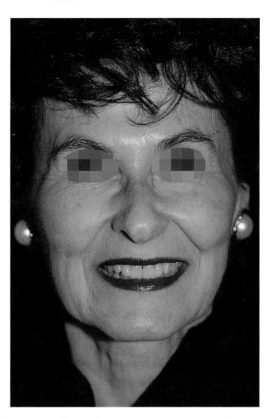

Figure 1.5 *Female patient who avoided sun exposure throughout her life. Her skin reflects only minimal signs of photoaging*

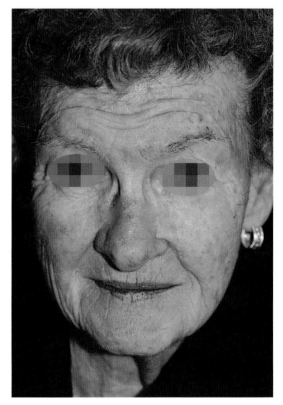

Figure 1.6 *Female patient with a history of extensive sun exposure in her life. Her skin reflects extensive photodamage with dyspigmentation and extensive wrinkle formation*

CHAPTER 2 | Topical Treatment Options

MECHANISM OF ACTION

- Sunscreen
  - The ultraviolet (UV) wavelengths of light associated with cutaneous damage are UVB (290–320 nm) and UVA (320–400 nm) light.
  - UVB absorption by DNA results in a p53 tumor suppressor gene mutation resulting in pyrimidine dimer formation, which is mutagenic and linked to cutaneous carcinogenesis.
  - Acute UVB exposure results in a sunburn (Fig. 2.1).
  - Repeat acute UVB exposures over time have been associated with the formation of basal cell carcinoma and melanoma.
  - Chronic UVB exposure has been linked to the development of actinic keratoses and squamous cell carcinoma.
  - UVA is unaffected by window glass, altitude, time of day, or season and can produce a tan and dyspigmentation without preceding erythema.
  - UVA light penetrates deeply into the dermis, producing many of the clinical findings associated with photo damage (Fig. 2.2).
  - UVA absorption by DNA results in formation of oxygen free radicals, thought to contribute to carcinogenesis. It causes immunosuppression through the depletion of Langerhans' cells and reduced antigen presenting cell activity.
  - UVA exposure has been linked to the development of melanoma in animal models.

Chemical sunscreen (Table 2.1)—absorbs light in the UV wavelength of light (UVB 290–320 nm) and UVA

TABLE 2.1 ■ Chemical Sunscreen: Active Ingredients

Avobenzone
  Cinoxate
Dioxybenzone
  Homosalate
Methyl anthranilate
  Mexoryl SX
  Mexoryl XL
  Octocrylene
Octyl methoxycinnamate
  Octyl salicylate
  Oxybenzone
  Padimate O
Para-aminobenzoic acid (PABA)
Phenyl benzimidazole sulfonic acid
  Sulisobenzone
  Trolamine salicylate

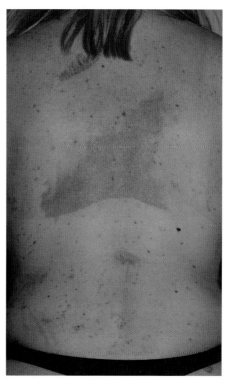

Figure 2.1 *Patient with an acute sunburn. There is marked swelling and redness present. The upper back scar is the site of a previous superficial spreading melanoma (Courtesy of Richard Johnson, MD)*

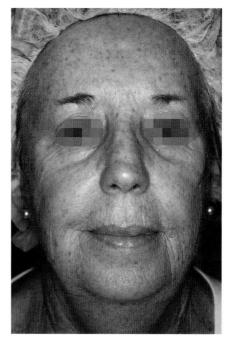

Figure 2.2 *Patient with marked photodamage due to chronic sun exposure. The patient was an avid golfer and reported only occasional sunscreen use*

320–400 nm), transforming this light into harmless long wave radiation and re-emitting as heat energy.

Physical screen (Table 2.2)—scatters or reflects UV radiation. Can also absorb UV light and release it as heat.

TABLE 2.2 ■ Physical Sunscreen: Active Ingredients

Titanium dioxide
  Zinc oxide

Sun protective factor—optimally a sunscreen would provide protection against the full spectrum of UV radiation. The sun protective factor (SPF) is the only internationally standardized measure of a sunscreen's ability to filter UV radiation. It is the ratio of the UV energy needed to produce a minimal erythema dose (MED) on sunscreen-protected skin to the UV energy required to produce an MED on unprotected skin. The American Academy of Dermatology currently recommends the daily use of sunscreen with SPF 30 or greater.

• Antioxidants—theoretically work to reduce and neutralize free radicals that damage DNA, cytoskeletal structures, and cellular proteins. They also possess anti-inflammatory effects and many play a role in pigment reduction.

 – In order to be biologically effective, these products must be able to penetrate into the skin and remain biologically active long enough to exert the desired benefits. A majority of the currently available antioxidant products are very unstable, with oxidation making them chemically inactive. Molecular formation and packaging are key factors in the stabilization of these products.

 – Antioxidants may work synergistically to provide their greatest benefit.

 – Vitamin C—the only antioxidant to date to have proven benefit for wrinkle improvement due to its ability to increase collagen formation rather than its antioxidative effects.

 – Vitamin E—demonstrated to inhibit UV-induced erythema and edema in animals. It has high contact dermatitis risk.

 – Coenzyme Q10—naturally occurring nutrient added to many over-the-counter products. Currently there are no studies available to document its long-term benefits on skin aging.

 – Idebenone—synthetic analog of Coenzyme Q10.

• Retinoic acid—retinoids are naturally occurring derivatives of β-carotene and labeled as vitamin A and its derivatives. Included are retinol, retinaldehyde, retinyl esters, and retinoic acid (Fig. 2.3). Its benefits are both preventative and reparative.

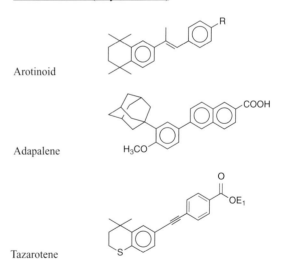

Figure 2.3 *Chemical structures of retinoic acids. The addition of aromatic rings has made third-generation retinoids more stable for more targeted therapy with less potential side effects. (Reproduced, with permission, from Baumann L. Cosmetic Dermatology: Principles and Practice, 2nd ed. New York: McGraw-Hill; 2009)*

– UVB exposure results in the up-regulation of several collagen-degrading matrix metalloproteinases, including collagenase, gelatinase, and stromelysin, which cause collagen degradation. Retinoids act to inhibit the induction of these metalloproteinases.

– UVB exposure also decreases collagen production. Retinoids work to inhibit this loss of pro-collagen synthesis.

– Tretinoin—a first-generation retinoid which was the first available topical retinoid. It is a nonselective retinoid, activating all retinoic acid pathways. It is not photo-stable. It is available in a generic form, as well as in brand formulations such as Renova and Avita. Currently Renova is FDA approved for photoaging. Tretinoin is also available in combination as tretinoin 0.025% with clindamycin for patients seeking benefits for both acne and photoaging and as tretinoin 0.25% in combination with 4% hydroquinone and 0.05% fluocinolone acetonide for hyperpigmentation.

– Retinol—this product must be converted to retinaldehyde and then to all-trans-retinoic acid within the keratinocyte in order to become active, thus displaying less activity than tretinoin. It is thought to be approximately 20% less potent than retinoic acid. It is not as frequently associated with irritation or erythema. It is primarily found in over-the-counter products at various concentrations.

– Adapalene—a third-generation retinoid with selective affinity for specific retinoic acid receptors, which allows for more targeted benefit and reduction of potential side effects. It is more chemically stable than tretinoin and does not break down in the presence of light. Currently available as Differin in a 0.1% and a 0.3% concentration. It is currently FDA approved for topical acne therapy.

– Tazarotene—a third-generation retinoid with selective affinity for specific retinoic receptors for more targeted benefit. Has been associated with significantly higher irritation than other retinoids. It is available in 0.1% and 0.05% gels and in 0.1% and 0.05% creams. It is currently FDA approved for topical acne therapy and plaque psoriasis.

• Skin lightening agents—these products act to inhibit one or more steps in the melanin biosynthesis pathway. The main target is tyrosinase, which is the rate-limiting step in melanin production (Table 2.3).

– Hydroquinone—phenolic compound found naturally in many plants, coffee, tea, bear, and wine.

  ◦ Inhibits conversion of tyrosinase to melanin.

  ◦ Decreases tyrosinase activity by 90%.

  ◦ May inhibit DNA synthesis.

  ◦ May inhibit RNA synthesis.

TABLE 2.3 ■ Skin Lightening Agents

• Tyrosinase inhibitors
  Hydroquinone
  Aloesin
  Arbutin
  Ascorbic acid
  Flavonoids
  Gentisic acid
  Hydroxycoumarins
  Kojic acid
  Licorice extract
  Mulberry extract
• Melanocyte transfer inhibition
  Lecithins
  Niacinamide
  Soybean/milk extracts
• Melanocyte cytotoxic agents
  Azelaic acid
  Mequinol
  Monobenzone
• Skin turnover acceleration
  Glycolic acid
  Lactic acid
  Linoleic acid
  Retinoic acid

○ Can be cytotoxic to melanocytes producing irreversible cell damage with monobenzyl ether of hydroquinone.

○ Concern regarding carcinogenic potential—currently heavily regulated and/or banned in Europe, Asia, and several African countries.

○ Available in over-the-counter products up to 2% and by prescription in 3% to 4% concentrations. Can be compounded up to 10% concentration.

○ Currently available in combination with topical retinoid acid and topical steroid and with other skin lightening agents.

– Retinoic acid

○ Accelerate epidermal turnover resulting in increased keratinocyte shedding leading to pigment loss

○ May inhibit tyrosinase induction

○ May result in keratinocyte pigment dispersion

○ May interfere with keratinocyte pigment transfer

– Natural cosmeceuticals

○ Kojic acid—derived from various fungal species such as *Aspergillus* and *Penicillium*. Primarily used as a food preservative and to promote the reddening of unripe strawberries. Generally used in 1% to 4% concentration. Noted to have high sensitizing potential.

○ Licorice extract—derived from the root of *Glycyrrhiza glabra linneva*. Its main active ingredient is glabridin. It inhibits tyrosinase activity with associated cytotoxicity. It has been shown to be 16× more efficacious than hydroquinone.

○ Azelaic acid—derived from Pityrosporum ovale. Its mechanism of action in not fully understood. It works best on active melanocytes.

○ Aloesin—derived from aloe vera. It acts as a competitive inhibitor on DOPA oxidation and noncompetitive inhibitor on tyrosine. When used in combination with arbutin, it has been demonstrated to inhibit UV-induced melanogenesis.

○ Arbutin—derived from the bearberry. It acts to inhibit melanosomal tyrosinase activity. Available as a mono treatment or in 1% concentration with other depigmenting agents.

○ Paper mulberry—derived from the roots of an ornamental tree, *Broussonetia papyrifera*.

○ Soy—acts to inhibit keratinocyte melanosome phagocytosis, thus reducing melanin transfer. Cosmeceutical effect noted only with fresh soy milk.

○ Niacinamide—acts to inhibit melanocyte transfer. Also exhibits anti-inflammatory and anti-oxidant properties.

Table 2.4 ■ Use of the "teaspoon rule" for sunscreen application can be beneficial in educating patients on the proper of amount of sunscreen that should be applied with each application.

Use of more than half a teaspoon each on:
• Head and neck region
• Right arm
• Left arm

Use of more than a teaspoon each on:
• Anterior torso
• Posterior torso
• Right leg
• Left leg

(Data from Draelos ZD. Procedures in Cosmetic Dermatology Cosmeceuticals. Saunders, 2005.)

○ Ascorbic acid—acts at various oxidative steps in melanin synthesis by interacting with copper ions at the tyrosinase active site and reducing dopa-quinone.

○ Glycolic acid—has an epidermal discohesive effect, resulting in increased epidermal turnover for increased shedding of pigmented keratinocytes. Should be used in lower concentrations to avoid skin irritation.

INDICATIONS

- Reduce the occurrence of actinic keratoses and non-melanoma skin cancer
- Reduce the formation of skin aging
- Rhytides
- Ephelides
- Lentigines
- Melasma
- Postinflammatory hyperpigmentation

PRETREATMENT EVALUATION

- Evaluation of pre-existing allergies to any active ingredient
- Past product use and response

IDEAL CANDIDATE

- All patients benefit from the daily application of a topical sunscreen, SPF 30 or greater
- Patients with realistic expectations that topical medications may provide preventative benefits and are less likely to reduce moderate to deep rhytides

LESS THAN IDEAL CANDIDATE

- Unrealistic patient expectations
- Patients with markedly dry or sensitive skin—topical treatments may exacerbate condition

CONTRAINDICATIONS

- Pre-existing allergy to active ingredient
- Use of topical tretinoin, salicylic acid, and skin lightening agents in pregnant and lactating women

APPLICATION TECHNIQUES

- A sunscreen should be applied a minimum of 30 minutes prior to sun exposure.

- Approximately 35 mL is the average amount of sunscreen that should be applied to the average-sized adult with each application. This translates to a teaspoon (approximately 6 mL) ot sunscreen to each leg, back, and chest and half a teaspoon (approximately 3 mL) applied to the arms, face, and neck for full coverage (Table 2.4).
- Topical retinoic acid products should be applied sparingly to treatment areas 30 minutes after washing to minimize potential for irritation.
- Bleaching creams should be applied to hyperpigmented treatment areas only, with efforts made to avoid uninvolved skin.

COMPLICATIONS

- Contact allergic dermatitis
- Contact irritant dermatitis
- Acne flare
- Skin peeling
- Xerosis
- Erythema
- Photoallergic reaction
- Phototoxic reaction
- Theoretical reduction in vitamin D absorption with sunscreen use
- Hyperpigmentation with bleaching cream use
- Exogenous ochronosis with bleaching cream
- Hypopigmentation with bleaching cream
- Potential carcinogenic risk of hydroquinone use

POSTTREATMENT CARE

- Strict photoprotection should be followed daily, including sun avoidance as much as possible, the use of a daily sunscreen SPF 30 or greater, use of a wide-brimmed hat, and sun protective clothing

PEARLS FOR TREATMENT SUCCESS

- Minimize the number of products applied daily to avoid the potential for irritation.
- Check the expiration dates of all products applied. This is particular key for sunscreens, as the active ingredients may not provide benefit beyond the recommended date of use.
- Topical retinoic acid products should be discontinued 2 weeks prior to facial procedures such as waxing or tweezing in order to avoid skin desquamation.

- Bleaching agents should be discontinued if redness or irritation develops, as they may worsen existing pigmentation.
- It is useful to discontinue the use of a hydroquinone cream every 3 to 4 months to decrease the risk of exogenous ochronosis and to prevent side effects.

BIBLIOGRAPHY

Bruce S. Cosmeceuticals for the attenuation of extrinsic and intrinsic dermal aging. *J Drugs Dermatol*, 2008; 7(2 Suppl):s17-s22.

Colven RM, Pinnell SR. Topical vitamin C in aging. *Clin Dermatol*. 1996;14:227-234.

Dreher F, Maibach H. Protective effects of topical antioxidants in humans. *Curr Probl Dermatol*. 2000;29:157-164.

Fisher GJ, Talwar HS, Lin J, et al. Molecular mechanisms of photoaging in human skin in vivo and their prevention by all-trans retinoic acid. *Photochem Photobiol*. 1999;69: 154-157.

Gensler HL, Aickin M, Peng YM, et al. Importance of the form of topical vitamin E for prevention of photocarcinogenesis. *Nutr Cancer*. 1996;26:183-191.

Guevara IL, Panda AG. Melasma treated with hydroquinone, tretinoin and a fluorinated steroid. *Int J Dermatol*. 2001;30:212-215.

Kang S, Voorhees JJ. Photoaging therapy with topical tretinoin: An evidence-based analysis. *J Am Acad Dermatol*. 1998;39:S55-S61.

Kligman AM. The growing importance of topical retinoids in clinical dermatology: A retrospective and prospective analysis. *J Am Acad Dermatol*. 1998;39:S2-S7.

Lin HW, Naylor M, Honigmann H, et al. American Academy of Dermatology Consensus Conference on UVA protection of sunscreens, summary and recommendations. *J Am Acad Dermatol*. 2000;44:505-508.

Naylor M, Boyd A, Smith D, et al. High sun protection factor sunscreens in the suppression of actinic neoplasia. *Arch Dermatol*. 1995;131:170-175.

Ogden S, Samuel M, Griffiths SE. A review of tazarotene in the treatment of photodamaged skin. *Clin Interv Aging*. 2008;3(1):71-76.

Picard M, Carrera M. New and experimental treatments of chloasma and other hypermelanoses. *Dermatol Clin*. 2007;25:353-362.

Schneider J. The teaspoon rule of applying sunscreen. *Arch Dermatol*. 2002;138:838-839.

Solano F, Briganti S, Picardo M, et al. Hypopigmenting agents: An updated review on biological, chemical and clinical aspects. *Pigment Cell Res*. 2006;19:550-571.

| CHAPTER 3 | Soft Tissue Augmentation |

MECHANISM OF ACTION

Use of a synthetic or biological product or surgical restructuring for the replacement of volume loss and enhancement of dermal, subcutaneous, and muscular deficiencies that result from trauma, surgical defects, lipoatrophic conditions, photoaging, or chronological aging.

IDEAL FILLER (Table 3.1)

- Biocompatible
- Nonimmunogenic
- Noncarcinogenic, nonteratogenic
- Nonresorbable
- Nonmigratory
- Inexpensive
- Easily obtained and stored
- Easy to administer
- Provides reproducible cosmetically beneficial results
- FDA approved if not autologous
- Demonstrates multipurpose use
- No side effects
- Easy to remove in the event of a poor cosmetic outcome

TABLE 3.1 ■ Commonly Used Filling Agents

Name	Composition	FDA approval	Skin testing required	Longevity
Adatosil 5000 (Dow-Corning, Midland, MI)	Silicone	No	No	Permanent
Alloderm (Life Cell Corp., Branchburg, NJ; Obaji Medical, Chicago, IL)	Acellular processed human cadaveric dermal allograft	Yes	No	1–2 yr
Aquamid (Contura International, Soebora, Denmark)	Poly-acrylamide gel	No	No	Permanent
Artefill (Canderm Pharma, Inc., Quebec, Canada; Medical International BV, Breda, The Netherlands)	Bovine collagen with poly(methyl methacrylate) beads	No	Yes	Permanent
Belotero Soft; Belotero Basic (Merz Pharma, Frankfurt, Germany)	Non-animal hyaluronic acid derived from bacterial fermentation	No	No	4–6 mo
Bio-Alcamid (Brindis, Italy)	Poly-acrylamide	No	Yes	Permanent
Captique™ (Inamed Corp, Santa Monica, CA)	Non-animal-stabilized hyaluronic acid(NASHA) derived from plant	Yes	No	4–6 mo
Cosmoderm™, Cosmoplast™ (Allergan, Irvine, CA)	Recombinant human collagen	Yes	No	4–6 mo
Cymetra Life Cell Corp., Branchburg, NJ; Obaji Medical, Chicago, IL	Acellular processed lyophilized human cadaveric tissue		No	4–6 mo

(continued)

TABLE 3.1 ■ Commonly Used Filling Agents *(Continued)*

Name	Composition	FDA approval	Skin testing required	Longevity
Fascian (Fascia Biomaterials, Beverly Hills, CA)	Human cadaveric preserved particulate fascia lata		No	3–4 mo
Fat, subcutaneous	Autologous	N/A	No	9–12 mo
Hylaform® (Biomatrix Inc., Ridgefield, NJ; Inamed Corp., Santa Monica, CA)	Hyaluronic acid derived from domestic fowl coxcombs	Yes	No	4–6 mo
Isolagen (Isolagen Inc., Houston, TX)	Autologous fibroblasts	Yes	No	1–2 yr
Juvederm™ Ultra, Ultra XC, Ultra Plus, Ultra Plus XC (Allergan, Inc., Irvine, CA)	Non-animal–stabilized hyaluronic acid (NASHA) derived from bacterial fermentation. XC formulations with 0.3% lidocaine	Yes	No	6–9 mo
Prevelle Silk (Mentor Corporation, Santa Barbara, CA)	Non-animal-derived hyaluronic acid with 0.3% lidocaine	Yes	No	4–6 mo
Radiesse™ (Bioform Medical, San Mateo, CA)	Synthetic calcium hydroxylapatite	Yes	No	9–12 mo
Restylane, Restylane-L, Perlane, Perlane L™ (Q-Med AB, Sweden; Medicis, Phoenix, AZ)	Non-animal-stabilized hyaluronic acid (NASHA) derived from bacterial fermentation. L formulations with 0.3% lidocaine	Yes	No	6–9 mo
Silikone-1000, Adatosil-5000 (Alcon Labs, Inc, Fort Worth, TX)	Silicone	No	No	Permanent
Softform (McGhan Medical, Santa Barbara, CA)	Gore-Tex	N/A	No	Permanent
Sculptra™ (Biotech Industry, SA, Luxembourg; Dermik, Berwyn, PA)	Lyophilized poly-L-lactic acid	Yes	No	1–2 yr
Zyderm®, Zyplast® (Allergan, Irvine, CA)	Bovine collagen	Yes	Yes	3–4 mo

PREOPERATIVE EVALUATION

- Identify the appropriate patient and treatment region
  - Significant past medical history, including history of bleeding or clotting disorders; keloid formation; existing drug allergies; immunocompromised state
  - Current medication use; past or current isotretinoin use
  - Past surgical interventions, year, and treatment response
  - Clinical evaluation to determine if the desired treatment areas are amenable to correction; outline baseline structural irregularities
  - Discuss line softening versus volume replacement for filler selection
  - Discuss medications to avoid 10 days preoperatively when medically safe, including aspirin, nonsteroidal medications, vitamin E supplements, St. John's Wort, and other herbal medications that have an anticoagulative effect

- Discuss the risks and benefits of the treatment
  - Allergic reaction, localized versus systemic
  - Procedural and postoperative discomfort
  - Postoperative edema
  - Postoperative bruising
  - Scar formation
  - Infection
  - Reactivation of herpes simplex virus
  - Incomplete augmentation
  - Irregular contour/texture
- Identify contraindications to treatment
  - Active infection at the treatment site
  - Nondistensible, rigid, or icepick scars
  - Extensive jowl formation, prominent folds, and furrows
  - Underlying connective tissue disorder
  - Immunologic disease
  - Prior allergic reaction to filler/related filler/positive skin test
  - Use of isotretinoin within the preceding 6 to 12 months
  - Pregnancy
  - Unrealistic expectations
- Outline the predicted outcome and limitations to the treatment
  - Duration of correction
  - Postoperative recovery period
  - Tissue source
  - Expense

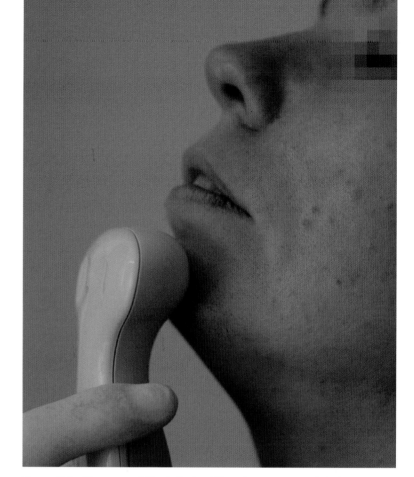

Figure 3.1 *Massager utilized during filler placement to minimize treatment discomfort*

SKIN TESTING (WHEN APPLICABLE)

- Initial test dose-two skin tests recommended
  - Injected in tuberculin manner into volar forearm
  - Four-week observation period for first test
  - Repeat skin test placed in opposite forearm
  - Two-week observation period for second test
- Retest dose—single test recommended
  - For new patients who have received treatment by another physician or patients who have not received treatment for more than 1 year
  - Two-week observation period recommended
- Positive filler reaction
  - Swelling, induration, tenderness, or erythema that persists or occurs 6 hours or longer after test implantation
  - A positive skin test is an absolute contraindication to filler use

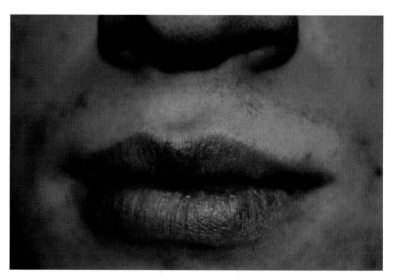

Figure 3.2 *Clinical findings after EMLA application to skin. Expected blanching lasts approximately 2 to 3 hours after application*

ANESTHESIA

- Injection of soft tissue fillers may be painful, especially with treatment of the lips. Most patients require some form of anesthesia to minimize treatment discomfort.

- "Talkesthesia," hand-holding, vibratory massager near the treatment site are useful for patient distraction (Fig. 3.1).

- Topical anesthesia can be utilized for small treatment areas. Commonly used agents include Betacaine Enhanced Gel (Canderm, Quebec, Canada), Betacaine Plus (Canderm, Quebec, Canada), L-M-X-4 and 5 (Ferndale Labs, Ferndale, MI), EMLA (AstraZeneca, Boston, MA), and ice (Fig. 3.2).

- Lidocaine integrated directly into the filler may eliminate the need for alternate forms of anesthesia.

- Regional nerve blocks are easily administered prior to treatment. The patient should avoid extremely hot or cold beverages and foods for 2 to 3 hours after mental and/or infraorbital nerve blocks to avoid mucosal injury due to inability to detect temperature accurately.

- Localized tumescent anesthesia is utilized for fat extraction with autologous fat transfer.

- Infiltrative anesthesia is to be avoided to obviate tissue distortion of the treatment site.

PROCEDURAL MEDICATIONS

- Valtrex 500 mg BID × 5 to 7 days initiated 1 day prior to the procedure for patients with a history of herpes simplex virus in or near the treatment site

- Keflex 500 mg BID × 7 days initiated 1 day prior to the procedure for patients undergoing autologous fat transfer or Gore-Tex implantation

- Diazepam 5 to 10 mg can be offered to anxious patients 30 minutes prior to the procedure

LEVEL OF INJECTION (Fig. 3.3)

- Superficial dermis: fine lines; vermilion border lip augmentation

Zyderm I, II; Cosmoderm I, II; Restylane Fine Line; Hylaform Fine Line

- Mid to deep dermis: superficial to moderate rhytides, scars, and defects; lip augmentation

Captique; Cosmoderm II, Cosmoplast; Hylaform; Juvederm Ultra; Prevelle Silk; Restylane; Zyderm II, Zyplast

- Deep dermis, subcutaneous fat, and muscle: deeper, more substantial defects and rhytides (Fig. 3.4)

Autologous fat transfer; Gore-Tex; Hylaform Plus; Juvederm Ultra Plus; Perlane; Radiesse; Sculptra

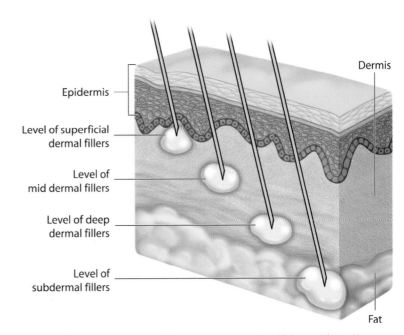

Figure 3.3 *Recommended filler injection depths. (Adapted from Keyvan N, Susana L-K, eds. Techniques in Dermatologic Surgery. United Kingdom: Mosby; 2003.)*

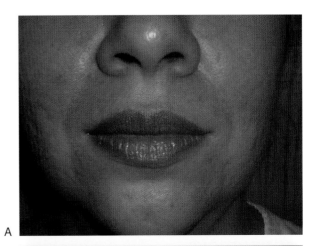

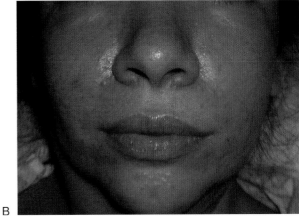

Figure 3.4 (A) *Prominent nasolabial folds prior to augmentation with hyaluronic acid.* **(B)** *Softening of folds after 3 c hyaluronic placed into treatment sites*

- Combination dermal, subcutaneous, and muscle: defects with both a superficial and a deep component utilize both a superficial and deep fixer for optimal augmentation (Fig. 3.5)

INJECTION TECHNIQUE (Fig. 3.6)

- Serial puncture: closely spaced punctures created along lines, folds (Fig. 3.7).
- Linear threading: withdrawal of filler along the length of the facial defect as a continuous thread of material (Fig. 3.8).
- Fanning: similar to linear threading. Needle direction is continually changed without withdrawing the needle tip. Useful for oral commissures, upper nasolabial folds.
- Cross-hatching: similar to linear threading. Material is injected at right angles to the first injections. Used for shaping facial contours.

DEGREE OF CORRECTION

- Dependent on the filler used. In general, overcorrection is not recommended. The most common technique error is under-correction.
- Multiple treatment sessions are generally required for volume replacement agents, including silicone and poly-L-lactic acid.

DURATION OF CORRECTION

Dependent on the material implanted, implantation technique, and amount implanted, the type of defect and mechanical stresses at the implantation sites.

ADVERSE REACTIONS

■ Hypersensitive

- Prolonged erythema and edema at injection sites
- Cyst/abscess formation—long-lasting; can persist for more than 2 to 3 years
- Granuloma formation
- Anaphylaxis

■ Non-Hypersensitive

- Biofilm
- Bruising
- Infection—includes reactivation of herpes simplex virus and bacterial infection

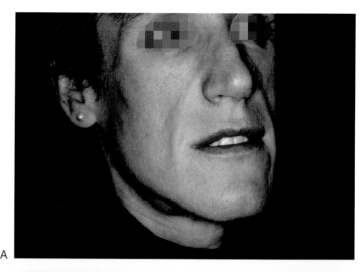

A

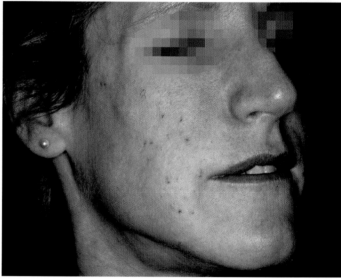

B

Figure 3.5 (A) *Facial lipoatrophy with "sunken cheek appearance" prior to Cymetra treatment.* **(B)** *Improvement of cheek volume after Cymetra treatment, 2.0 cc total volume*

- Necrosis—due to vascular compromise at the treatment site
- Nodule formation/beading
- Partial vision loss—due to vascular compromise at the treatment site
- Ulceration

■ Technique Complications

- Irregular texture—due to uneven placement
- Beading due to too superficial placement (Fig. 3.9)
- Implant rejection—due to too superficial placement
- Necrosis—due to vascular injection or vascular compression

PEARLS FOR TREATMENT SUCCESS

- With fillers, the affected treatment sites should be fully augmented to ensure an even, complete augmentation. Under-correction will lead to an inadequate augmentation and patient dissatisfaction. With most temporary fillers, this is obtained at the first treatment. Permanent fillers require repeat treatments for correction completion.
- With temporary fillers, patients must understand that the treatment response is variable and can last less than or greater than the average expected time. Repeat treatment will be required over time.
- Patient expectations must be tempered to minimize unrealistic expectations about filler benefits. Patients must be aware that the treatment endpoint is a softening of the affected areas.
- Postoperative beading is generally responsive to localized massage over 5 to 7 days. Persistent beading can be corrected by injecting 2 mg/mL of triamcinolone acetonide into the bead or by 11-blade incisional extraction of the filler material.
- A thorough preoperative evaluation is necessary to ensure that there are no contraindications to filler use, especially when using permanent fillers.
- Conservative augmentation of the glabellar region is critical to avoid vascular necrosis.

BIBLIOGRAPHY

Beer K, Solich N. Hyaluronics for soft tissue augmentation: Practical considerations and technical recommendations. *J Drugs Dermatol.* 2009;8(12):1086-1091.

Clark DP, Hanke CW, Swanson N. Dermal implants: Safety of products injected for soft tissue augmentation. *J Am Acad Dermatol.* 1989;21:992-998.

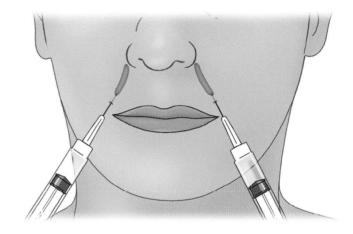

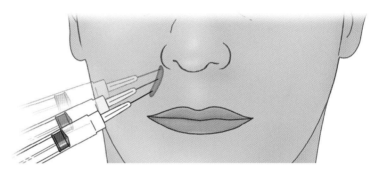

Figure 3.6 *Injection techniques A. Linear threading technique B. Serial puncture technique. (Adapted from Keyvan N, Susana L-K, eds. Techniques in Dermatologic Surgery. United Kingdom: Mosby; 2003.)*

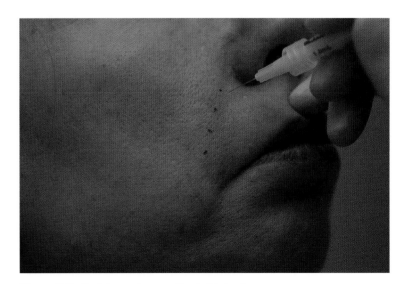

Figure 3.7 *Serial puncture method of injection*

Cohen JL. Understanding, avoiding and managing dermal filler complication. *Dermatol Surg.* 2008;(34 Suppl 1):S92-S93.

Coleman SR. Facial recontouring with liposculpture. *Clin Plast Surg.* 1997;24(2):347-367.

Glaich AS, Cohen JL, Goldberg LH. Injection necrosis of the glabella: Protocol for prevention and treatment after use of dermal fillers. *Dermatol Surg.* 2006;32(2):276-281.

Jones DH. Semipermanent and permanent injectable fillers. *Dermatol Clin.* 2009;27(4):433-444.

Matarasso SL. Injectable collagens: Lost but not forgotten—a review of products, indications and injection techniques. *Plast Reconstruct Surg.* 2007;120(6 Suppl): 17S-26S.

Schuller-Petrovic S. Improving the aesthetic aspect of soft tissue defects on the face using autologous fat transplantation. *Facial Plast Surg.* 1997;13(2):19-24.

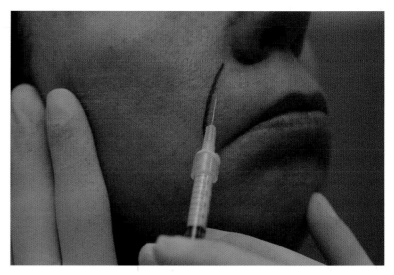

Figure 3.8 *Linear threading method of injection*

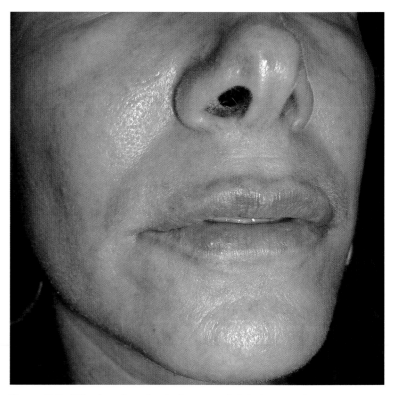

Figure 3.9 *Filler beading due to too superficial placement*

CHAPTER 4 | Botulinum Toxin

PHARMACOLOGY

Botulinum toxin is a protein produced by the bacterium *Clostridium botulinum*. Seven serotypes exist, designated as A, B, C_1, D, E, F, and G. Each one of them is a protease with a light chain linked to a heavy chain by a disulfide bond.

Each is antigenically distinct. However, botulinum toxin A (BTX-A), B (BTX-B), and F are the only serotypes currently available for clinical use (Table 4.1).

TABLE 4.1 ■ Botulinum Toxin Preparations

Type	Units toxin/bottle	Dosing equivalents	Dilution
Botox Cosmetic (Allergan Inc., Irvine, CA)—type A	100 U lyophilized powder	1 U Botox = 4 U Dysport	Average 1—4 mL in preservative-free or preserved saline
Reloxin (Medicis Esthetics, Scottsdale, AZ), Dysport (Ipsen Limited, Berkshire, UK)—type A	500 U in lyophilized powder	1 U Botox = 2.5—4 U	
Reloxin/Dysport	Average 1—2.5 mL in preservative-free or preserved saline		
Myobloc (Soltice Neurosciences, San Francisco, CA)—type B	2,500, 5,000, and 10,000 U/mL aqueous solution	Not well established for cosmetic use	May be used as is or dilute with saline
Xeomin (Merz Pharmaceuticals, Frankfurt, Germany)—type A	100 U vial	Reported 1 U Botox = 1 U Xeomin	Not well established
Neuronox (Medy-Tox, Inc, Seoul, South Korea)—type A	100 U vial	Reported 1 U Botox = 1 U Neuronox	Not well established
Prosigne (Lanzhou Institute of Biological Products, Lanzhou, China)—type A	50 U vial and 100 U vial	Not well established	Not well established

MECHANISM OF ACTION

Inhibition of acetylcholine release at the neuromuscular junction resulting in muscular flaccid paralysis. Receptor site binding is mediated by the heavy chain portion of the toxin, is specific for the toxin serotype, and is irreversible. Once bound, the receptor–neurotoxin complex is internalized into the nerve terminal and the toxin light chain acts as a protease to cleave specific synaptic protein peptide bonds required for acetylcholine formation. The target of BTX-A is the synaptasome-associated protein of 25 kDa, SNAP-25. BTX-B and BTX-E cleave the vesicle-associated membrane protein, synaptobrevin.

DILUTION

BTX-A is stored in lyophilized vials. It can be reconstituted in preserved saline or preservative-free saline. Dilutions vary according to physician preference and experience with BTX. A dilution ranges from 1 mL (10 U/0.1 cc) to 4 mL (2.5 U/0.1 cc). Dysport diluted to 2.5 mL will attain a concentration of 20 U/0.1 cc. The injected volume must be sufficiently small to provide accurate toxin delivery without an excessive volume effect or delivery of toxin to surrounding muscles other than the targeted muscles. The volume must be sufficiently large to permit accurate injection into the targeted muscles.

CONTRAINDICATIONS

■ Absolute

• Underlying neuromuscular condition such as myasthenia gravis or amyotrophic lateral sclerosis

• Pregnancy/breast-feeding—pregnancy category C

• Active infection in treatment area

• Unrealistic patient expectations

■ Relative

• Calcium channel blockers use—may potentiate effect

• Aminoglycoside antibiotic use—may potentiate effect

• Patients who are dependent on facial expression for their livelihood (eg, actors)

• Prominent eyelid ptosis, heavy brow or ectropion

PREOPERATIVE EVALUATION

• Patient expectations must be defined and matched with the expected treatment outcomes

• Patient medical history

• Past treatment history and outcome

• Clinical evaluation

• Determine location and extent of involvement of the treatment site

• Document asymmetries noted; presence of ptosis/lid laxity/brow prominence

■ Lower Eyelid "Snap Back" Test to Assess Lower Lid Laxity

The middle of the lower lid is grasped between the index finger and the thumb and pulled forward and upward. The lid is then released and allowed to "snap" back

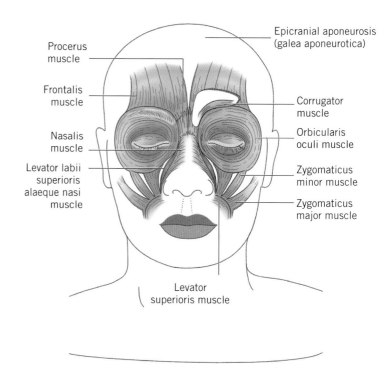

Figure 4.1 *Anatomical illustration of the upper and midfacial musculature*

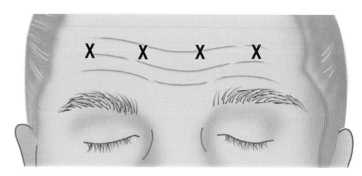

Figure 4.2 *Approximate injection sites for the forehead to obtain a more horizontal brow. This pattern is most frequently used to create a more masculine brow*

against the globe. A quick return to its normal state indicates minimal laxity. Botulinum toxin to this region can provide benefit. A slow return of skin to its natural position indicates significant laxity. Botulinum toxin should not be used in these patients, as it may accentuate the lines present.

PROCEDURE

- Patient consent obtained
- Preoperative pictures taken at rest and with targeted muscle groups contracted
- Pretreatment with topical anesthetic or ice for pain reduction
- Patient placed upright
- Treatment areas wiped with alcohol
- Injections administered. Use of 1 mL syringes with a 30 to 32 gauge needle is frequently utilized. Use of insulin syringes with an integrated 30-gauge syringe and a hubless system may help to reduce toxin volume loss

MUSCLE GROUPS

A thorough knowledge of the facial musculature and facial anatomy is required for the proper use and placement of botulinum toxin (Fig. 4.1).

▣ Forehead—Frontalis Muscle (Figs. 4.2 and 4.3)

Insertion: Originates at frontal bone galea aponeurotica and inserts into fibers of the procerus, corrugator, and orbicularis oculi

Function: Opposes depressor muscles of the glabellar complex and brows to elevate the brow and forehead

Lines noted: Horizontal lines across the forehead

Injection technique: 2 to 3 units (U) added at 1.5-cm intervals across the midforehead, a minimum of 2 cm above the upper brow

Dose injected: Average 12 to 20 U

Avoid:

- Excess treatment of this muscle; unopposed depressor function will result in loss of upper facial expression, a "tired" appearance, and risk of brow ptosis.
- Treatment of this muscle if the frontalis is supporting a ptotic upper eyelid or if the patient has low-set brows and/or excess upper eyelid skin.
- Inject 1 cm above the eyebrows to reduce the risk of brow ptosis. Patient must be aware that residual lines will be present after the treatment if low forehead wrinkles are present.

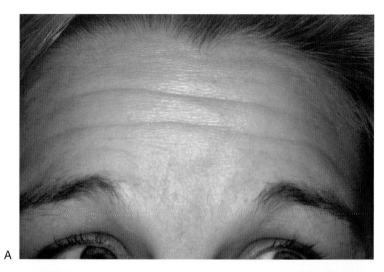

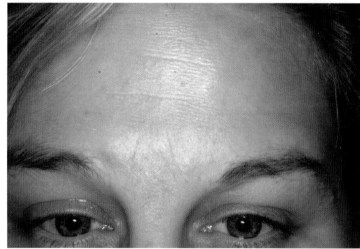

Figure 4.3 (A) *Forehead lines prior to BTX-A treatment.* **(B)** *Forehead lines 1 month following BTX-A treatment*

• Injection too close to the medial orbital rim; toxin diffusion through the orbital septum to the levator palpebrae superioris and orbicularis muscles may lead to diplopia.

■ Glabellar Complex—The Corrugator Supercilii, the Procerus, Medial Orbicularis Oculi, and Frontalis Muscles (Figs. 4.4 and 4.5)

Insertion: Originates at the nasal process of the frontal bone and extends laterally and upward to insert into the middle third of the eyebrow

Function: Opposes elevator muscles of the frontalis for brow adduction and brow/skin downward and medial movement

Lines noted: Frown lines; "angry" or "worried" appearance

Injection technique: Females have arched eyebrows; males have flatter or horizontal eyebrows; technique tailored to match the brow shape; 3 to 10 U into the procerus; 4 to 6 U in the inferior and superior bellies of the corrugators; 2 to 3 U into the medial orbicularis oculi

Dose injected: 15 to 40 U (dependent on muscle mass)

Avoid:

• Undertreatment of this region

• Too low of an injection resulting in toxin diffusion into the orbital septum and orbit with resultant lid ptosis. Palpation of the superior bony orbital rim with injection 1 cm or more above this landmark helps to minimize this risk

• Concurrent treatment of the forehead if a heavy brow is noted

■ Periorbital Region—Orbicularis Oculi (Figs. 4.6 and 4.7)

Insertion: Encircles the periorbital region and inserts into the medial and lateral canthal tendons as well as into the fibers of the frontal, procerus, and corrugator supercilii muscles

Function: Forceful closure of the eyes and depression of the brows and eyelids

Lines noted: Lateral canthal lines; "crows feet"

Injection technique: 3 to 5 U are injected into three points in a vertical line 1 cm from the lateral canthus; if a strong snap test is noted, 2 to 4 U can be placed 3 cm below the midpupillary line

Dose injected: 22 to 38 U

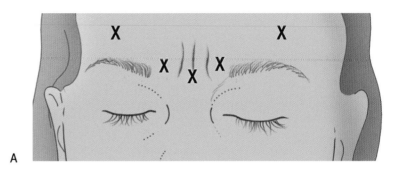

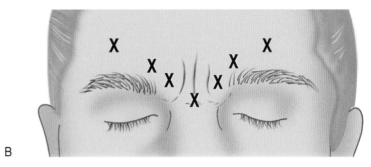

Figure 4.4 *Approximate injection sites for the glabellar frown lines.* **(A)** *Female brow.* **(B)** *Male brow*

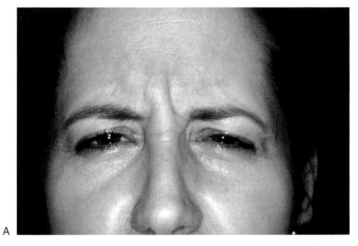

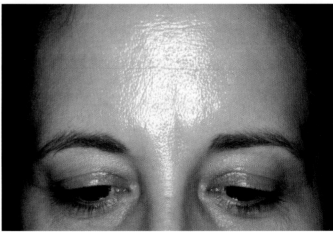

Figure 4.5 (A) *Glabellar complex before BTX-A injection and* **(B)** *3 weeks following BTX-A injection*

Avoid:

- Injection of the infraorbital region if a delayed snap test is noted; ectropion of the injected lid may develop
- Overtreatment of this area; improper eye closure, brow ptosis, or lid ptosis may ensue
- An injection aimed too low at the lower periorbital wrinkles. Weakening of the levator labii superioris muscles with an upper lip droop and abnormal smile may be observed

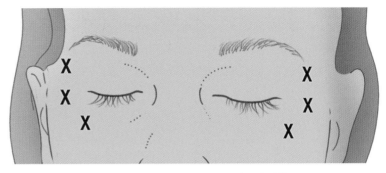

Figure 4.6 *Approximate injection sites for periorbital lines*

◼ Upper Nasal Root (Fig. 4.8)

Insertion: Encircles the periorbital region and inserts into the medial and lateral canthal tendons as well as into the fibers of the frontal, procerus, and corrugator supercilii muscles

Function: Nasal wrinkling

Lines noted: Upper nose fanning rhytides; "bunny lines"

Injection technique: 2 to 4 U is injected into each lateral nasal wall into the belly of the upper nasalis as it traverses the dorsum of the nose

Dose injected: 4 to 8 U

Avoid: Injection into the upper nasofacial groove may result in lip ptosis

Use of botulinum toxin in the lower face is minimally beneficial. Other treatment modalities are likely to be more beneficial with fewer potential side effects. A strong understanding of the lower face and neck anatomy is critical for injection placement (Fig. 4.9).

◼ Nasolabial Fold (Figs. 4.10 and 4.11)

It is key to weigh the limited benefit of BTX-A in this region compared with the increased risk of complications. Filling agents may provide greater benefit with fewer side effects.

Insertion: Result of skin laxity, gravitational ptosis, and subcutaneous fat loss overlying the cutaneous attachment in the zygomaticus major and minor, levator labii superioris, and levator labii superioris alaeque nasi muscles

Function: Associated with mouth and lip movement

Lines noted: Prominent crease, medial cheek; "gummy show"

Injection technique: 1 to 2 U injected into the upper aspect of the nasolabial fold 2 to 3 mm lateral to its insertion with the nose

Dose injected: 2 to 4 U

Avoid:

- Complete relaxation of this area; upper lip ptosis creating a sad appearance may occur

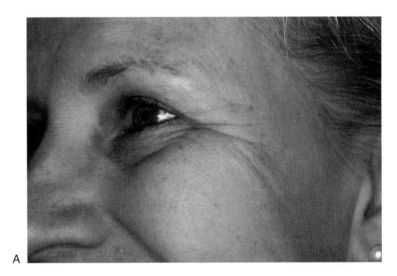

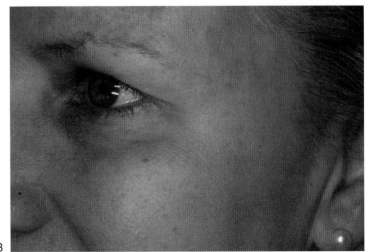

Figure 4.7 (A) *Periorbital lines prior to treatment with BTX-A.* **(B)** *Periorbital lines 6 weeks following BTX-A treatment*

• Uneven paralysis; an asymmetric smile or disproportionate lip may be seen

■ Perioral Region—Orbicularis Oris with Contributing Fibers from the Buccinator, Caninus, and Triangularis Muscles; Depressor Anguli Oris; Mentalis Muscle (Figs. 4.12 and 4.13)

Insertion: Orbicularis oris originates from the maxillary alveolar border running circumferentially around the mouth to the overlying cutaneous attachments; depressor anguli oris (DAO) arises from the mandibular oblique line, inserting into the angle of the mouth. It is continuous with the platysma muscle; mentalis muscle originates from the mandibular incisive fossa and descends to a cutaneous insertion

Function: Opposition and protrusion of the lips; mouth angle depression; lower lip protrusion and chin dimpling

Lines noted: Deep and superficial rhytides, upper and lower lip; prominent angular folds, "sad appearance"; chin wrinkling

Injection technique: 0.5 to 1.0 U injected 2 to 3 mm above the vermilion border in four areas each for the upper and lower lip; 1 to 2 U injected at the intersection of a line drawn from the nasolabial fold and an area 1 cm above the jawline angle; 5 to 10 U into the inferior mid-chin

Dose injected: 4 to 8 U for the upper and lower lips; 2 to 4 U for the DAO; 5 to 10 U for the mentalis muscle

Avoid:

• Overtreatment of this area; speech difficulties, an asymmetric smile, inability to close the mouth, drooling and altered facial expressions may ensue

• Deep injections; increased risk of side effects

• Too high of an injection for the DAO; inability to raise the corner of the mouth may develop

■ Neck—Platysma Muscle Complex (Fig. 4.14)

Insertion: Originates on the fascia of the upper pectoralis major and deltoid muscles and proceeds upward and medially along the sides of the neck. Fibers are inserted into the mandible, subcutaneous tissue of the lower face, perioral muscle, and skin

Function: Facial animation; lower jaw depression; lower lip depression

Lines noted: Neck wrinkling; central bands

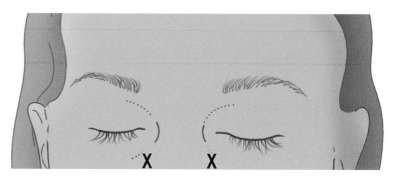

Figure 4.8 *Approximate injection sites for upper nasal root rhytides*

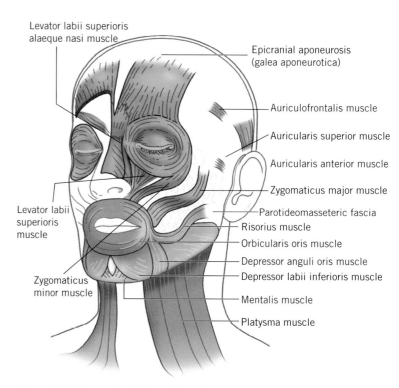

Levator labii superioris alaeque nasi muscle

Epicranial aponeurosis (galea aponeurotica)

Auriculofrontalis muscle

Auricularis superior muscle

Auricularis anterior muscle

Zygomaticus major muscle

Parotideomasseteric fascia

Risorius muscle

Orbicularis oris muscle

Depressor anguli oris muscle

Depressor labii inferioris muscle

Mentalis muscle

Platysma muscle

Levator labii superioris muscle

Zygomaticus minor muscle

Figure 4.9 *Anatomical illustration of the musculature of the lower face and neck*

Injection technique: 2 to 5 U injected from the superior to inferior portion of each platysmal band at 1 to 1.5 cm intervals with the patient's teeth clenched to contract the muscle during injection

Dose injected: 20 to 100 U

Avoid: Too deep an injection; neck weakness, laryngeal muscle weakness, or dysphagia may develop

POSTOPERATIVE CONSIDERATIONS

- Ice or cold compresses may be applied to reduce possible bruising and edema
- Active contraction of the treated muscles for 20 to 30 seconds every 30 minutes for 4 hours after treatment may expedite toxin uptake
- Physical activity should be limited for 4 hours after treatment to avoid the theoretical possibility of untoward toxin diffusion

COMPLICATIONS

- Transient pain
- Eyelid ptosis
- Eyebrow ptosis
- Bruising
- Headache
- Incomplete or asymmetric chemical denervation
- Diplopia
- Dry eyes
- Ectropion
- Asymmetrical smile
- Drooling
- Decreased pucker
- Dysphagia
- Punctate keratitis
- Mask-like expressionless face
- Antibody resistance
- Flu-like symptoms

TREATMENT BENEFITS

Recovery from BTX-A paralysis generally begins at 3 to 4 months after injection. Patients who routinely receive BTX-A may note the recovery time to extend to 4 to 6 months over time. Side effects including eyelid and eyebrow ptosis and bruising generally resolve within 2 to 3 weeks of onset. Treatment benefits may be lengthened with concomitant conservative use of a filler for soft tissue augmentation.

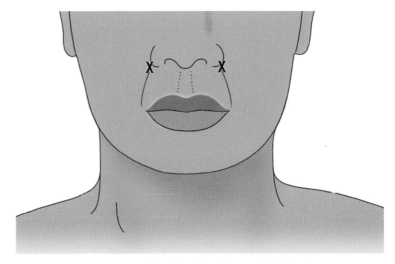

Figure 4.10 *Approximate injection sites for nasolabial folds*

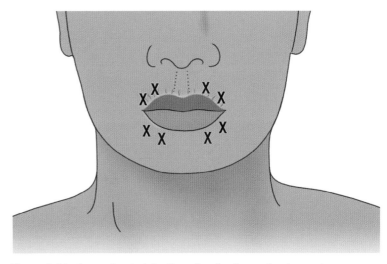

Figure 4.11 *Approximate injection sites for the perioral muscles*

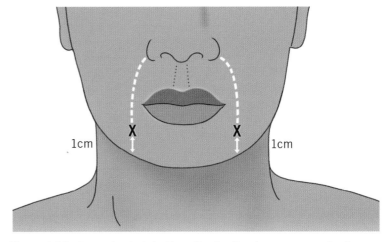

Figure 4.12 *Approximate injection sites for the depressor anguli oris muscle*

PEARLS FOR TREATMENT SUCCESS

• Patients with known neutralizing antibodies against Botox-A may respond to Myobloc given the lack of significant cross reactivity between the two toxins.

• Only FDA-approved botulinum products should be utilized. Unlicensed botulinum toxin may result in severe, life-threatening botulism.

• In the event of an eyelid ptosis, use of (α-adrenergic agonist eyedrops such as apraclonidine hydrochloride 0.5% eyedrops (Iopidine, Alcon, Fort Worth, TX) may be used to provide temporary lid elevation.

• Patients should be informed that the maximum benefit of Botox can take up to 4 weeks to develop.

• Deep furrows will only partially respond to botulinum treatment. Combination therapy with a filler substance may provide the best clinical endpoint.

• It should be emphasized to patients that a single botulinum treatment will not be completely effective in eliminating all treated lines and wrinkles. As well, it should be explained that some residual muscular movement is the desired treatment endpoint.

BIBLIOGRAPHY

Alam M, Dover JS, Arndt KA. Pain associated with injection of botulinum A exotoxin reconstituted using isotonic sodium chloride with and without preservative: A double-blind, randomized controlled trial. *Arch Dermatol.* 2002;138:510-514.

Alster T, Lupton, J. Botulinum toxin type B for dynamic glabellar rhytides refractory to botulinum toxin type A. *Dermatol Surg.* 2003;29(5):516-518.

Blitzer A, Binder WJ, Aviv JE, et al. The management of hyperfunctional facial lines with botulinum toxin. A collaborative study of 210 injection sites in 162 patients. *Arch Otolaryngol Head Neck Surg.* 1997;123:389-392.

Brandt FS, Bocker A. Botulinum toxin for the treatment of neck lines and neck bands. Dermatol Clin. 2004;22:159-166.

Carruthers A, Bogle M, Carruthers JD, et al. A randomized, evaluator-blinded two-center study of the safety and effect of volume on the diffusion and efficacy of botulinum toxin type A in the treatment of lateral orbital rhytides. *Dermatol Surg.* 2007;33:567-571.

Carruthers A, Kiene K, Carruthers J. Botulinum A exotoxin use in clinical dermatology. *J Am Acad Dermatol.* 1996;34:788-797.

Carruthers J, Carruthers A. Botulinum toxin A in the mid and lower face and neck. *Dermatol Clin.* 2004;22:151-158.

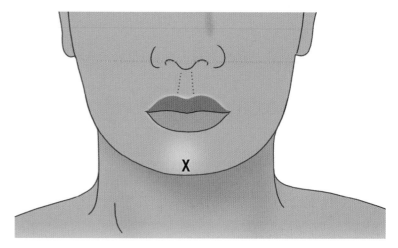

Figure 4.13 *Approximate injection site for the mentalis muscle*

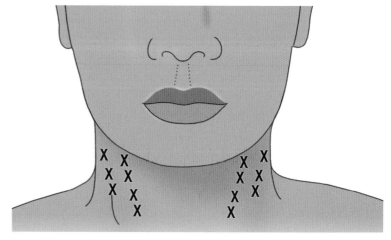

Figure 4.14 *Approximate injection sites for the platysma muscle complex*

Carruthers J, Matarraso S; Botox Consensus Group. Consensus recommendation on the use of botulinum toxin type A in facial aesthetics. *Plastic Reconstruct Surg.* 2004;114:1S-22S.

Chertow DS, Tan ET, Maslanka SE, et al. Botulism in 4 adults following cosmetic injections with an unlicensed, highly concentrated botulinum preparation. *JAMA.* 2006;296:2476-2479.

Hsu TS, Dover JS, Arndt KA. Effect of volume and concentration on the diffusion of botulinum exotoxin. *Arch Dermatol.* 2004;140:1351-1354.

LeLouarn C. Botulinum toxin A and facial lines: The variable concentration. *Aesth Plast Surg.* 2001;25:73-84.

Zimbler MS, Holds JB, Koloska MS, et al. Effect of botulinum toxin pretreatment on laser resurfacing results: A prospective, randomized, blinded trial. *Arch Facial Plast Surg.* 2001;3:165-169.

CHAPTER 5   Chemical Peels

MECHANISM OF ACTION

The application of a wounding agent to induce epidermal and/or dermal sloughing.

INDICATIONS

- Epidermal defects—ephelides, melasma
- Epidermal and dermal defects—melasma, lentigines, post-inflammatory hyperpigmentation, actinic keratoses, superficial rhytides, acne vulgaris
- Dermal defects—deep rhytides, acne scarring, scars

PREOPERATIVE EVALUATION

Peeling agents are selected based on the patient's lifestyle, defect depth, skin characteristics, and defect location (Tables 5.1–5.3).

- Past medical history
  - Past radiation history—decreased adnexal structures likely
  - History of oral herpes simplex virus—reactivation may occur
  - Pregnancy—peels contraindicated with the exception of glycolic acid
  - History of keloid formation—moderate and deep-depth peels should be avoided

TABLE 5.1 ■ **Clinical Indications and Peel Types**

Indication	Peel type	Peel depth/treatment endpoint
Acne vulgaris	Superficial when active	Localized epidermal peeling required; lesional improvement
Ephelides; lentigines	Superficial or medium	Total epidermal peeling required for complete removal; lightening with superficial application
Post-inflammatory inflammation	Superficial or medium	Total epidermal peeling required; lightening with either strength
Melasma	Superficial or medium	Total epidermal peeling required; lightening with either strength; inconsistent response
Superficial rhytides	Superficial	Localized epidermal peeling required; softening
Moderate rhytides	Medium or deep	Total epidermal and papillary dermal peeling required; softening
Deep rhytides	Deep	Total epidermal to reticular dermal peel required; softening
Actinic keratoses	Medium	Total epidermal to papillary dermal peeling required; lesional clearance
Depressed scars	Medium or deep	Lesional edges targeted; total epidermal and partial dermal peeling required; lesional flattening; variable response

TABLE 5.2 ■ **Wounding Depth of Superficial, Medium-Depth, and Deep-Depth Strength Peels**

Superficial peel	Medium-depth peel	Deep peel
α-Hydroxy acid	Glycolic acid and TCA	Baker's Gordon phenol, unoccluded
Modified Unna's resorcinol paste	Jessner's and TCA	Baker's Gordon phenol, occluded
Jessner's	Solid carbon dioxide and TCA	
Salicylic acid	50% TCA	
Solid carbon dioxide slush	Pyruvic acid	
Tretinoin	88% Full-strength phenol	
10%–25% TCA; 35% variable		

TABLE 5.3 ■ **Peeling Agent Characteristics**

Peel type	Color endpoint	Application	Healing time	Safe for
Glycolic acid	Confluent erythema	1–2 coats	1–2 h	All skin types
Jessner	Pale white	Coats are applied singly and endpoint monitored for 3–4 min prior to repeat application	4–5 d; mild epidermal desquamation noted	All skin types
TCA (30% or greater)	Solid white	Single even application; localized applications for lighter white areas may be considered	10–14 d; severe sunburn-like peeling observed	I and II; caution with III and IV
Phenol	Gray white	Single even application; can be conservatively reapplied	10–14 d; superficial burn appearance	I and II

- Past surgical history

  - Prior cosmetic procedures—prior face lift, blepharoplasty, carbon dioxide resurfacing, or dermabrasion may affect peel outcome. Increased ectropion risk present.

- Medication use

  - Previous isotretinoin use and year

  - Topical medications such as tretinoin and α-hydroxy acids may potentiate peel penetration

  - Coumadin use

- Fitzpatrick skin phototype
  - Skin phototypes I–III patients respond to all peel types.
  - Skin phototypes IV and V patients also respond to all peel types, but the risk of post-treatment dyspigmentation is greater.
  - A test site may be warranted for darker skin types to evaluate peel outcome.
- Degree of actinic damage and photoaging
  - A white line of demarcation between peeled and unpeeled skin may be prominent in the presence of moderate to severe dermatoheliosis.
- Wood's lamp evaluation
  - Helpful in ascertaining pigmentation type present
  - Epidermal origin: lesional color enhancement (Fig. 5.1)
  - Dermal or combination epidermal and dermal: no lesional color enhancement to light
  - Examination does not accurately predict clinical peel response
  - Epidermal pigment may respond better to peeling agents compared with dermal or combination pigment deposition
- Medical clearance
  - A recent electrocardiogram is necessary to serve as a baseline for phenol peels in the event of cardiotoxicity.
  - Liver function and renal function tests should be evaluated to ensure adequate hepatorenal function for phenol peels.

IDEAL CANDIDATE

- Skin phototype I or II
- Actinic damaged skin
- Static rhytides associated with sun exposure

LESS IDEAL CANDIDATE

- Dynamic rhytides—achieved benefits are temporary in nature
- Extensive gravitational folds and furrows—likely to require surgical intervention in conjunction with chemical peels
- Deep rhytides
- Boxcar acne or moderate depth atrophic scarring

CONTRAINDICATIONS

- Unrealistic patient expectations
- Patient unable to perform necessary postoperative care

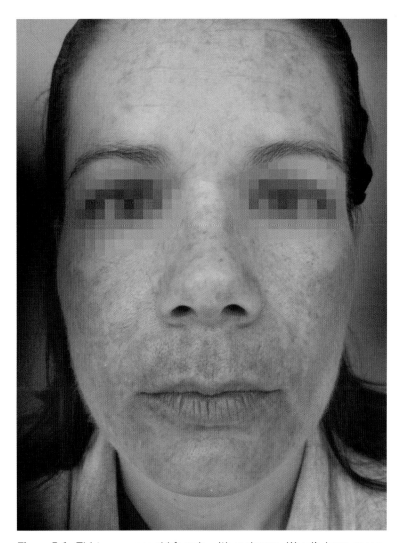

Figure 5.1 *Thirty-one-year-old female with melasma. Wood's lamp accentuated her facial pigmentation*

- Patients with icepick scars or deep atrophic scars
- Patients with dilated, large pore size
- History of oral isotretinoin use within 1 year prior to procedure
- History of keloid formation
- Patient with underlying cardiac arrhythmias (for deep peels)
- Coumadin use (for deep peels)
- Skin phototypes III–VI (for deep peels)

MEDICATIONS

- Preoperative antiviral medications are recommended. Valtrex 500 mg BID or Acyclovir 400 mg TID initiated on the day of procedure and continued for 5 to 14 days is administered depending on peel depth.
- Topical retinoic acid and α-hydroxy acid products are discontinued 48 hours prior to a glycolic acid peel and 1 week prior to a deeper peel and not reinitiated for 1 week post treatment.

WOUND DEPTH

Determined by multiple factors.

- Anatomic considerations
- Facial skin differs from non-facial skin in the relative number of pilosebaceous units per cosmetic unit and thickness. Prominent adnexal structures are required to promote re-epithelialization post treatment.
  - The nose and forehead have more sebaceous glands than do the cheeks or temples.
  - The face has more sebaceous glands than the non-facial areas including the neck.
  - More actinically damaged skin is thinner with fewer pilosebaceous units present.

Body location and presence of actinically damaged skin significantly affects the selection of the wounding agent. The peeling agent may be more destructive in areas with fewer adnexal structures and thinner skin; therefore a less aggressive peeling agent should be utilized in these areas.

- Prepeel skin defatting—use of acetone to defat the treatment area results in a deeper penetrating peel
- Wounding agent strength—an increased strength will result in deeper skin peeling
- Amount of agent applied—deeper skin penetration with each peel layer applied

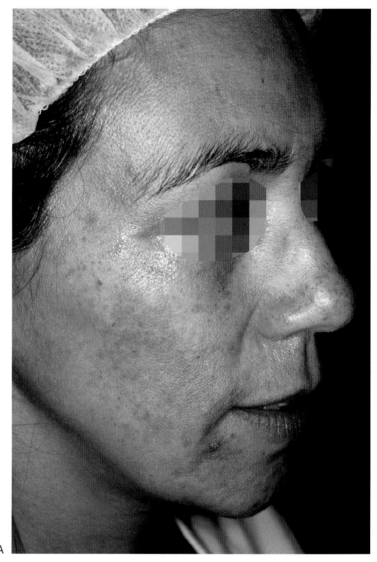

A

Figure 5.2 (A) *Epidermal melasma unresponsive to topical bleaching creams.*

PEEL TYPES

- Superficial peels—partial or complete epidermal injury; may extend into the papillary dermis (Fig. 5.2A and B)

- Medium-depth peels—injury extends into the papillary to upper reticular dermis (Fig. 5.3A and B)

- Deep peels—injury extends into the mid-reticular dermis

PROCEDURE

- Preoperative written consent obtained.

- Preoperative pictures taken.

- Patient's makeup removed and face cleansed with an antiseptic wash (eg, chlorhexidine).

- Scrub the treatment area with acetone on cotton gauze for 2 to 3 minutes.

- The peeling agent should be poured into a glass cup.

- The peeling agent is applied to the treatment site.

  - A paintbrush or cotton ball may be used to apply glycolic acid.

  - A sable brush is recommended for Jessner peel for increased penetration.

  - Cotton-tipped applicators or cotton gauze may be used to apply trichloroacetic acid (TCA) peeling agents.

  - One or two small cotton-tipped applicators are used for phenol application.

  - A round toothpick or wooden portion of a broken cotton-tipped applicator may be used to treat individual rhytides and icepick acne scars.

  - The number of applicators used and the pressure applied to the treatment site with agent application will affect solution delivery and depth of penetration (Figs. 5.4 and 5.5).

- A fan is required to help reduce the associated patient discomfort.

- Pretreatment with Jessner or glycolic acid prior to a TCA peel allows for deeper peel penetration.

- Feathering into the hairline and at the jawline conceals the possible line of demarcation. Feathering should also be performed when the perioral area is treated alone to prevent lines of demarcation (Fig. 5.6).

- The periorbital tissue should be treated first with TCA peels, followed by the nose, cheeks, perioral area, and forehead for best patient tolerance. The upper and lower eyelids may be treated. Extension 2 to 3 mm onto the perioral vermillion is beneficial for rhytides reduction.

- A saline syringe should be available in the case of inadvertent introduction of the peeling agent into the eye.

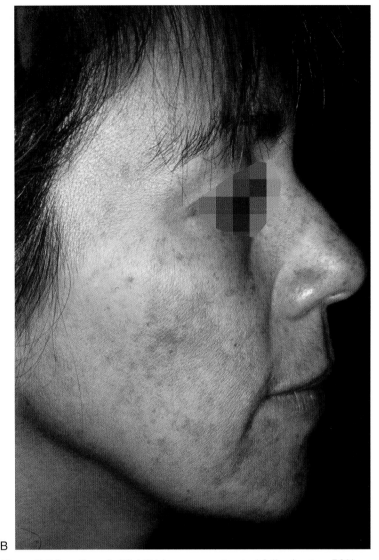

B

Figure 5.2 (*continued*) **(B)** *Mild improvement noted following two 50% glycolic acid peels*

• The applicator should be wrung out and semi-dried to prevent dripping. The glass container should be held away from the patient to avoid direct spilling onto the patient.

• Jessner peel, TCA, and phenol peels are self-neutralizing. Glycolic acid peels must be neutralized with water or bicarbonate solution.

• Cool washcloth is applied to the treated areas.

• Vaseline is applied to the treatment site for Jessner, TCA, and phenol peels. Glycolic acid peels require a light moisturizer.

• Deep peels have inherent cardiac, renal, and hepatic toxicities. Full-face application requires intravenous fluids, sedation, cardiac monitoring, pulse oximeter, and blood pressure monitoring.

COMPLICATIONS

• Greater depth of peel provided than expected (Fig. 5.7)

• Infection—viral, bacterial, fungal

• Temporary or permanent hyperpigmentation or depigmentation

• Prolonged erythema

• Scarring—atrophic, hypertrophic, keloidal; ectropion, delayed healing

• Contact dermatitis

• Textural changes

• Acne

• Milia

• Cardiac arrhythmias (deep phenol peel)

• Laryngeal edema (deep phenol peel)

POSTOPERATIVE CARE

• A light moisturizer is applied twice daily for glycolic acid peels.

• Vaseline is kept on round the clock with twice daily cleansing soap and water, Jessner, TCA, and phenol peels.

• Strict photoprotection is stressed for a minimum of 1 month after a glycolic acid peel and 2 to 3 months for the remainder of peels.

• Patients are instructed to allow natural sloughing of the treated skin. The skin must not be manually removed.

PEARLS FOR TREATMENT SUCCESS

• Careful patient selection and peel selection is necessary for treatment success. It is best to undertreat with a less potent peeling agent in non-facial areas to minimize the risk of scar formation.

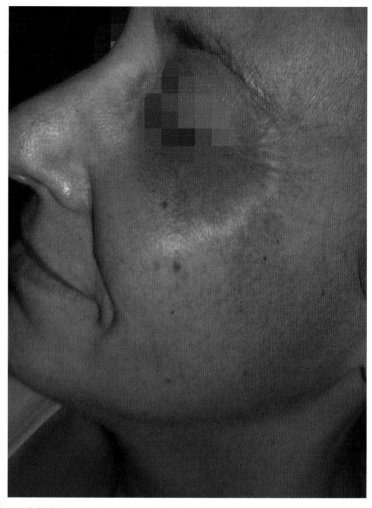

A

Figure 5.3 (A) *Pseudo-ochronosis. The pigmentary changes persisted despite discontinuation of the inciting medication.*

- Patients must be aware of the expected recovery time with each chemical peel and the necessary postoperative wound care they will need to perform to expedite healing. Although one deep peel may provide the greatest benefit, lifestyle or work constraints make serial superficial or medium-depth peels a better long-term goal.

- The margin of safety is much narrower and the risk of complications much greater with increased peel strengths.

- Patients with skin phototypes III and IV have a greater risk of developing pregnancy-induced hypertension after a chemical peel. Consideration of a test site is warranted for medium-depth peels.

- Chemical peels will not alter pore size and may in fact increase their size.

BIBLIOGRAPHY

Baker TJ, Gordon HL, Mosienko P, et al. Long-term histological study of skin after chemical facial peeling. *Plast Reconstr Surg.* 1974;53:522-525.

Brody HJ. Medium-depth chemical peeling of the skin: A variation of superficial chemosurgery. *Adv Dermatol.* 1988;3:205-220.

Grimes PE. Melasma: Etiologic and therapeutic considerations. *Arch Dermatol.* 1997;131:1453-1457.

Gross D. Cardiac arrhythmia during phenol face peeling. *Plast Reconstr Surg.* 1984;73:590-594.

Kligman AM, Baker TJ, Gordon HL. Long-term histologic follow-up of phenol face peels. *Plast Reconstr Surg.* 1985;75:652-659.

Landau M. Combination of chemical peelings with botulinum toxin injections and dermal fillers. *J Cosmet Dermatol.* 2006;5(2):121-126.

MacKee GM, Karp FL. The treatment of post-acne scars with phenol. *Br J Dermatol.* 1952;64(12):456-459.

Matarasso SL, Glogau RG. Chemical face peels. *Dermatol Clin.* 1991;9:131-150.

Monheit G. The Jessner's-trichloroacetic acid peel. *Dermatol Clin.* 1995;13(2):277-283.

Murad H, Shamban AT, Premo PS. The use of glycolic acid as a peeling agent. *Dermatol Clin.* 1995;13(2):285-307.

Que SK, Bergstrom KG. Hyperpigmentation: Old problem, new therapies. J *Drugs Dermatol.* 2009;8(9):879-882.

Rullan P, Karam AM. Chemical peels for darker skin types. *Facial Plast Surg Clin North Am.* 2010;18(1):111-131.

Szzchowicz EH, Wright WK. Delayed healing after full-face chemical peels. *Facial Plast Surg.* 1989;6(1):6-13.

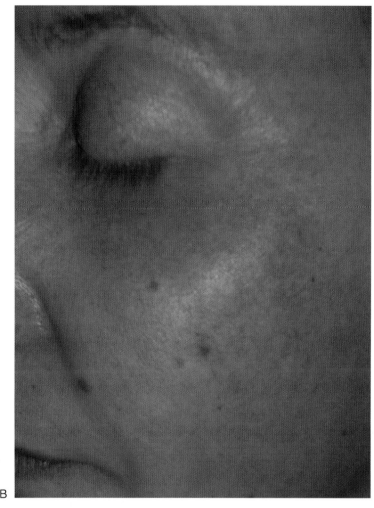

B

Figure 5.3 (*continued*) (B) *Marked pigment lightening after three Jessner 35% TCA peels*

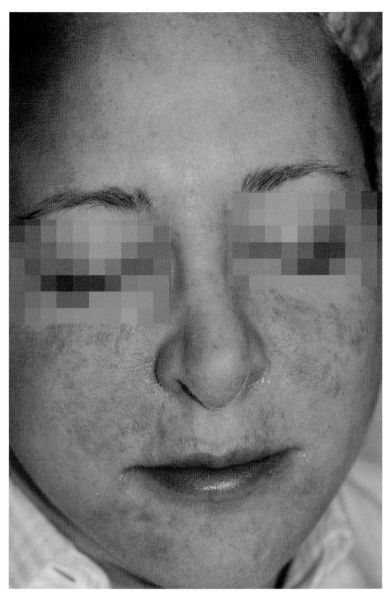

Figure 5.4 *Fine white color immediately following a 20% salicylic acid peel*

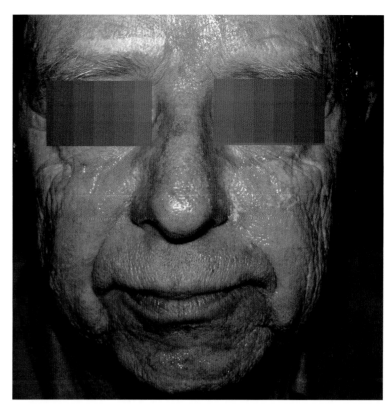

Figure 5.5 *Pale white color immediately following a Jessner peel*

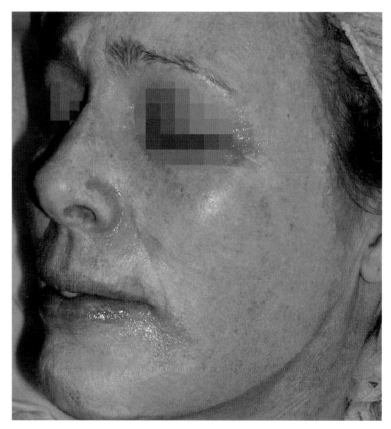

Figure 5.6 *Solid white color immediately following a Jessner/35% TCA peel*

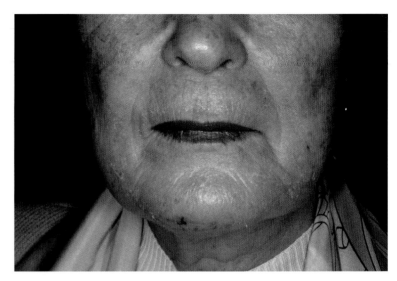

Figure 5.7 *Patient with line of demarcation between the Jessner/35% TCA peel treated perioral area and untreated skin. Patient appears hypopigmented in the treatment site. A subsequent medium-depth peel to the remainder of the face resulted in a more even facial appearance*

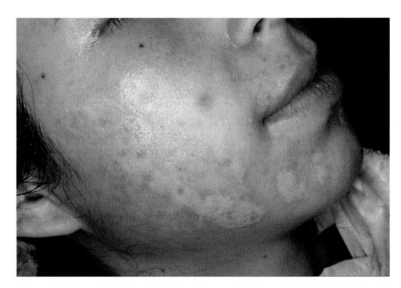

Figure 5.8 *Localized frosting following application of a 50% glycolic acid peel. The localized peel resulted in some mild desquamation for 3 days*

CHAPTER 6 | Nonablative Laser Resurfacing

INTRODUCTION

There are multiple laser and light source treatments for photoaging. These treatments range in efficacy and side effects. Typically, there is a trade-off between clinical improvement and a concomitant increase in side effects and downtime from work and social activities. Other chapters have focused on such treatments as nonablative fractional resurfacing, ablative fractional resurfacing, and traditional resurfacing. This chapter examines nonablative laser resurfacing and, in particular, the use of mid-infrared lasers. Other devices such as intense pulsed light, nonablative fractional resurfacing lasers, and vascular lasers also achieve nonablative benefits, and are addressed in detail in other chapters.

Photoaging encompasses all the changes produced by exposure to ultraviolet (UV) radiation, including telangiectasias, rhytides, poor skin texture, and tone as well as skin laxity (see Dermatoheliosis chapter). Nonablative rejuvenation treats sun-damaged skin by heating dermal collagen with the aim of stimulating new collagen growth. It is also effective in the treatment of acne scars. Epidermal cooling is provided to ensure that thermal heating is targeting the dermis, and not the epidermis. The best advantage of nonablative treatments is that they require little, if any, downtime from work and social activities. This is in contrast to ablative and fractional ablative treatments. In skilled hands, side effects are typically mild and temporary (Fig. 6.1).

Often, they produce subtle or mild benefits, even after multiple treatments. Unfortunately, the predictability of improvement is uncertain. Some patients do not experience any discernible benefit even after multiple treatments. In the past few years, nonablative fractional lasers have produced enhanced results from other forms of nonablative resurfacing, with multiple treatments. These lasers have also proven to be safe in skilled hands. With the advent of nonablative fractional lasers, traditional nonablative laser resurfacing has declined in popularity.

In addition to intense pulsed light sources and vascular lasers, there are many nonablative devices that utilize visible, near-infrared, and mid-infrared wavelengths with epidermal skin cooling. These wavelengths target the water that is abundant in dermal tissue. The skin cooling protects against epidermal damage. These lasers produce deeper dermal penetration, greater absorption, and dermal thermal injury than vascular lasers. Further, there is significantly decreased risk of pigmentary changes in darker skin phototypes at these wavelengths. While the best candidates for treatment are those with mild to moderate static rhytides, the degree of improvement after treatment is difficult to quantify.

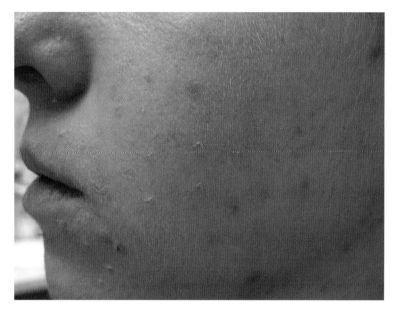

Figure 6.1 *Vesicles appeared 1 day after treatment with a 1450-nm diode laser with a Fitzpatrick skin type 1 patient. These vesicles completely cleared without sequelae 3 days later*

Nonablative lasers

- Subtle improvement of rhytides, particularly when compared to ablative devices

  - Best for patients with mild to moderate photodamage, skin laxity, and skin coarseness

- Requires multiple treatments to provide mild improvement of skin texture, tone, and rhytides

- Little to no postoperative downtime compared to traditional ablative devices

- Patient can return to work or social activities the same day as the procedure

- Can treat cosmetic units effectively without lines of demarcation

INDICATIONS

- Indications

  - Mild rhytides

  - Photodamage, including skin texture and tone

  - Acne scars, including boxcar, atrophic, rolling scars

  - Subtle benefit

  - Mild improvement in skin laxity

  - Not effective for dynamic or deeper rhytides

PREOPERATIVE EVALUATION

- Skin type (can treat darker skin types with mid-infrared lasers, but requires caution with skin cooling)

- Sun exposure

- History of keloids

- Isotretinoin use in past 6 months

- Patients with unrealistic expectations

A consultation is required before this treatment to assess the patient as well as appropriately prepare the patient for the procedure. The patient should be fully educated as to the risks and benefits of the procedure. It is imperative that expectations are set realistically in terms of the mild degree of improvement that will often be seen for rhytides. The patient should also be informed that the benefits of rhytid treatment accrue 3 to 6 months after treatment.

PROPHYLAXIS/ANESTHESIA

May include any of the following:

- Antiviral prophylaxis

- Topical anesthetic

  - 23% Lidocaine/7% tetracaine

  - 7% Lidocaine/7% tetracaine

  - Eutectic mixture of local anesthetic (EMLA)

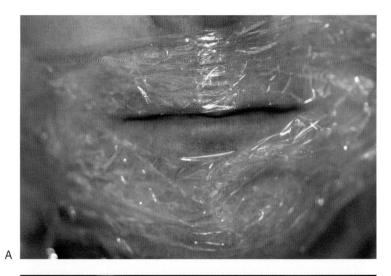

A

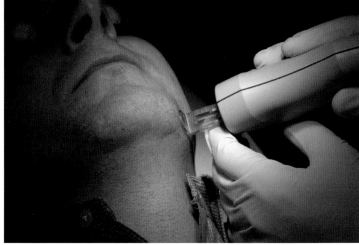

B

Figure 6.2 **(A)** *Patient with EMLA under occlusion prior to treatment of acne scars.* **(B)** *Treatment with 1450-nm diode laser with DCD cooling*

Because some of mid-infrared laser treatments can be painful, some form of anesthesia is often required. It will vary according to the aggressiveness of treatment, the particular susceptibilities of the patient, and the physician's comfort with various anesthetic regimens.

■ Mid-infrared Lasers

The 1320-nm Nd:YAG laser (Cooltouch Inc., Roseville, CA) features a thermal feedback system that measures epidermal temperature to more precisely target dermal collagen. Thus, the laser surgeon can control heating with more precision. It is theorized that new collagen stimulation is caused by inflammatory cytokines after dermal heating.

The 1450-nm diode laser (Smoothbeam, Candela Corp., Wayland, MA) also targets dermal water, while protecting the epidermis with a cryogen spray device (Fig. 6.2). There is no temperature feedback device. With either device, aggressive cooling can produce temporary pigmentary changes.

LASER SAFETY

• Eye protection: metal eye goggles

   – All personnel present at the time of treatment must wear safety glasses/goggles to avoid inadvertent corneal damage.

ADVERSE SIDE EFFECTS

Adverse side effects: far less common than ablative procedures, but do occur with higher fluences as well as inadvertent pulse stacking (ie, firing twice in rapid succession over the same area)

• Scarring

• Bullae (Fig. 6.2)

• Postinflammatory hyperpigmentation (usually from overly aggressive skin cooling)

■ Postoperative Care (Fig. 6.1)

• Little postprocedure pain.

• Any erythema is mild and resolves shortly after treatment.

• There is no requirement for a follow-up visit after treatment.

• No postoperative care is required.

• Patient should be instructed to call if erythema persists or if vesicles or bullae develop (Fig. 6.1).

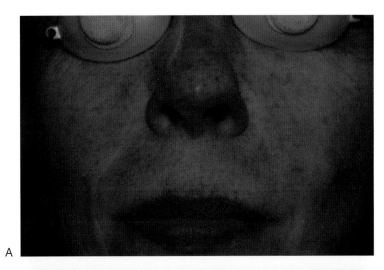

A

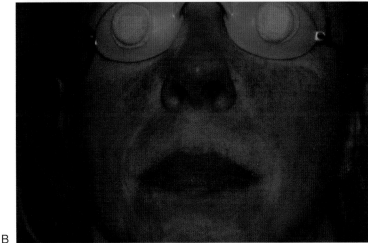

B

Figure 6.3 *Pretreatment and immediate posttreatment photos of non-bruising pulsed dye laser treatments. There is mild erythema after treatments. Many patients note an improvement in the texture and tone of skin after a series of treatments*

- Postoperative erythema resolves quickly. Strict sun avoidance is recommended.

The following practices all significantly increase the risk of scar:

- Aggressive treatments increase risk of scar
- Poor technique, ie, excessive overlap (pulse stacking)

In sum, nonablative laser resurfacing procedures offer the advantage of quick, safe treatments that produce mild improvement of photodamaged skin. Usually, they can be performed on the same day as work and social obligations. Nonetheless, the treatment has its drawbacks such as

- Results are usually modest.
- Duration of benefit, if any, is not known.
- Best results often require more multiple treatments.

Because the improvement is often subtle and unpredictable, even after multiple treatments, other procedures such as nonablative fractional resurfacing have increasingly supplanted the appeal of traditional nonablative procedures.

BIBLIOGRAPHY

Tanzi EL, Williams CM, Alster TS. Treatment of facial rhytides with a nonablative 1450-nm diode laser: A controlled clinical and histologic study. *Dermatol Surg*. 2003;29(2):124-128.

Tanzi EL, Alster TS. Comparison of a 1450-nm diode laser and a 1320-nm Nd:YAG laser in the treatment of atrophic facial scars: A prospective clinical and histologic study. *Dermatol Surg*. 2004;30(2 Pt 1):152-157.

| CHAPTER 7 | Ablative Laser Resurfacing |

MECHANISM OF ACTION

Utilizing the principles of selective photothermolysis, ablative removal of skin in a precisely controlled fashion with resultant minimal surrounding thermal damage is achieved. The depth of tissue penetration is dependent on selective absorption of water. Immediate tissue effects are dependent on the spot size and power utilized as well as the speed of treatment administration. The time of laser–tissue interaction is the critical factor for residual thermal damage. Epidermal obliteration and(or partial ablation or coagulation of the upper dermis is the endpoint. Re-epithelialization results from the migration of cells that arise from surrounding follicular adnexae. Normal compact collagen and elastic fibers replace the amorphous elastotic dermal components, and normal, well-organized epithelial cells replace the disorganized photodamaged epidermis. Collagen remodeling is noted both intraoperatively via thermal shrinkage and contraction and postoperatively within the remodeling phase of wound healing.

■ Carbon Dioxide Laser (CO$_2$ Resurfacing)

Continuous wave (10,600 nm), super-pulsed, and scanned CO$_2$ lasers are utilized for resurfacing. A relatively bloodless surgery with reduced swelling is achieved via the photocoagulative effect on blood vessels and lymphatics. The risk of scarring, unpredictable level of thermal damage, and delayed healing of the continuous wave laser limit its clinical use. The scanned and pulsed CO$_2$ lasers deliver high peak fluences in less than 0.001 seconds to achieve tissue vaporization of 20 to 30 μm per pass. Approximately 40 to 120 μm of residual thermal damage is noted per pass (Fig. 7.1).

■ Erbium:Yttrium-Aluminum Garnet Laser (Er:YAG)

A laser of wavelength 2,490 nm is utilized for more superficial resurfacing. It is 16× more selectively absorbed by water. It achieves tissue vaporization of 1 to 5 μm per pass. It results in a narrower zone of residual thermal damage (5–30 μm). As a zone of thermal damage of 50 μm or greater is required for photocoagulation, Er:YAG treatment results in a slightly bloody surgical field. The thermal damage is also insufficient to produce immediate collagen contraction. Long-term collagen remodeling is limited (Fig. 7.2).

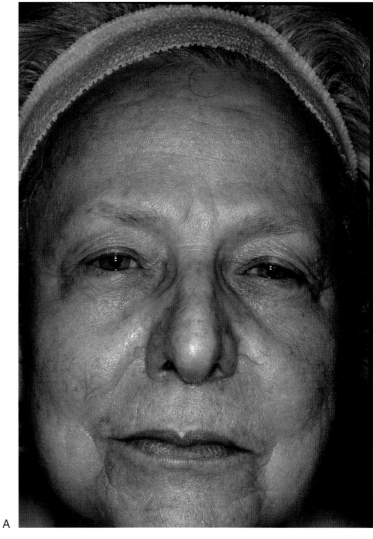

A

Figure 7.1 (A) *A 58-year-old woman with extensive actinic damage.*

INDICATIONS

Ablative lasers have been utilized as a cutting tool and vaporizing tool to treat epidermal and superficial dermal lesions.

- Cutting tool: keloids, acne keloidalis nuchae, cyst removal, basal carcinoma, burn, and ulcer debridement; hair transplantation; blepharoplasty; other incisional surgeries where controlled hemostasis is desired or where epinephrine is contraindicated or a pacer precludes use of electrosurgery.

- Vaporizing tool: treatment of numerous conditions including static and dynamic rhytides, boxcar, crateriform and hypertrophic acne scars, pox scars, warts, lentigines, adenoma sebaceum, angiokeratomas, pyogenic granuloma, lymphangioma circumscriptum, Bowen's disease, erythroplasia of Queyrat, oral florid papillomatosis, actinic cheilitis, actinic keratoses, epidermal nevi, syringomas, granuloma faciale, neurofibromas, xanthelasma, and tattoos.

- Not indicated for the treatment of icepick acne scars.

PREOPERATIVE EVALUATION

Significant past medical history includes a history of herpes labialis; underlying autoimmune disease or immune deficiency; underlying koebnerizing/infectious conditions including psoriasis, verrucae, and molluscum; history of keloid or hypertrophic scar formation; underlying cardiac or pulmonary conditions that may be exacerbated by the use of anesthetic medications; existing drug allergies; tobacco use; active acne vulgaris.

Significant past surgical history includes prior surgical treatments to the treatment sites, surgical dates, and patient response.

The patient must be aware of the lengthy recovery period that will require extensive hands-on patient care for optimal treatment results. Re-epithelialization requires 7 to 10 days with associated pain, edema, and erythema. Postoperative erythema resolves over an average period of 3 to 5 months. Strict sun avoidance must be followed for a minimum of 1 year postoperatively to avoid pigmentary changes and photosensitivity. Realistic expectations are the most important determinants of treatment success. The patient must be aware that the treatment will improve but does not eliminate all or even most rhytides or scars and that dynamic rhytides are likely to recur within a few months postoperatively.

Procedural risks to emphasize include temporary and/or permanent hyperpigmentation and depigmentation, infection (viral, bacterial, yeast), and scar (atrophic, hypertrophic, keloidal) formation; acne flare; eczema lasting 1 to 2 months. Predictable side effects include procedural and postoperative discomfort; edema, oozing,

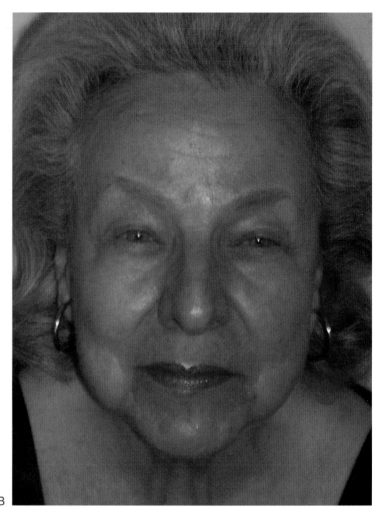

B

Figure 7.1 (*continued*) **(B)** *A marked reduction in rhytides and dyspigmentation is noted 2 months after full-face carbon dioxide resurfacing*

and crusting lasting 1 to 2 weeks; erythema, skin tightness, and pruritus lasting up to 3 to 4 months.

IDEAL LASER CANDIDATE

- Fair skin type (Fitzpatrick phototypes I–II)
- Laser-amenable lesions
- Minimal associated dyspigmentation of neck and chest
- Able to tolerate extended period of convalescence postoperatively
- Able to follow and execute necessary postoperative skin care regimen
- Realistic treatment expectations

LESS THAN IDEAL LASER CANDIDATE

- Darker skin type (Fitzpatrick phototypes III, IV, and V); treat with caution, due to significant risk of temporary and/or permanent pigmentary alterations
- Moderate associated dyspigmentation of neck and chest
- Unable to follow and execute necessary postoperative skin care regimen
- Prior facial surgical procedures performed
- Prominent facial pore pattern—laser treatment may exacerbate their appearance

ABSOLUTE CONTRAINDICATIONS

- Use of oral tretinoin within 1 year of surgery
- Skin phototypes V and VI
- Active cutaneous infection
- Preexisting ectropion
- Poor patient compliance
- Unrealistic patient expectations

RELATIVE CONTRAINDICATIONS

- Extensive underlying dyspigmentation of face and surrounding neck and chest-risk of demarcation line/difference in skin color of treated versus untreated skin
- Skin phototypes III and IV
- Underlying connective tissue
- Underlying koebnerizing condition
- Underlying immunologic disease
- Previous lower lid and/or blepharoplasty (for infraorbital resurfacing)

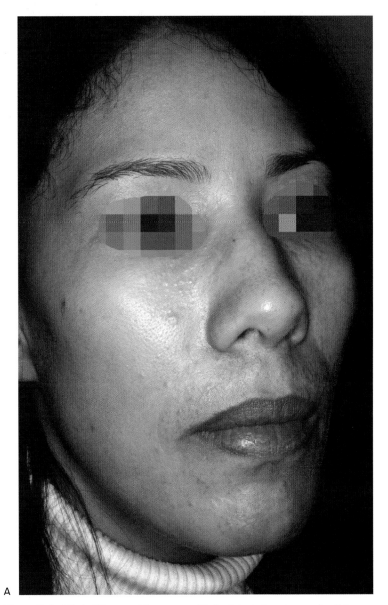

A

Figure 7.2 (A) *A 45-year-old woman with facial photoaging and mild acne scarring.*

- Previous ablative resurfacing, dermabrasion, cryosurgery; facelift or phenol peel
- History of facial radiation treatment

MEDICATIONS

- Antibacterial therapy: to avoid impetiginization and bacterial infection of the treatment sites, prophylactic antibiotics are initiated 1 day preoperatively.

  - Dicloxacillin 500 mg PO BID or Keflex 500 mg PO BID for 10 to 14 days is prescribed.

  - In penicillin-allergic individuals, Ciprofloxacin 500 mg PO BID × 10 to 14 days or azithromycin 500 mg PO × 1 day followed by 250 mg daily for 5 days is recommended.

- Antiviral therapy: laser resurfacing may trigger a herpes simplex outbreak that can spread to the treatment sites with an increased risk of scar formation.

  - Prophylactic antiviral medications are initiated 1 day preoperatively.

  - Valacyclovir 500 mg PO BID for 14 days or acyclovir 400 mg PO TID for 14 days is recommended.

- Topical tretinoin

  - Use of tretinoin prior to CO_2 laser resurfacing has been shown clinically and via biochemical analysis to not provide enhanced collagen formation, accelerated re-epithelialization, or quicker resolution of postoperative erythema.

  - Use of this medication is optional.

  - Use of this medication postoperatively should be postponed until all associated erythema and inflammation have resolved.

- Bleaching creams: no published, controlled trials have demonstrated the benefits of preoperative bleaching creams to reduce the risk of postinflammatory hyperpigmentation. To possibly reduce this risk, patients with skin phototypes III and IV are prescribed a bleaching cream to be applied twice daily for 6 to 7 weeks prior to treatment. As well, strict sun avoidance is mandatory.

ANESTHESIA

- Cold-air cooling (Zimmer) may be adequate for localized or single-pass CO_2 treatment or Er:YAG treatment.

- Topical anesthesia may be adequate for localized or single-pass CO_2 treatment or Er:YAG treatment.

- Regional nerve blocks with supplemental infiltrative anesthesia are generally administered for multiple-pass CO_2 treatment.

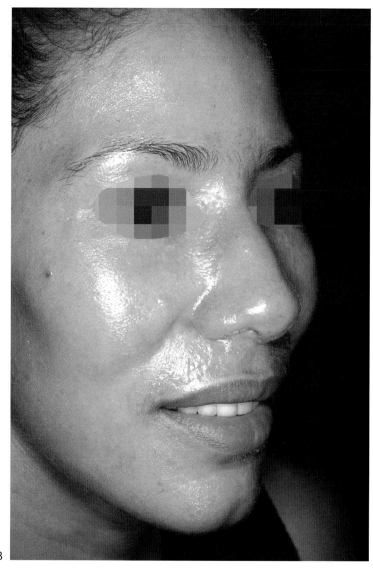

B

Figure 7.2 (*continued*) **(B)** *Improvement of photoaging 3 weeks after full-face erbium treatment*

- Site-dependent blocks include supraorbital, supratrochlear, infraorbital, and mental blocks.

- Lidocaine (1%) with 1:100,000 or 1:200,000 epinephrine, a total of 0.5 to 1.0 mL is administered per site.

- Supplemental infiltrative anesthesia consisting of an equal mixture of 1% lidocaine, 0.5% bupivacaine, and 1:10 sodium bicarbonate is generally required, especially for the jawline, upper eyelids, and temples.

- Hyaluronidase (Wydase) 75 U for tissue diffusion may be added to the infiltrative anesthesia.

- Treatment is delayed 10 to 15 minutes to allow for complete anesthetic effect.

• Conscious intravenous sedation and general anesthesia have been employed by trained physicians in certified facilities in patients unable to tolerate the injections or for larger procedures.

SAFETY MEASURES

• Eye protection

- One or two drops of 0.05% topical proparacaine (Alcaine) or 0.05% topical tetracaine (Pontocaine) are placed into each eye of the patient, followed by the application of topical erythromycin ointment or ophthalmic lubricant (eg, Lacri-Lube) and nonreflective metallic ocular shields (eg, Byron Medical, Tucson, AZ; Oculo-Plastik, Montreal, Canada).

- All personnel must wear clear plastic safety glasses to avoid inadvertent corneal damage.

• Operative field

- All reflective surfaces and windows must be covered to avoid inadvertent treatment of a reflective surface.

- The treatment room door must be labeled properly to warn others not to enter during laser treatment.

- All flammable materials and anesthetic gases must be kept away from the operative field.

- Wet drapes and sponges are placed around the surgical site to prevent accidental irradiation of surrounding skin and to minimize potential fire risk.

- A nonflammable ointment (eg, Surgilube; KY Jelly) must be placed over the exposed hairline and eyebrows to avoid hair singeing. Surgilube should not be used over the eyelashes to avoid the risk of corneal keratitis.

- All surgical tools utilized must possess a nonreflective or roughened black coating to prevent laser beam deflection.

- A laser smoke evacuator that filters particles as small as 0.12 m in diameter and laser-grade surgical masks must be used to reduce potential spread of infectious particles in the laser plume.

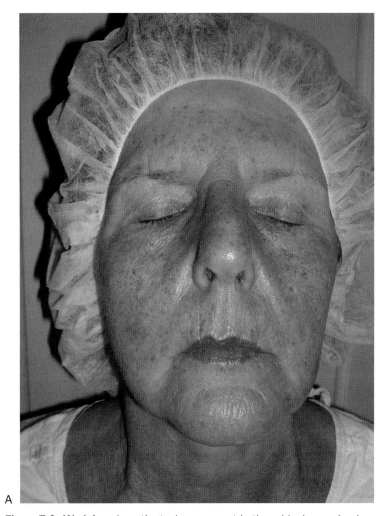

A

Figure 7.3 (A) *A female patient who was most bothered by her perioral rhytides, but was also noted to have moderate dermatoheliosis with numerous lentigines and actinic damage of the remainder of her face.*

– Use of Hibiclens, isopropyl alcohol, and acetone is prohibited due to their flammable nature. All makeup and hairspray are to be removed, as they are potentially flammable.

– The laser should be kept in the standby mode at all times other than active treatment to avoid accidental firing.

– Oxygen should be avoided, but if needed, should be closely monitored and only used in conjunction with a closed gas system that includes either endotracheal intubation of laryngeal mask airway.

PROCEDURE

• A thorough review of the risks and benefits is performed.

• Patient written consent is obtained.

• Representative preoperative pictures are obtained.

• Pretreatment preparation is performed.

• The choice of laser and laser parameters varies, depending on the clinical situation.

– The CO_2 laser is preferable for deeper lines and scarring processes and for fair-skinned patients (Fig. 7.1).

– The Er:YAG laser is beneficial for superficial lines and dyspigmentation and for darker skinned patients (Fig. 7.2).

– The patient's postoperative considerations also affect the choice of laser. The CO_2 laser will have an expected longer recovery compared with the Er:YAG laser.

• In general, treatment of a cosmetic unit or full face is best to minimize the risk of textural mismatch between nontreated and treated areas. In an isolated treatment, one must treat the entire lesion or line to their end rather than remain within a cosmetic unit.

• The vermilion border can be treated conservatively to minimize lipstick "bleeding."

• Treatment should extend beyond the anatomical unit being treated with a feathering technique (decreased fluence) employed to blend into the untreated skin.

• For depressed scars, additional passes with a smaller spot size on the defect edge allow for more significant flattening of the scar.

• Scar contraction will occur with healing. To avoid atrophic scar formation, administer treatment to the level of near normal adjacent skin only.

• Ablative resurfacing of dynamic rhytides provides only temporary benefit. Consideration of combination therapy with botulinum toxin or a filler substance should be entertained to achieve maximum benefit.

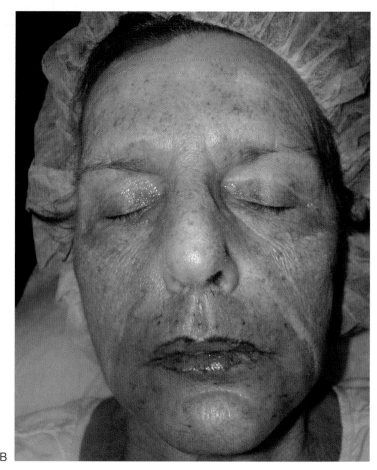

B

Figure 7.3 (*continued*) **(B)** *Same patient immediately after perioral carbon dioxide laser resurfacing and a Jessner/35% trichloroacetic acid peel to the remainder of her face.*

- Minimal mechanical trauma technique: fewer CO_2 passes performed with retainment of the last pass eschar to expedite healing and minimize scar risk and pigmentary changes. This technique is optimal for younger patients with more superficial lesions and for darker skin types.

- With any treatment modality, the presence of larger collagen bundles herald entry into the deep reticular dermis and warn of the possibility of scar formation. Treatment should be discontinued immediately.

- Resurfacing of nonfacial rhytides is associated with a high risk for textural and pigmentary changes due to the reduction in adnexal structures and poor vascularity in comparison to the face. The CO_2 laser should not be utilized for the treatment of nonfacial rhytides. The Er:YAG laser should be utilized with extreme caution.

- Combination therapies of carbon dioxide resurfacing and chemical peels, botulinum toxin, or soft tissue augmentation may provide the greatest benefit (Fig. 7.3).

POSTOPERATIVE CARE

- An open wound technique or closed technique may be followed.

- Postoperative discomfort is characterized by moderate burning within the first 24 hours. This is minimized with the use of an occlusive dressing. It can generally be controlled with ice packs, cold compresses, and acetaminophen, as well as frequent wound care.

- Postoperative edema develops 24 to 48 hours postoperatively and can be controlled with ice packs and head elevation. Oral steroids are employed when marked swelling develops intraoperatively or immediately postoperatively.

- Re-epithelialization occurs within 3 to 10 days and is dependent on the laser utilized, the number of laser passes executed, and the surgical candidate. Younger patients, patients who undergo Er:YAG treatment, and fewer passes show faster healing. Delayed healing is observed in older patients, smokers, and increased laser passes.

- Topical antibiotics and Aquaphor Healing Ointment should be avoided due to the risk of allergic contact dermatitis.

- Close follow-up is mandatory to ensure proper care and healing of the treated sites (Figs. 7.4 and 7.5).

- Prophylactic antibiotics and antiviral medications are continued for 10 to 14 days postoperatively to avoid infection.

- Strict sun avoidance is maintained for 1 year postoperatively to avoid photosensitivity and to minimize the risk of postinflammatory hyperpigmentation.

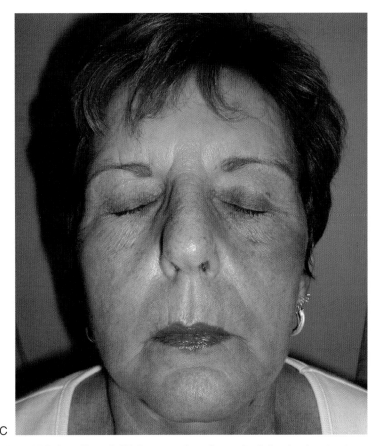

C

Figure 7.3 (*continued*) (C) *Same patient 6 months following her treatment. A marked reduction in both her rhytides and dyspigmentation is appreciated.*

PEARLS FOR TREATMENT SUCCESS

- Preoperative wound care instructions are critical for treatment success. The patient and significant others must be prepared for the extensive care that will be required for expedient and safe healing. Patients should be shown postoperative pictures to prepare them for how they will appear. Postoperative supplies, including wound care supplies and desired camouflage foundation, should be obtained prior to the treatment date. Patients with younger children must prepare them for the significant changes that will be noted during the healing period. Any postoperative assistance the patient may require should be arranged prior to treatment if possible.

- Patients require frequent postoperative evaluation for the first 14 days to ensure proper wound care is being employed, predicted healing is noted, and no side effects such as scar formation or infection occur. Patients should be evaluated on postoperative day 2, postoperative day 5 to 7, and postoperative day 10 to 14 and anytime the patient expresses a concern of need for evaluation.

- Patients' expectations must be tailored to the expected benefits. Patients should be informed that the greatest benefits will not be appreciated for 6 to 12 months postoperatively.

- Strict photoprotection and sun protection are critical in reducing the occurrence of postinflammatory hyperpigmentation and sunburn and should be followed for a minimum of 1 year after treatment.

- Treated skin is sensitive to a majority of facial products, perfumes, and topical medications for an average of 12 weeks posttreatment. Bland products, including a sun block, are recommended during this healing time.

- Persistent areas of erythema should raise concern regarding scar formation or infection. A culture is recommended to rule out bacterial or yeast infection. Use of a potent topical corticosteroid and/or pulsed dye laser is crucial with close follow-up to ensure resolution.

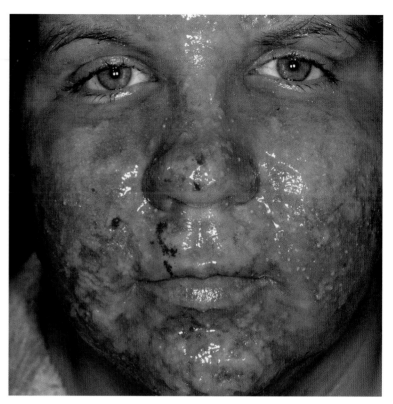

Figure 7.4 *Under aggressive wound care. A substantial amount of crusting is observed. Proper wound care was demonstrated in-office and with repeat written instructions reviewed*

BIBLIOGRAPHY

Alster TS. Cutaneous resurfacing with CO_2 and erbium:YAG lasers: Preoperative, intraoperative and postoperative considerations. *Plast Reconstr Surg.* 1999;103:619-634.

Anderson RR, Parrish JA. Selective photothermolysis: Precise microsurgery by selective absorption of pulsed radiation. *Science.* 1983;220:524-527.

Carruthers J, Carruthers A, Zelichowska A. The power of combined therapies: Botox and ablative laser resurfacing. *Am J Cosmet Surg.* 2000;17:129-131.

David I, Ruiz-Esparza J. Fast healing after laser skin resurfacing. The minimal mechanical trauma technique. *Dermatol Surg.* 1997;23:359-361.

Dover JS, Hruza GJ, Arndt KA. Lasers in skin resurfacing. *Semin Cutan Med Surg.* 1996;15:177-188.

Duke D, Grevelink JM. Care before and after laser skin resurfacing. A survey and review of the literature. *Dermatol Surg.* 1998;24:201-206.

Fitzpatrick RS, Goldman MP, Satur NM, Tope WD. Pulsed carbon dioxide laser resurfacing of photoaged facial skin. *Arch Dermatol.* 1996;132:395-402.

Fitzpatrick RE, Tope WD, Goldman MP, et al. Pulsed carbon dioxide laser, trichloroacetic acid, Backer–Gordon phenol and dermabrasion: A comparative clinical and histologic study of cutaneous resurfacing in a porcine model. *Arch Dermatol.* 1996;132:469-471.

Nanni CA, Alster TS. Complications of carbon dioxide laser resurfacing: An evaluation of 500 patients. *Dermatol Surg.* 1998;24:315-320.

Orringer JS, Kang S, Johnson TM, et al. Tretinoin treatment before carbon-dioxide laser resurfacing: A clinical and biochemical analysis. *J Am Acad Dermatol.* December 2004;51(6):940-946.

Raulin C, Grema H. Single-pass carbon dioxide laser skin resurfacing combined with cold-air cooling: Efficacy and patient satisfaction of a prospective side-by-side study. *Arch Dermatol.* 2004;140(11):1333-1336.

Ruiz-Esparza J, Barba Gomez JM, Gomez de la Torre OL. Wound care after laser skin resurfacing. A combination of open and closed methods using a new polyethylene mask. *Dermatol Surg.* 1998;24:79-81.

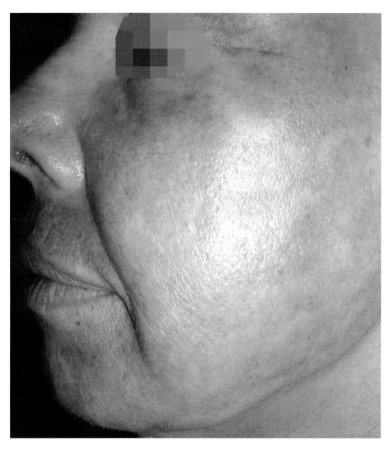

Figure 7.5 *Postinflammatory hyperpigmentation 6 weeks after perioral carbon dioxide resurfacing. This pigmentation resolved with the use of 4% hydroquinone twice daily for 2 months*

| CHAPTER 8 | Nonablative Fractional Laser Resurfacing |

MECHANISM OF ACTION

Nonablative fractional resurfacing (NAFR) is a novel concept of skin rejuvenation that can target both epidermal and dermal conditions. NAFR produces a unique thermal damage pattern consisting of multiple columns of thermal coagulative damage, referred to as microthermal treatment zones (MTZs) (Fig. 8.1). NAFR characteristically spares the tissue surrounding each MTZ, thus allowing fast epidermal repair due to microscopic size of the wounds and short migratory distance for the viable keratinocytes present at the MTZ epidermal margins. Only a fraction of the skin of the surface area is treated.

DERMATOPATHOLOGY

MTZ reveals homogenized columns of dermal matrix and the formation of microscopic epidermal necrotic debris (MEND) (Fig. 8.2). MEND formation is thought to represent the process of elimination of the thermally damaged epidermis containing pigment by the rapidly migrating viable keratinocytes at the MTZ margins. MEND may also contain dermal structures such as the elastic fibers. Vessels in the MTZ regions can be thermally destroyed in a nonselective manner. Higher energies result in deeper and wider MTZs. Higher energies result in deeper and wider MTZs. NAFR can be helpful in the treatment of epidermal pigmentation such as melasma and lentigines due to the process of MEND formation. NAFR can also be helpful in improving rhytides and scarring due to the process of collagen remodeling and new collagen formation, induced by the dermal thermal damage.

INDICATIONS

NAFR can be an effective treatment of fine-to-moderate rhytides; acne scars, surgical, traumatic, and burn scars; melasma; dyschromia; and dermatoheliosis (Fig. 8.3).

PREOPERATIVE EVALUATION

- Significant past medical history includes history of herpes labialis, keloid or hypertrophic scar formation, oral tretinoin intake (date last course completed), topical retinoid use, tobacco use, and known drug allergies including lidocaine allergy.
- Significant past surgical history includes prior surgical treatments to the treatment sites, the dates of the procedures, the patient's response, and the associated side effects.

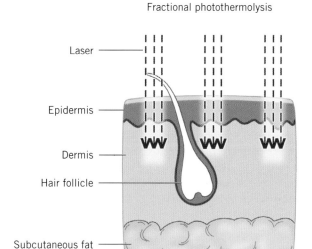

Fractional photothermolysis

Figure 8.1 *Schematic of microscopic treatment zones (MTZ) created by fractional resurfacing laser (note the characteristic sparing of the surrounding tissue between the treatment zones)*

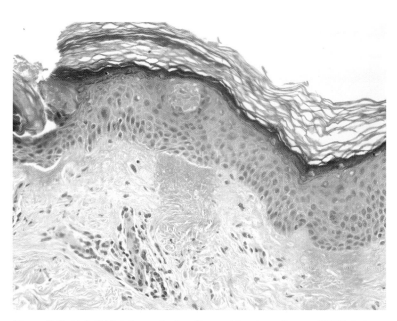

Figure 8.2 *H & E histology of microthermal treatment zone (MTZ) 1 day after fractional resurfacing treatment (note the microscopic epidermal necrotic debris (MEND) overlying a column of homogenized dermis)*

- The patient should be aware of the following:
  - Procedural discomfort.
  - Sunburn-like sensation for several hours after the procedure.
  - Sunburn-like postoperative erythema that may persist for 3 to 7 days (Fig. 8.4).
  - Postoperative edema, generally mild, that usually resolves within 2 to 3 days.
  - Postoperative bronzing that is generally noted on the third postoperative day and often persists for 3 to 4 days.
  - Postoperative superficial peeling that is often mild and is noted to start on the third postoperative day and to persist for 3 to 4 days.
  - Realistic expectations for the procedure: the patient should be aware that the treatment will improve fine-to-moderate wrinkles, pigmentation, and superficial scars but does not eliminate moderate-to-deep rhytides. A modest benefit may be noted for deeper wrinkles.
  - Procedural risks: although these adverse events are uncommon and are much less frequent than those associated with ablative resurfacing, they still exist. They include temporary postinflammatory hyperpigmentation (Fig. 8.5), blistering, crusting, milia (Fig. 8.6), acneiform eruption, pinpoint hemorrhage (Fig. 8.7), herpes simplex reactivation, and rarely hypertrophic scarring. This is in addition to the predictable side effects that include procedural discomfort, postoperative erythema, bronzing, and edema. There is usually no associated oozing or crusting unless very high energies and/or high densities are utilized.
- The ideal candidate is a fair-skin patient (Fitzpatrick phototypes I–III). However, NAFR can be safe and effective in darker skin types (Fitzpatrick phototypes IV and V). It is also safe to use on nonfacial areas including the neck, trunk, and extremities, provided that decreased fluences and densities are utilized.

CONTRAINDICATIONS

- Oral tretinoin use within 6 months to 1 year of surgery
- Active cutaneous infection
- Unrealistic patient expectations
- Pregnant or lactating woman

MEDICATIONS

- Antibacterial therapy: prophylactic antibiotics are generally not required

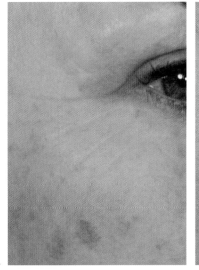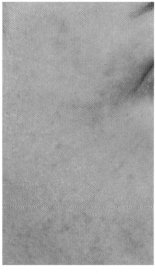

A   B

Figure 8.3 *Periorbital rhytides* **(A)** *following one fractional resurfacing treatment and* **(B)** *following four fractional resurfacing treatments. An appreciable softening is noted (Courtesy of R. Fitzpatrick, MD)*

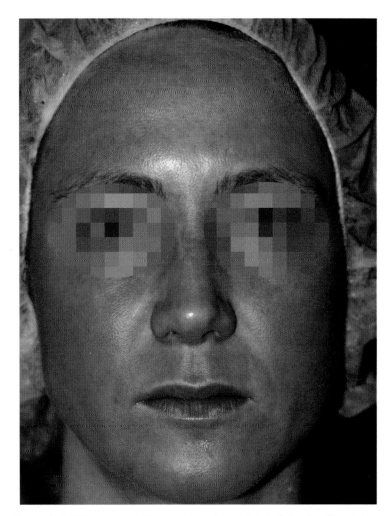

Figure 8.4 *Mild sunburn-like erythema immediately following Fraxel laser treatment with 6 to 8 mJ, 250 MTZ/cm², eight passes. This erythema may persist for 3 to 7 days*

- Antiviral therapy
  - Fractional resurfacing may trigger reactivation of herpes simplex that can spread to the treatment sites.
  - Prophylactic antiviral medications are initiated 1 day prior to the procedure. Valacyclovir 500 mg PO BID or acyclovir 400 mg PO TID for 7 days is usually recommended. An alternative is valacyclovir 2 PO BID for 1 day to be started the morning of the procedure.
- Tretinoin: it is advised to discontinue tretinoin cream at several days before NAFR to prevent skin irritation at the treatment sites.

ANESTHESIA

- Cold-air cooling (Zimmer) is very effective in decreasing the procedural discomfort.
- Topical anesthesia (oil or cream base) applied at least 1 hour before the procedure is generally adequate, especially in combination with cold-air cooling (Zimmer).
- Regional nerve blocks can be effective to reduce the discomfort for patients with low pain thresholds, especially when utilizing higher fluences and densities. Infraorbital and mental blocks can be helpful when treating perioral wrinkles, but are usually not necessary.

PREOPERATIVE PREPARATION

- Explain the risks and benefits of the procedure.
- Obtain the patient's written consent.
- Wash the area to be treated with soap and water.
- Obtain preoperative pictures.
- Apply a thick layer of topical anesthetic in an oil or cream base to the treatment site.
- Wait at least 60 minutes to achieve optimal anesthetic effect.
- Wipe off the topical anesthetic with a damp cloth.

PROCEDURAL TIPS

- The laser parameters are chosen according to the clinical target.
  - For epidermal conditions such as photodamage, lentigines, melasma, and dyschromia: lower fluences and higher densities are usually utilized.
  - For deeper processes such as rhytides or acne scarring: higher fluences are utilized.
- Lower percent coverage of skin surface area; that is, lower densities are indicated in darker skin types to avoid postinflammatory hyperpigmentation.

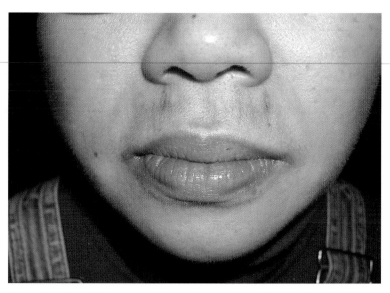

Figure 8.5 *Postinflammatory hyperpigmentation following fractional resurfacing treatment to the upper lip*

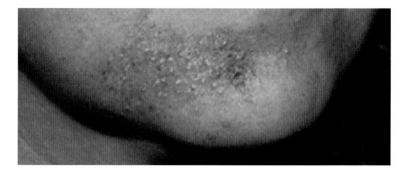

Figure 8.6 *Milia on the chin 1 day after NAFR*

- Caution should be exerted when treating smaller areas such as upper lip, nose, and temple in order to avoid bulk heating that can result in blistering and scarring.
  - Allow adequate time between passes for the heat to dissipate and the skin to cool down before the next pass.
  - When treating the upper lip, alternate the treatment between the right side and the left side, and start each pass from the same point.
- Three to six treatment sessions (depending on the indication for treatment) are administered 3 to 4 weeks apart. Longer period between treatments is advised in darker-skin patients to avoid or decrease the incidence of postinflammatory hyperpigmentation (PIH).

POSTOPERATIVE CARE

- Postoperative discomfort is generally mild and transient. The patient will experience a sunburn sensation for several hours.
- Patients may apply makeup immediately after the treatment.
- Patients are encouraged to use mild moisturizers for several days after the procedure.
- Postoperative edema is usually minimal but can be controlled with ice packs and head elevation. In rare instances of marked swelling, oral prednisone can be prescribed for 3 to 7 days.
- Sun avoidance is maintained for at least 4 to 6 weeks after the procedure to minimize the risk of postinflammatory hyperpigmentation. Sunscreens with a minimum SPF of 30 are recommended.
- Typically, patients can return to work on the first postoperative day.

PEARLS FOR TREATMENT SUCCESS

- Patient selection is the key. Treating rhytides or scars that are too deep will prove disappointing to the patient and physician. The patient must be aware of the need for multiple treatments to obtain the desired clinical benefit.
- NAFR can result in serious side effects such as scarring when used at very high fluencies by inexperienced physicians or health care workers. Caution should be taken to stay within the recommended parameters and apply appropriate overlapping technique to avoid potential complications.
- Patients must be aware that benefits may be short lasting and may require maintenance treatments for continued clinical benefit.

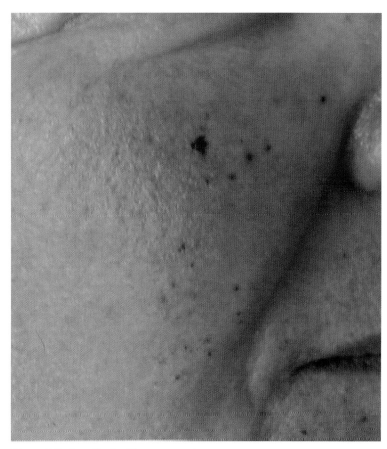

Figure 8.7 *A patient with rosacea who developed pinpoint hemorrhage 1 day after Fraxel Restore treatment. Pinpoint hemorrhage can occur with higher energies and usually resolves in few days with no sequelae*

- Effective NAFR treatment in patients with skin phototypes III to V can be achieved. An increased incidence of postinflammatory hyperpigmentation is generally noted. Patients must be aware of the possibility of PIH with each treatment. Decreasing the density of treatment reduces the risk of PIH.

DEVICES

The most commonly used NAFR devices that are available in the market are Fraxel Restore (Solta Medical, Inc., Hayward, CA), Lux 1,540 nm laser (Palomar Medical Technologies, Burlington, MA), and Affirm 1,440 nm Nd:YAG laser (Cynosure, Westford, MA) (Table 8.1). Fraxel Restore utilizes the scanning technology whereas Lux 1,540 nm and Affirm 1,440 nm lasers utilize the stamping technology and do not usually require topical anesthesia or disposable tips.

TABLE 8.1 ■ Nonablative Fractional Lasers

Company	Laser device	Laser wavelength (nm)	Mode	Tip diameter (mm)	Max energy/MTZ or microbeam (mJ)	Density delivered (cm^2)
Solta Medical	Fraxel Restore (Fraxel SR 1,500)	1,550	Scanning	7 15	70	12–4,000 (5–48%)
Palomar	Lux 1,540	1,540	Stamping	10 15	100 15	100 320
Cynosure	Affirm 1,440 Nd:YAG	1,440	Stamping	10	8 J/cm^2/pulse	1,000

BIBLIOGRAPHY

Laubach HJ, Tannous Z, Anderson RR, Manstein D. Skin responses to fractional photothermolysis. *Lasers Surg Med.* 2006;38(2):142-149.

Manstein D, Herron GS, Sink RK, Tanner H, Anderson RR. Fractional photothermolysis: A new concept for cutaneous remodeling using microscopic patterns of thermal injury. *Lasers Surg Med.* 2004;34(5):426-438.

Narurkar VA. Nonablative fractional laser resurfacing. *Dermatol Clin.* 2009;27(4):473-478, vi.

Tannous Z. Fractional resurfacing. *Clin Dermatol.* 2007; 25(5):480-486.

CHAPTER 9 | Ablative Fractional Laser Resurfacing

INTRODUCTION

Treatments for photoaging range from nonablative laser resurfacing to ablative laser resurfacing. Both of these techniques are described in detail in previous chapters.

Put simply, the most effective lasers, carbon dioxide and erbium ablative resurfacing lasers, provide the most dramatic benefit for photoaging and other skin conditions, but also carry the highest risk for adverse effects. They remain the gold standard treatment for photodamaged skin. Dramatic results, however, can be seen with one treatment. Side effects include prolonged erythema (for months), permanent hypopigmentation, temporary hyperpigmentation, infection, and scar. Additionally, downtime from work and social activities is significant. For this reason, the popularity of ablative lasers has decreased dramatically over the past several years among patients and physicians.

By contrast, nonablative lasers, with multiple treatment sessions, provide a safe method for providing mild improvement of mild-to-moderate photodamage with little risk of side effects. Unfortunately, the predictability of improvement is uncertain. Some patients do not experience any discernible benefit even after multiple treatments. In the past 5 years, nonablative fractional lasers have produced enhanced results from other forms of nonablative resurfacing with multiple treatments. These lasers have also proven to be safe in skilled hands. Still, their efficacy is limited, especially when compared to ablative laser resurfacing.

More recently, fractional ablative lasers, both carbon dioxide and erbium variants, have been developed to provide enhanced results with relatively good safety. The concept is to provide the more aggressive technology of ablation, but to confine potential downtime and side effects by employing a fractional pattern of tissue damage, which encourages more rapid healing times with fewer side effects. Only a fraction of the skin is ablated at each treatment, as opposed to traditional ablative resurfacing procedures. Further, the depth of ablation is deeper than with traditional ablative resurfacing procedures.

Advantages of fractional ablative lasers are as follows:

- Better improvement of deeper rhytides than nonablative devices
- Significant benefit with one treatment
- Can provide some improvement for skin laxity, pigmented lesions, and vascular dyschromia as well
- Significant reduction in postoperative downtime compared to traditional ablative devices

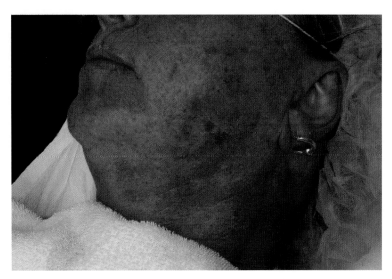

Figure 9.1 *Immediate endpoint of pixilated damage pattern with an erbium fractional ablative device*

• Can treat cosmetic units effectively without lines of demarcation often seen with traditional ablative procedures, that is, perioral/periorbital areas

INDICATIONS

• Rhytides, especially moderate-to-severe perioral and periorbital rhytides

• Photodamage, including skin texture and tone

• Acne scars, including boxcar, atrophic, rolling scars

• Surgical and burn scars

• Mild improvement in skin laxity

• Not effective for dynamic rhytides

PREOPERATIVE EVALUATION

• Skin type (I–III are best candidates)

• Sun exposure

• History of keloids

• Systemic infections

• Prior plastic surgery, especially neck lifting procedures and face lifts

• Isotretinoin use in past 6 months

• Patients with unrealistic expectations

A consultation is required before this treatment to assess the patient as well as appropriately prepare the patient for the procedure. The patient should be fully educated as to the risks and benefits of this procedure. The patient must be aware of the recovery period of 4 to 7 days (on average). The patient should be shown postoperative pictures to prepare them for how they will appear. Any postoperative assistance the patient may require should be arranged prior to treatment if possible. The patient should also be informed that the benefits of the treatment accrue 3 to 6 months after treatment. A patient who is unable to follow and execute necessary postoperative skin care regimen should not be treated.

PROPHYLAXIS/ANESTHESIA

May include any of the following:

• Antiviral and antibiotic prophylaxis

• Topical anesthetic

  – 23% Lidocaine/7% tetracaine

• Oral pain medication and anxiolytic

  – Vicodin/acetaminophen/ativan/nothing

• Nerve blocks/IM Toradol

• General anesthesia

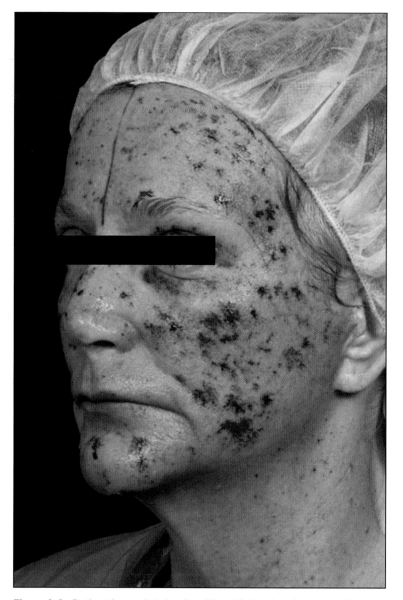

Figure 9.2 *Patient immediately after CO_2 ablative fractional resurfacing treatment. Note erythema, edema, and pinpoint hemorrhage*

Because this procedure is painful, some form of anesthesia is required. It will vary according to the aggressiveness of treatment, the particular susceptibilities of the patient, and the physician's comfort with various anesthetic regimens. Regional nerve blocks with supplemental infiltrative anesthesia are generally helpful. Site-dependent blocks include supraorbital, infraorbital, and mental blocks. Lidocaine (1%) with 1:100,000 or 1:200,000 epinephrine, at a total of 0.5 to 1.0 mL can be injected at each site.

LASER SAFETY

- Eye protection: metal eye shields

  - One or two drops of 0.05% topical proparacaine (Alcaine) or 0.05% topical tetracaine (Pontocaine) are placed into each eye of the patient, followed by the application of topical erythromycin ointment or ophthalmic lubricant (eg, Lacri-Lube) and nonreflective metal ocular shields.

  - All personnel present at the treatment must wear safety glasses/goggles to avoid inadvertent corneal damage.

Due to the pain, bleeding, and pain medications associated with this treatment, it is imperative that the patient be accompanied by a friend, spouse or relative who can drive or accompany the patient home after the procedure.

■ Postoperative Care (Fig. 9.1)

- Interestingly, little postprocedure pain (Fig. 9.2)
- Best explanation: heat release through ablated channels
- Imperative to give oral and written wound care instructions to patient
- Gauze soaks and emollients immediately postoperative
- Room temperature sterile water soaks for 20 minutes, every 3 to 4 hours followed by Aquaphor/Vaseline application for 2 to 3 days

■ Follow-up at 48 to 72 hours (Fig. 9.3)

- Re-epithelialization is usually complete.
- Erythema, edema, and residual pinpoint hemorrhagic crusting are expected.
- Milia are common and often clear within a few days.
- Assess for vesicles, bullae, pustules.
- Emollients twice daily for 3 to 7 days.
- Instructions to call if any concerns or changes in wound healing.

Postoperative erythema resolves over a period of weeks. Strict sun avoidance must be followed for a

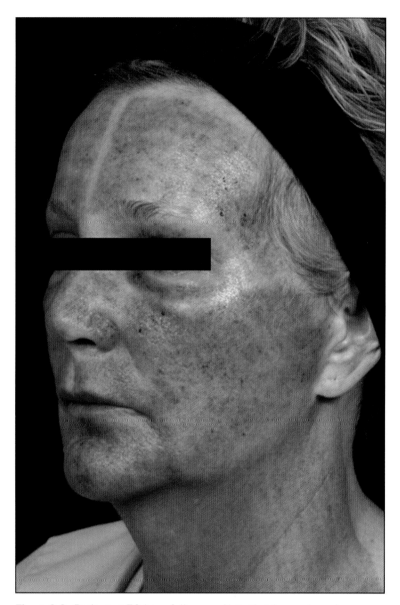

Figure 9.3 *Patient at 72-hour follow-up. Note that hemorrhage is no longer present, but edema and erythema persist*

minimum of 3 months postoperatively to avoid pigmentary changes and photosensitivity.

■ Adverse Side Effects

• Delayed onset hypopigmentation

• Scarring

• Postinflammatory hyperpigmentation

• Persistent erythema

• Infection

The side effects for fractional ablative resurfacing are the same as those for traditional ablative resurfacing procedures, albeit far less frequent or severe in skilled hands. As with nonablative fractional resurfacing, post-inflammatory hyperpigmentation (PIH) is more likely to occur with higher treatment densities, particularly in darker skin phototypes (Fig. 9.4). Hypertrophic scarring of the neck is a significant and potentially permanent complication of fractionated CO_2 laser resurfacing (Fig. 9.5). Caution is required for these procedures.

The following practices all significantly increase the risk of scar:

• Aggressive treatments increase risk of scar

• Poor technique, that is, excessive overlap

• Postoperative wound infection

• History of facelift or neck lifting procedures

• Treatment of nonfacial skin, especially the neck

■ Infection (Fig. 9.6)

The key to treating infection is to recognize it at its inception. Infections are diagnosed clinically. Cultures can confirm a diagnosis. Empiric antibiotics and close clinical follow-up are the keys to treatment. Persistent areas of erythema should raise concern regarding scar formation or infection. A culture is recommended to rule out bacterial or yeast infection. Do not perform these procedures if you cannot recognize and treat bacterial, viral, fungal infections.

■ Nonfacial Skin

Nonfacial skin is more vulnerable to thermal energy due to underprivileged wound healing capabilities. There are fewer pilosebaceous units on the neck and more limited cutaneous vasculature to support wound healing. This is especially true where there is a history of prior plastic surgery. Face/neck lifting procedures place neck skin onto the face; thus, you may be treating "neck" skin on the face. If there is a history of prior plastic surgery, it is best to treat at lower settings.

Because of the risks of serious side effects, it is strongly advised that fractional ablative resurfacing

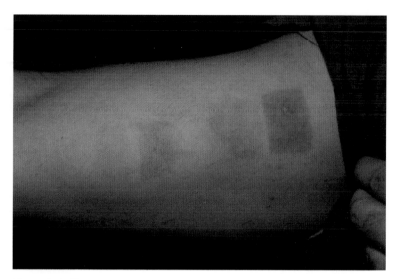

Figure 9.4 *Test spot treatments with a CO_2 ablative fractional resurfacing device in a young male with Fitzpatrick skin type 5. The test spots are not arranged in order of aggressiveness. The darker areas of PIH coincide with increased treatment density. Increasing pulse energies do little to worsen PIH*

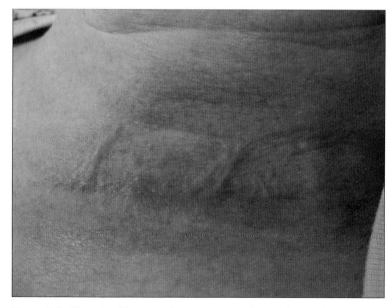

Figure 9.5 *Hypertrophic scar after treatment with a CO_2 fractional ablative device*

should only be performed by an appropriately trained physician experienced in postoperative wound care following resurfacing procedures.

In sum, ablative fractional resurfacing procedures offer the advantage of good results with one treatment as well as offering significant improvement where nonablative fractional and nonfractional devices do not, such as moderate and severe rhytides. At the same time, it offers the flexibility of treating smaller areas than traditional resurfacing procedures because it does not typically leave lines of demarcation. Additionally, there is significantly reduced clinical and social downtime compared to full surface ablative procedures. Nonetheless, the treatment has its drawbacks such as

- Tightening is usually modest.
- Duration of benefits is not known.
- Best results often require more than one treatment.
  - Especially acne scars.
  - Requires 1 week away from work and social activities.
  - Series nonablative treatments may be more tolerable and practical for many patients.

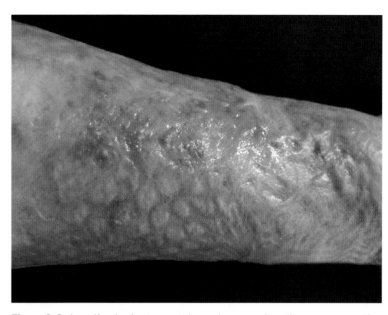

Figure 9.6 *Localized minute pustules, edema, and erythema representing a localized pseudomonas infection in the setting of post-CO_2 fractional ablative resurfacing for a burn scar. It cleared fully without sequelae after oval antibiotic treatment.*

CHAPTER 10 | Tissue Tightening

There have been a variety of noninvasive devices that purport to lift and tighten "loose" necks, jawlines, and eyes. These devices work by delivering monopolar, bipolar, or infrared energy to the deep dermis and subcutaneous tissue, resulting in tightening and lifting of skin and creation of new collagen. The chief obstacle for these devices has been inconsistent clinical results. Some patients have had dramatic results in comparison to traditional invasive surgery and others have seen little or no improvement. Patients who understand the risks before the procedure are happy with excellent results and not disappointed by lack of improvement.

MECHANISM OF ACTION

There are different radiofrequency (RF) technology and infrared devices that deliver volumetric heat to the deep dermis and subcutaneous tissue which tightens existing collagen and helps create new collagen.

CANDIDATE SELECTION

As with all procedures, candidate selection is vital to the success of the procedure. These devices will not treat epidermal changes of aging such as lentigo, telangiectasia, or rough skin. Candidates should have deep cutaneous signs of aging such as "sagging" skin in the neck, jaw, or around the eyes. Some physicians have reported good success in treating areas off the face including upper arms, abdomen, and breasts. All patients must be aware that the amount of clinical improvement is highly variable not predictable before the procedure. Patients that do not understand this should not undergo the procedure.

THE PROCEDURE

When first introduced the chief complaint with RF devices was intolerable pain. The procedure was done with a single pass at high energy settings. Over the years the trend has been toward more passes with lower fluencies. This has greatly reduced the pain associated with the procedure. Multiple passes, lower fluencies, and different spot sizes have resulted in greater immediate tissue tightening observed in patients and a higher percentage of patients with improvement after 6 months.

■ Preprocedure Checklist

• Remove all makeup.

• Remove all jewelry.

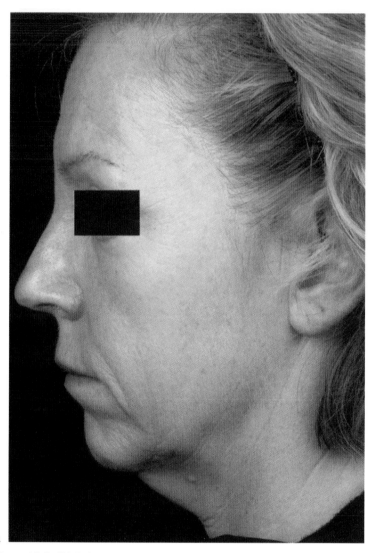

A

Figure 10.1 (A) *Prior to treatment skin laxity is observed in the jowl region.*

- No pacemaker or defibrillator.
- All patients with facial implants should have the material of the implant identified before the procedure. If it is unknown, do not treat directly over the implant.
- Apply thick layer of topical anesthetic 30 minutes before procedure.
- Determine appropriate spot size and fluence.
- Keep the hand piece even with the skin throughout the procedure.
- After the procedure patients can resume regular activities immediately.
- Patients should communicate with their physician in case of any questions or concerns.
- Improvement occurs for up to 6 months after the procedure.

SIDE EFFECTS

The amount of serious side effects has been reduced over the years as treatment protocols have been refined. With lower fluences the risk of side effects has been substantially reduced.

◼ Potential Side Effects

- Atrophoderma which may be temporary or permanent
- Burn
- Erosion/ulcer
- Scar
- Dyschromia
- Nerve damage
- Ocular damage

CLINICAL PEARLS

- All patients should be warned before any procedure that the amount of clinical improvement varies from person to person. Improvement can range from dramatic to NO improvement at all. Any patient who does not understand the potential for no improvement should not have the procedure performed.
- While treating each patient continuously, observe the skin and ask the patient to inform the physician if there is a particular spot with increased pain or unusual symptoms. If a patient complains of unusual pain or symptoms, stop the procedure and reevaluate the settings.
- Make sure a uniform amount of energy is delivered with each pulse. This is done by using the appropriate spot size and applying uniform gentle but firm pressure to the skin.
- Do not perform the procedure on a patient with active sunburn or tan.

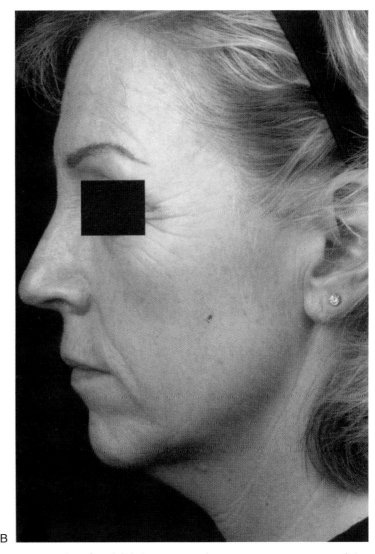

B

Figure 10.1 (*continued*) **(B)** *Six months after treatment appearance of the jowl and neck is improved slightly. (Reproduced, with permission, from Hirsch R, Sadick N, Cohen JL. Aesthetic Rejuvenation: A Regional Approach. New York: McGraw-Hill, 2009:97.)*

CHAPTER 11	Dermatochalasis

Dermatochalasis is a condition characterized by upper and/or lower eyelid skin, muscle redundancy and laxity, and fat pad herniation. It is mainly attributable to chronological aging and chronic sun exposure.

EPIDEMIOLOGY

Incidence: very common

Age: most frequently observed in individuals older than 50 years

Sex: no predilection

Race: most common in fair-skinned individuals (skin phototypes I and II); less common in darker-skinned individuals (skin phototypes IV–VI)

Precipitating factors: chronological aging; chronic sun exposure; thyroid disease

PATHOGENESIS

Upper and/or lower eyelid skin and muscle hypertrophy and prolapse; fat pad descension.

PHYSICAL EXAMINATION

Early findings include a double lid crease with only modest hooding. Severe findings include prominent eyelid hooding with upper and lateral visual field obstruction. Coexisting brow ptosis may further compromise the peripheral vision.

Tests for lower lid laxity help determine if a lid-tightening procedure is needed.

Lower lid horizontal laxity is measured by the distraction test that requires pulling the lower lid anteriorly away from the globe. A greater than 7-mm lid excursion indicates laxity.

Orbicularis oculi tone is measured by the snap test that is performed by pulling the lower lid inferiorly. If the lid does not spontaneously return to the normal position prior to the next blink, the test is positive indicating lower lid laxity.

DIFFERENTIAL DIAGNOSIS

Blepharochalasis (recurrent idiopathic eyelid inflammation with resultant relaxation of the upper lid skin); upper eyelid hooding secondary to eyebrow ptosis.

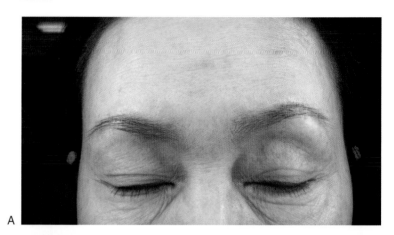

A

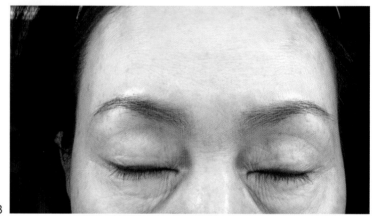

B

Figure 11.1 (A) *A 59-year-old female concerned about her sunken eyes and forehead wrinkles.* **(B)** *Improvement of the blepharloptosis, sunken eyes, and forehead wrinkles 9 months following upper lid blepharoplasty and leavator aponeurotica advancement. (Reproduced, with permission, from Harue Suzuki, MD, Kyoto, Japan.)*

DERMATOPATHOLOGY

Epidermal acanthosis with flattening of the dermal–epidermal junction; dermal collagen breakdown with formation of amorphous masses and increase in glycosaminoglycans.

COURSE

- Chronic progressive course; visual eye fields may be affected.

KEY CONSULTATIVE QUESTIONS

- Any associated symptoms including visual obstruction, dry eyes, excessive tearing
- Underlying medical conditions, especially eye disease and thyroid conditions
- Prior treatment and response

MANAGEMENT

- Prevention: strict sun avoidance
- Control underlying thyroid disease

TREATMENT

- Topical therapy: daily sunscreen application with UVB/UVA coverage
- Surgical therapy
  - Coronal browlift—upper face rejuvenation
  - Trichophytic browlift—upper face rejuvenation
  - Blepharoplasty—upper and lower eyelid rejuvenation (Fig. 11.1)
- Laser therapy
  - Placement of protective eye shields prior to laser treatment if paramount.
  - Conservative treatment is necessary to avoid ectropion formation and/or scar formation.
  - Carbon dioxide laser resurfacing.
  - Erbium:YAG laser.
  - Fractionated ablative carbon dioxide laser resurfacing.

PITFALLS TO AVOID

- A conservative approach to surgical removal of this skin is vital to prevent a "startled" appearance or ectropion.

- Retention of all or portions of any herniated fat pads helps minimize the skeletonized appearance often noted to develop with age and loss of facial volume.
- Direct visualization of the inferior oblique muscle is vital to avoid muscle injury.
- Treatment with lubricants and taping lids may help prevent keratoconjunctivitis.

BIBLIOGRAPHY

Ancona D, Katz BE. A prospective study of the improvement in periorbital wrinkles and eyebrow elevation with a novel fractional CO_2 laser—the fractional eyelift. *J Drugs Dermatol.* 2010;9(1):16-21.

Carter S, Seiff S, Choo P. Lower eyelid CO_2 laser rejuvenation: A randomized prospective clinical study. *Ophthalmology.* 2001;108:437-441.

Codner MA, Wolfli JN, Anzarut A. Primary transcutaneous lower blepharoplasty with routine lateral canthal support: A comprehensive 10-year review. *Plast Reconst Surg.* 2008;121:1241-1250.

Junzeker CM, Weiss ET, Geronemus RG. Fractionated CO_2 laser resurfacing: Our experience with more than 2000 treatments. *Aesthet Surg J.* 2009;29(4):317-322.

Korn BS, Kikkawa DO, Cohen SR. Transcutaneous lower eyelid blepharoplasty with orbitomalar suspension: Retrospective review of 212 consecutive cases. *Plast Reconstr Surg.* 2010;125(1):315-323.

Lee D, Law V. Subbrow blepharoplasty for upper eyelid rejuvenation in Asians. *Aesthet Surg J.* 2009;29(4):284-288.

Lemke BN, Stasior OG. The anatomy of eyelid ptosis. *Arch Ophthalmol.* 1932;100:981-986.

Levine MR. *Manual of Oculoplastic Surgrery.* Philadelphia: Butterworth Heinemann; 2003.

Shorr N, Enzer Y. Considerations in aesthetic eyelid surgery. *J Dermatol Surg Oncol.* 1992;1:1081-1095.

CHAPTER 12 | Poikiloderma of Civatte

Poikiloderma of Civatte (POC) is a condition that is attributable to chronic sun exposure of the neck and the chest. The severity of findings is dependent on the duration and intensity of sun exposure, constitutive skin color (Fitzpatrick skin type), and the capacity to tan.

EPIDEMIOLOGY

Incidence: common

Age: most frequently observed in persons older than 40 years

Sex: slight female predominance

Race: most common in fair-skinned individuals (skin phototypes I and II); rarely seen in darker-skinned individuals (skin phototypes IV–VI)

Precipitating factors: chronic sun exposure including intentional sun exposure since youth and occupational exposure; trauma; chronological aging

PATHOGENESIS

Ultraviolet B (UVB) is the most damaging UV radiation, with high dose ultraviolet A (UVA) contributing to the noted changes. In addition, visible and infrared radiations have been shown to augment the action of UVB.

PHYSICAL EXAMINATION

Telangiectases, mild atrophy, reticulated hyperpigmentation, and hypopigmentation affecting the lateral and posterior aspect of the neck, anterior chest, and jawline. Submental neck is spared. Perifollicular sparing noted (Figs. 12.1 and 12.2).

DERMATOPATHOLOGY

Epidermal acanthosis with flattening of the dermal–epidermal junction. Focal increase in epidermal basal cell melanocytes; irregular basal cell hyperpigmentation. Dermal collagen breakdown with formation of amorphous masses and increase in glycosaminoglycans. Telangiectasia noted.

DIFFERENTIAL DIAGNOSIS

Rothmund–Thomson syndrome; radiation dermatitis; Kindler syndrome; Bloom's syndrome; Ataxia-telangiectasia.

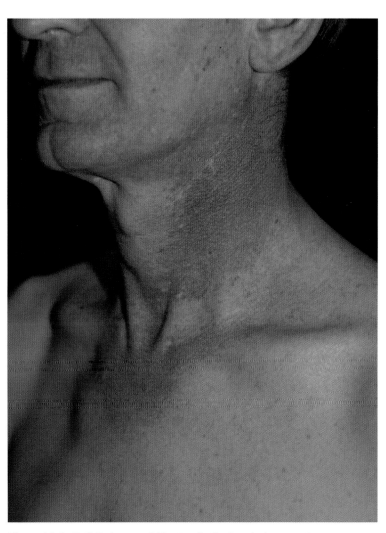

Figure 12.1 *Poikiloderma of Civatte. Reticulated pigmentation, erythema, and atrophy can be seen with characteristic sparing of the submental area. The erythematous component is more prominent in this patient. (Courtesy of Richard A. Johnson, MD.)*

COURSE

Chronic progressive course with continued sun exposure.

KEY CONSULTATIVE QUESTIONS

- Past and current sun exposure history
- Occupation
- Hobbies/sporting activities
- Underlying medical conditions
- H/o radiation therapy
- Past treatments and response

MANAGEMENT

Prevention: strict sun avoidance.

TREATMENT

- Topical therapy: daily sunscreen application with UVB/UVA coverage.
- Laser therapy: great caution must be followed with any laser treatment administered to minimize the risk of scar formation, dyspigmentation, "finger-printing" or treatment skip areas, and textural changes. The neck is particularly prone to scarring given fewer pilosebaceous units. A test site is recommended. Multiple sessions are generally required.

 Laser fluences should be lowered by approximately 25% to 30% of facial parameters to avoid adverse effects.

  - Pulsed dye laser-low fluences utilized (eg, Vbeam 595 nm, 0.45–1.0 ms, 4–6 J/cm^2, 7–10-mm spot, DCD 30/20). Improvement in telangiectasia and atrophy seen. Limited benefit for dyspigmentation.
  - Intense pulsed light (eg, StarLux, 20–30 ms, 28–34 J/dm^2, 10% pass overlap)—improvement of all components may be possible.
  - VersaPulse 532-nm laser—low fluences necessary (Fig. 12.3).
  - Fractionated nonablative and ablative laser—all components may be targeted. Can be safely utilized in affected body areas, though conservative laser parameters are required to avoid potential scarring.

PITFALLS TO AVOID

- A conservative approach must be followed with any treatment used for POC, given the significant risk of uneven removal of the pigmentation and erythema resulting in a "footprint"-like appearance (Fig. 12.4).

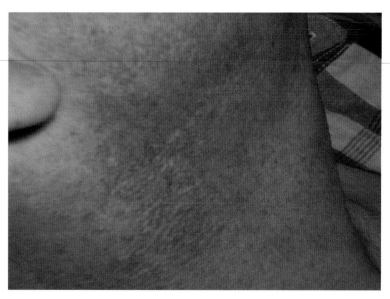

Figure 12.2 *Poikiloderma of Civatte—the pigmented component is more prominent in this patient.*

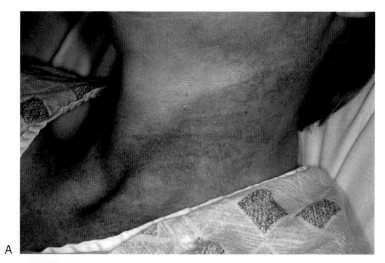

A

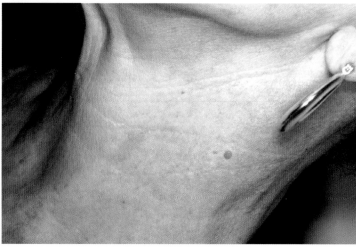

B

Figure 12.3 **(A)** *Poikiloderma of Civatte pretreatment.* **(B)** *Poikiloderma of Civatte following three VersaPulse 532-nm laser treatments. Marked reduction in erythematous component is observed.*

This mottled appearance can occur normally during the course of treatment. The patient must be aware of this possibility. Continued treatment to the residual lesions generally results in a resolution of this side effect.

- Patients must be aware of the difficulty in improving this condition. Multiple treatments are expected for end point of lightening. Textural changes are likely to persist.

- POC with a primary erythematous component typically responds better than POC with a primarily hyperpigmented component.

BIBLIOGRAPHY

Batta K, Hindson C, Cotterill JA, Foulds IS. Treatment of poikiloderma of Civatte with the potassium titanyl phosphate (KTP) laser. *Br J Dermatol.* 1999;140(6): 1191-1192.

Geronemus R. Poikiloderma of Civatte. *Arch Dermatol.* 1990;126(4):547-548.

Katoulis AC, Stavrianeas NG, Panayiotides JG, et al. Poikiloderma of Civatte: A histopathological and ultrastructural study. *Dermatology.* 2007;214(2):177-182.

Langeland J. Treatment of poikiloderma of Civatte with the pulsed dye laser: A series of seven cases. *J Cutan Laser Ther.* 1999;1(2):127.

Rusciani A, Motta A, Fino P, Menichini G. Treatment of poikiloderma of Civatte using intense pulsed light source: 7 years of experience. *Dermatol Surg.* 2008;34(3):314-319.

Tierney EP, Hanke CW. Treatment of poikiloderma of Civatte with ablative fractional laser resurfacing: Prospective study and review of the literature. *J Drugs Dermatol.* 2009;8(6):527-534.

Tierney EP, Kouba DJ, Hanke CW. Review of fractional photothermolysis: Treatment indications and efficacy. *Dermatol Surg.* 2009;35(10):1445-1461.

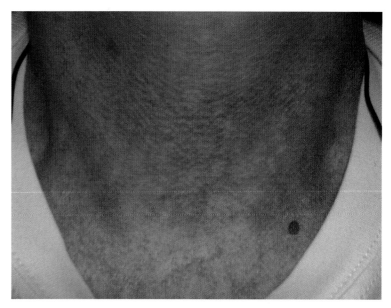

Figure 12.4 *"Footprinting" of the anterior neck after a single intense pulsed light (IPL) source treatment for Poikiloderma of Civatte. This subsequently resolved with continued IPL treatments*

SECTION TWO

Disorders of Sebaceous Glands

CHAPTER 13 Acne Vulgaris

Acne vulgaris is a chronic inflammatory disease of the pilosebaceous unit. Acne lesions favor the face, neck, upper back, chest, and upper arms. Multiple clinical variants exist and they include comedonal acne, papulopustular acne, nodulocystic acne, acne conglobata, and acne fulminans.

EPIDEMIOLOGY

Incidence and age: predominantly a disorder of adolescence; affects 85% of individuals between 12 and 24 years of age; may affect all age groups

Race: lower incidence in African-Americans and Asians

Sex: more severe forms in males

Precipitating factors: genetic predisposition, endocrine disorders, stress, mechanical factors (friction, pressure, occlusion), contact with acnegenic materials (oils, chlorinated hydrocarbons, cosmetics), and drugs (steroids, lithium, androgens, hydantoin)

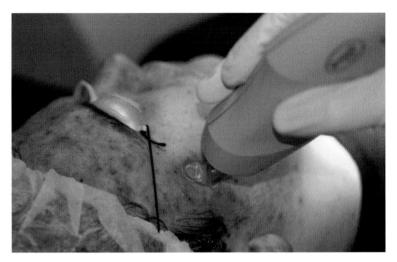

Figure 13.1 *An 18-year-old male with cystic acne being treated with 1,450-nm diode laser*

PATHOGENESIS

Many patients with nodulocystic acne have a first-degree relative with a history of severe acne. The primary pathophysiology involves altered follicular keratinization resulting in obstruction of sebaceous follicles, increased sebum production, hyperproliferation of Propionibacterium acnes, and increased production of chemotactic factors which result in inflammation.

PHYSICAL EXAMINATION

Comedones (closed and open), erythematous papules, pustules, nodules, and cysts. May resolve with residual hyperpigmentation or scarring.

DIFFERENTIAL DIAGNOSIS

Acne rosacea, steroid acne, acne mechanica, Pityrosporum folliculitis, and bacterial folliculitis.

LABORATORY DATA

■ Endocrine Studies

No routine studies are needed. If history and physical examination raise concerns then consider ordering—screen for free and total testosterone, dehydroepiandrosterone, and follicle stimulating hormone/lutenizing hormone (FSH/LH) ratios to exclude polycystic ovary syndrome or other hormonal abnormalities especially in women with moderate-to-severe acne, hirsutism, irregular menses, and weight gain. Diet *may* play a role in flares of acne. High glycemic diets may exacerbate acne. Further studies are needed.

■ Dermatopathology

Pathology of early lesion (comedone) reveals obstruction of the follicular infundibulum by cornified cells leading to dilatation. Later lesions reveal follicular rupture with lymphocytes, neutrophils, and macrophages. Scarring may be seen.

COURSE

This disease demonstrates a chronic course and remits spontaneously in the early-to-mid-third decade in the majority of patients. However, acne may persist much longer in some patients.

MANAGEMENT

Early treatment of acne is essential for the prevention of dyschromia or associated scarring (see scar treatment chapter 61). Many acne patients benefit from combination therapies. A thorough history and physical examination are paramount to administering a maximally effective plan. This should include current cosmetics and sunscreens, skin type, lifestyle, occupation, medications, past treatments and response, diet, menstrual and oral contraceptive history.

■ Topical Treatment

Topical treatment may be required for the duration of this condition. Topical formulations should be applied to the lesions as well as to the adjacent acne-prone clinically normal skin.

- Retinoids: tretinoin, adapalene, tazarotene
- Antibacterial agents: benzoyl peroxide, clindamycin, erythromycin
- Keratolytic agents: salicylic acid, hydroxy acid, azelaic acid, sodium sulfacetamide, and sulfur

■ Systemic Treatment

- Antibiotics: tetracycline, doxycycline, minocycline are most commonly used. Alternatives include erythromycin, azithromycin, and amoxicillin.
- Hormones: oral contraceptives or spironolactone for women with persistent acne on lower face, chin, and neck.

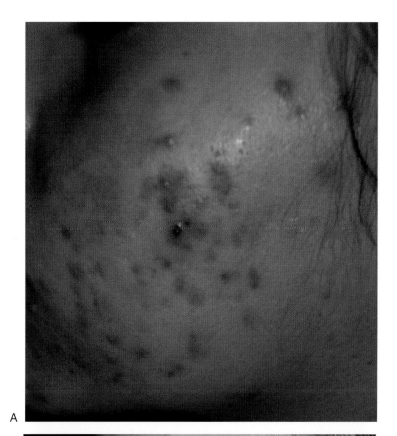

A

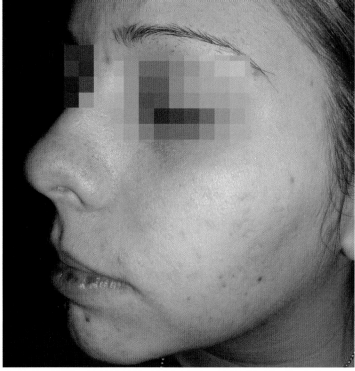

B

Figure 13.2 **(A)** *Facial inflammatory acne vulgaris unresponsive to multiple topical and oral treatment regimens.* **(B)** *Marked improvement of acne 6 months following five 1,450-nm diode laser treatments (Smoothbeam, Candela Corp., Wayland, MA), 6-mm spot, 14 J/cm² , DCD 30 ms*

• Isotretinoin: for severe nodulocystic acne that has failed other topical and systemic therapies.

■ Surgical Treatment

• Comedone extraction: expression of keratinous contents of open comedones by applying the comedone extractor to the comedones and applying pressure. A nick may be made to the overlying skin with a #11-blade or 18-gauge needle to ease in the extraction. The Schamberg, Unna, and Saalfield comedone expressors are most commonly utilized. Comedone extraction is contraindicated for inflamed comedones or pustules due to increased scar risk.

• Intralesional steroid injection: triamcinolone acetonide (2–3 mg/mL) is injected into inflamed cystic lesions using a 30-gauge needle. Maximum dose injected should not exceed 0.1 mL per lesion to avoid atrophy. Patients should be warned that atrophy from an inflammatory cystic lesion can occur with or without an intralesional steroid injection.

• Chemical peels: serial salicylic acid peels, glycolic acid peels (20–70%), and trichloroacetic acid (TCA) peels (10–20) have been utilized to reduce the number of comedones and improve postinflammatory hyperpigmentation and persistent erythema. Peels may be performed every 2 to 4 weeks, with increasing strengths and time applied as tolerated. Mild irritation may be observed. Adjunctive therapy is generally necessary.

• Microdermabrasion: this is primarily effective for comedonal acne. It is usually performed every 2 to 3 weeks. Multiple treatments are needed with variable improvement.

■ Light Treatment

• Lasers: lasers and light sources are not the first-line therapy for acne but can be an effective alternative or adjuvant to medical therapy when required.

– 1450-nm diode laser (Smoothbeam laser, Candela Corp., Wayland, MA): treatment fluencies from 8 to 14 J/cm^2, 6-mm spot size, and dynamic cooling device setting of 30–35 ms can result in mild to dramatic improvement of inflammatory trunk and facial acne with a significant reduction in lesion count after an average of three, separated by 4-to-6-week intervals (Figs. 13.1 and 13.2). It is important to deliver nonoverlapping pulses to reduce the risk of side effects. Topical lidocaine cream applied prior to treatment is needed to minimize the treatment-associated pain. It is vital to apply the cream over a limited body surface to limit any risk of lidocaine toxicity.

– Lower fluencies of 8 J/cm^2 with two full-face passes versus a single full-face pass at higher fluencies (10–14 J/cm^2) have been used to reduce pain.

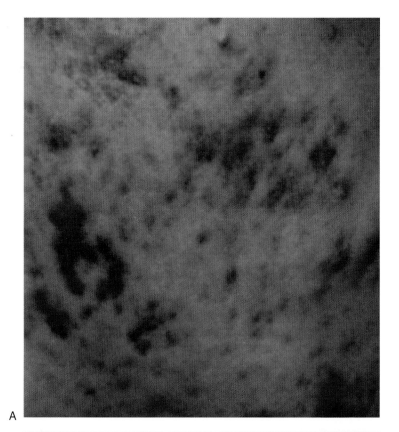

A

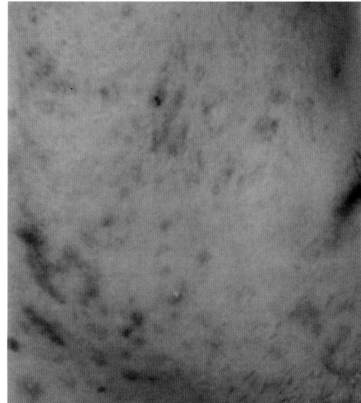

B

Figure 13.3 (A) *Severe acne before treatment.* **(B)** *After three treatments of photodynamic therapy with topical 5-aminolevulinic acid and pulsed dye laser, 7-mm spot, 6 J/cm^2, 6-ms pulse duration (Courtesy of Mark Nestor, MD, PhD)*

– Pulsed dye laser (PDL): studies examining the efficacy of PDL for inflammatory acne have produced conflicting data. Pulsed dye laser alone or in combination with long pulsed 1,064-nm YAG laser has been effective in reducing inflammatory acne. PDL can improve postacne erythema. Fluences of 5.5 to 7 J/cm^2, 7-mm spot size with pulse durations of 3 to 6 ms are most commonly employed. Several treatments are needed to achieve the greatest benefit.

• Phototherapy: multiple light sources have been reported to significantly improve acne with minimal side effects. These sources include high-intensity narrow-band blue light, high-intensity metal halide lamp, high-energy broad-spectrum blue light, as well as mixed blue and red light.

• Photodynamic therapy (PDT): PDT utilizing the topical administration of 5-aminolevulinic acid (ALA, Levulan Kerastick, DUSA Pharmaceuticals, Inc., Wilmington, MA) activated by light exposure is another potentially effective modality to treat acne (Figs. 13.3 and 13.4). Short contact ALA-PDT (15–60-minute drug incubation) was capable of improving acne significantly in a variety of clinical studies. Different light sources have been utilized including blue light (405–420 nm), red light (635 nm), long-pulsed 595-nm pulsed dye lasers, and intense pulsed light (430–1200 nm) (Fig. 13.5).

BIBLIOGRAPHY

Bowe WP, Joshi SS, Shalita AR. Diet and acne. *J Am Acad Dermatol.* 2010;63(1):124-141.

Friedman PM, Jih MH, Kimyai-Asadi A, Goldberg LH. Treatment of inflammatory facial acne vulgaris with the 1450-nm diode laser: A pilot study. *Dermatol Surg.* 2004;30(2 pt 1):147-151.

Hamilton FL, Car J, Lyons C, Car M, Layton A, Majeed A. Laser and other light therapies for the treatment of acne vulgaris: Systematic review. *Br J Dermatol.* 2009;160(6): 1273-1285.

Leheta TM. Role of the 585-nm pulsed dye laser in the treatment of acne in comparison with other topical therapeutic modalities. *J Cosmet Laser Ther.* 2009;11(2): 118-124.

Pollock B, Turner D, Stringer MR, et al. Topical aminolevulinic acid-photodynamic therapy for the treatment of acne vulgaris: A study of clinical efficacy and mechanism of action. *Br J Dermatol.* 2004;151(3):616-622.

Yeung CK, Shek SY, Yu CS, Kono T, Chan HH. Treatment of inflammatory facial acne with 1,450-nm diode laser in type IV to V Asian skin using an optimal combination of laser parameters. *Dermatol Surg.* 2009;35(4):593-600.

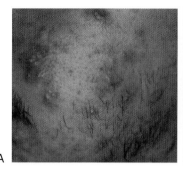
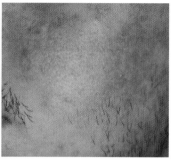

Figure 13.4 (A) *Facial inflammatory acne prior to photodynamic therapy.* **(B)** *Marked reduction of the inflammatory acne after three sessions of photodynamic therapy (Courtesy of Mark Nestor, MD, PhD)*

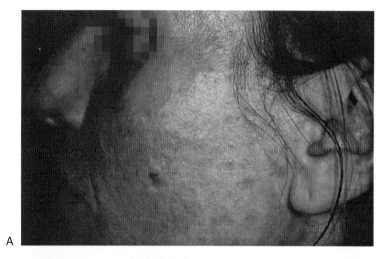
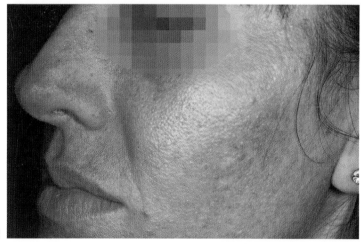

Figure 13.5 (A) *Mild acne scarring and dyschromia prior to Er:YAG laser resurfacing.* **(B)** *Four months after Er:YAG laser resurfacing utilizing a 5-mm spot at 1 J with four passes results in significant improvement (Reproduced, with permission, from Dover J, Arndt K, Geronemus R, et al. Illustrated Cutaneous & Aesthetic Laser Surgery. McGraw-Hill, Inc.; 2000)*

CHAPTER 14 | Rosacea

Acne rosacea is a chronic vascular and acneiform disorder of the pilosebaceous unit that affects predominantly the central face including the central cheeks, nose, and chin. The eyes and the eyelids can occasionally be involved. Typically, there is an increased reactivity of capillaries to heat, leading to flushing and ultimately telangiectasia. Subtypes of rosacea include (1) vascular rosacea (erythematotelangiectatic), (2) papulopustular rosacea, (3) sebaceous hyperplasia (phymatous rosacea) including rhinophyma (nasal sebaceous hyperplasia), and (4) ocular rosacea. Granulomatous rosacea is a variant of rosacea.

EPIDEMIOLOGY

Incidence: common

Age: 30 to 50 years; peak incidence between 40 and 50 years

Sex: female predilection; male predominance for rhino phyma

Race: most common in fair-skinned individuals (skin phototypes I and II); rarely seen in darker-skinned individuals (skin phototypes IV–VI)

Precipitating factors: excessive sun exposure, caffeine, spicy foods, hot foods and beverages, heat, alcohol, seborrhea, topical corticosteroid use, and underlying Parkinson's disease

PATHOGENESIS

Multiple factors are involved in the pathogenesis of rosacea including vascular hyperactivity, Demodex folliculorum mites, Helicobacter pylori, and hypersensitivity to Propionibacterium acnes.

PHYSICAL EXAMINATION

Variable clinical features can be present depending on the severity and the subtype of rosacea. Early features include transient and nontransient flushing, erythematous papules, and pustules. No comedones are noted. Late features include telangiectasias, sebaceous hyperplasia, nasal thickening and enlargement (rhinophyma), and lymphedema. Ocular involvement is frequently seen.

DIFFERENTIAL DIAGNOSIS

Acne vulgaris, seborrheic dermatitis, perioral dermatitis, steroid rosacea, systemic lupus erythematosus, and lupus miliaris disseminatus faciei.

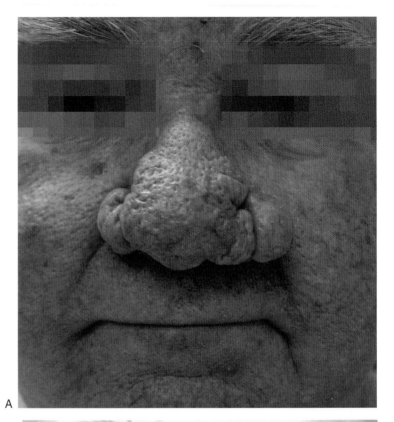

A

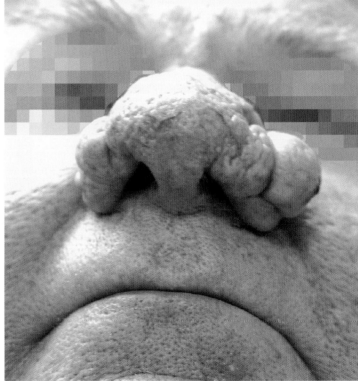

B

Figure 14.1 A&B *Severe rhinophyma prior to electrosurgery (Courtesy of Suzanne Olbricht, MD)*

DERMATOPATHOLOGY

Vascular ectasia as well as perifollicular and perivascular lymphohistiocytic infiltrates are the most common findings. Demodex folliculorum is usually detected in the follicles. Noncaseating epithelioid granulomas are seen in the granulomatous variant. Sebaceous hyperplasia and fibrosis are seen in rhinophyma.

COURSE

Chronic with frequent recurrences. May spontaneously resolve after several years.

MANAGEMENT

Prevention, reduction, or elimination of exacerbants; sun avoidance.

■ Topical Therapy

Metronidazole (0.75%–1%) once or twice daily, 10% sodium sulfacetamide with 5% sulfur once daily, and azelaic acid once daily, alone or in combination, are helpful in suppressing the papulopustular component of rosacea.

■ Systemic Therapy

- Tetracycline, 1,000 to 1,500 mg daily in divided doses, until clear; then taper to a maintenance dose of 250 to 500 mg daily.
- Minocycline and doxycycline, 50 to 100 mg twice daily, with a tapering to once daily use.
- Oral isotretinoin is reserved for severe cases not responding to oral antibiotics and requires close follow-up. A low-dose regimen may be effective.

■ Surgical Therapy

Rhinophyma

Multiple surgical modalities have been used to correct the hypertrophic changes of rhinophyma. It is important to examine a photograph of the patient prior to the onset of the rhinophymatous change in order to help guide the surgeon in the remodeling of the nose. A regional nerve block with additional local anesthesia is sufficient in the majority of cases for perioperative pain management. Direct injection of anesthesia requires multiple infiltrations and is less effective and far more painful.

- Electrosurgery: electrosection (cutting) is very effective in debulking and recontouring the rhinophymatous nose with the added advantage of a relatively bloodless field. It is similar in efficacy to CO_2 laser treatment and less expensive (Fig. 14.1).

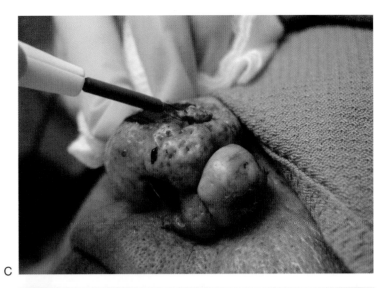

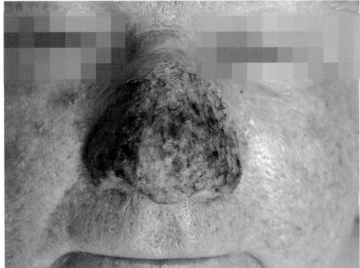

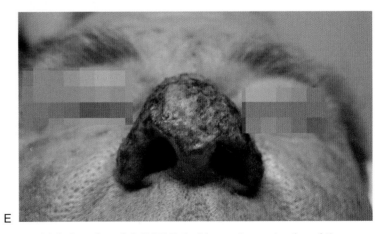

Figure 14.1 (continued) C, D,&E *Debulking and recontouring of the rhinophymatous nose in a relatively bloodless field utilizing large wire loop electrosurgery. Impressive flattening of the rhinophymatous nose after electrosurgery. The wound is left to heal by secondary intention (Courtesy of Suzanne Olbricht, MD)*

- The hypertrophied tissue is removed with care to preserve the pilosebaceous units.
- Overcorrection will produce scarring and contractures. Wound contracture with healing may pull the nasal tip upward.
- Permanent depigmentation may result from overvigorous treatment.
  - The Ellman Surgitron can be used with a large wire loop in blended waveform "fully rectified" mode which provides cutting with hemostasis, at a power control between 4 and 5.
  - A vacuum evacuator should be utilized for eliminating plumes of smoke.
  - Any remaining bleeding points can be coagulated at the end of the procedure by switching to the coagulation "partially rectified" mode.
  - The wound is allowed to heal by secondary intention.
  - The patients are instructed to keep the wound moist by multiple applications of petroleum jelly daily until re-epithelialization is complete approximately 2 weeks postop.
- Excision by the far-infrared lasers (ie, CO_2 or Er:YAG) followed by vaporization is also very effective with a relatively bloodless surgical field. A scanned CO_2 laser is the optimal device given the need to debulk large, thick areas of skin. The pulsed CO_2 laser can also be used in the continuous wave mode to remove the bulk of the rhinophyma and in the pulsed mode to sculpt and resurface the remainder of the nose.

Telangiectasias

Laser and flashlamp treatments based on selective light absorption by hemoglobin are usually very effective for removing telangiectasias and partially effective in inhibiting flushing. Patients must be aware that over time they are likely to develop more telangiectasias and background erythema.

- Laser treatment: multiple effective options are available.
  - Pulsed dye lasers (PDL) are the treatment of choice for facial telangiectasias.
    - The traditional PDL with a short pulse duration of 0.45 or 1.5 ms provides the most effective treatment for facial telangiectasias. However, posttreatment purpura occurs which generally lasts 10 to 14 days.
    - A variable-pulse PDL (595 nm, Candela V-beam, Wayland, MA) with stuttered pulse durations (ie, - 0.45, 1.5, 3, 6, 10, 20, 30, 40 ms) can provide a reduced purpura treatment of facial telangiectasias, but is somewhat less effective and usually requires multiple treatments.

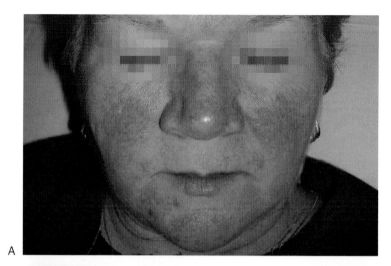

A

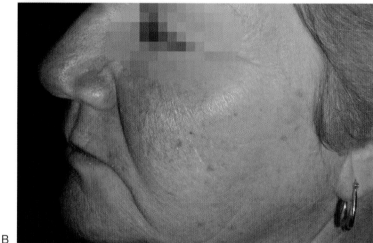

B

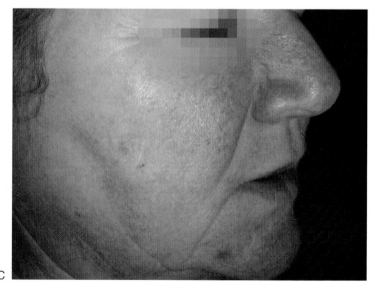

C

Figure 14.2 (A, B, C) *Prominent facial erythema prior to treatment with IPL.*

❑ Commonly, subpurpuric fluences of less than 10 J/cm² at pulse duration of 10 ms with a 7-mm spot size are utilized.

❑ Better efficacy of the variable-pulse PDL in treating facial telangiectasias can be achieved by utilizing purpuric fluences or with a pulse stacking of subpurpuric pulses (stacked 2–4 subpurpuric pulses at a 1.5-Hz repetition rate, 7.5 J/cm², 10-ms pulse duration, 10-mm spot size, DCD of 30/20).

❑ Facial edema, erythema, and discomfort can occur after extensive treatment with the purpura-free variable-pulse PDL. However, these undesired effects are generally better tolerated when compared to a purpura-inducing laser treatment.

– Intense pulsed light (IPL) can be highly effective in treating background erythema while PDLs work better for individual telangiectasia. IPL fluencies of 30 to 40 J/cm² with a 20 msec pulse duration are usually effective (Starlux Lux G handpiece, Palomar Medical Technologies, Burlington, MA). The treatment endpoint is immediate vessel clearance or selective vessel darkening. Multiple treatments may be required for the greatest treatment benefit.

– The variable pulse width 1,064-nm Nd: YAG laser has proven to be effective in the treatment of facial telangiectasias. Shorter pulse widths with higher fluences might be necessary for effective treatment of smaller vessels but have an *increased* risk of blister and scar formation.

– Frequency-doubled 532 nm Nd: YAG laser, also called potassium-titanyl-phosphate (KTP) laser, provides effective absorption of hemoglobin with a pulse duration of 1 to 50 ms making it ideally suited to treat superficial vessels without purpura formation. Tracing of individual vessels is a useful technique for patients with a countable number of discrete, visible vessels.

• Flashlamp (pulsed light) treatment: IPL provides another effective, purpura-free method for reducing facial telangiectasias and erythema (Figs. 14.2 and 14.3).

BIBLIOGRAPHY

Aferzon M, Millman B. Excision of rhinophyma with high-frequency electrosurgery. *Dermatol Surg.* 2002;28(8): 735-738.

Alam M, Dover JS, Arndt KA. Treatment of facial telangiectasia with variable-pulse high-fluence pulsed-dye laser: Comparison of efficacy with fluences immediately above and below the purpura threshold. *Dermatol Surg.* 2003;29(7):681-684. Discussion 685.

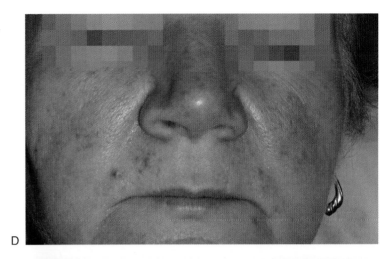

D

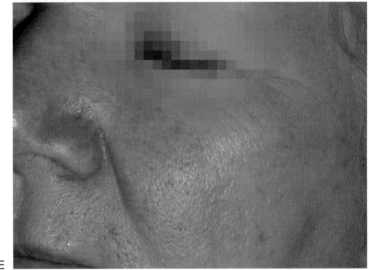

E

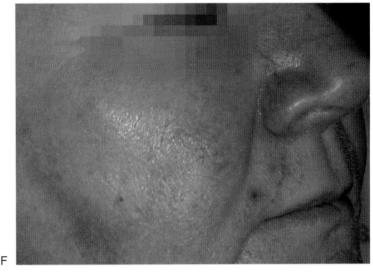

F

Figure 14.2 (*continued*) (D, E, F) *Reduction of the facial erythema after two treatments with IPL, Starlux Lux G handpiece*

Bernstein EF, Kligman A. Rosacea treatment using the new-generation, high-energy, 595 nm, long pulse-duration pulsed-dye laser. *Lasers Surg Med.* 2008; 40(4):233-239.

Del Rosso JQ. Anti-inflammatory dose doxycycline in the treatment of rosacea. *J Drugs Dermatol.* 2009;8(7): 664-668.

Jasim ZF, Woo WK, Handley JM. Long-pulsed (6-ms) dye laser treatment of rosacea-associated telangiectasia using subpurpuric clinical threshold. *Dermatol Surg.* 2004;30(1):37-40.

Mark KA, Sparacio RM, Voigt A, Marenus K, Sarnoff DS. Objective and quantitative improvement of rosacea-associated erythema after intense pulsed light treatment. *Dermatol Surg.* 2003;29(6):600-604; 163-167. Discussion 167.

Neuhaus IM, Zane LT, Tope WD. Comparative efficacy of nonpurpuragenic pulsed dye laser and intense pulsed light for erythematotelangiectatic rosacea. *Dermatol Surg.* 2009;35(6):920-928.

Sarradet DM, Hussain M, Goldberg DJ. Millisecond 1064-nm neodymium: YAG laser treatment of facial telangiectases. *Dermatol Surg.* 2003;29(1):56-58.

Thiboutot DM, Fleischer AB, Del Rosso JQ, Rich P. Related Articles 7: A multicenter study of topical azelaic acid 15% gel in combination with oral doxycycline as initial therapy and azelaic acid 15% gel as maintenance monotherapy. *J Drugs Dermatol.* 2009;8(7):639-648.

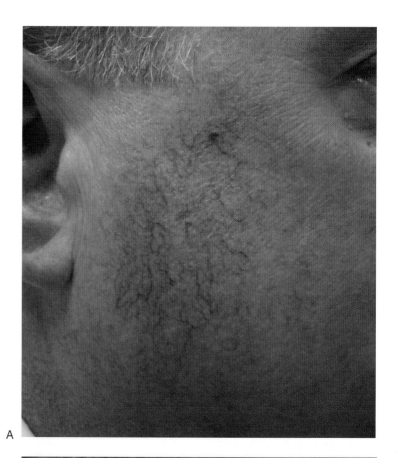

A

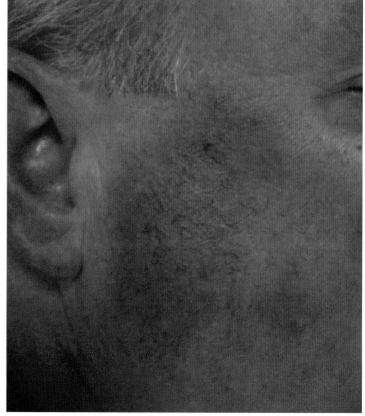

B

Figure 14.3 **(A)** *Prominent facial telangiectasias prior to treatment with IPL.* **(B)** *Posttreatment erythema immediately after IPL treatment*

CHAPTER 15 Sebaceous Hyperplasia

Sebaceous hyperplasia appears as 1-to-3-mm yellow umbilicated papules with overlying telangiectasias on the face of middle-aged individuals (Fig. 15.1). They represent a benign proliferation of sebaceous glands. The lesions are sometimes mistaken for basal cell carcinoma.

EPIDEMIOLOGY

Incidence: very common

Age: most commonly middle age and elderly but can appear in young individuals as well

Race: more common in Caucasians

Sex: equal

Precipitating factors: organ transplantation is a rare precipitant

PATHOGENESIS

Unknown.

PATHOLOGY

Increased numbers of large, mature sebaceous lobules are clustered around a central duct in the upper dermis. The lobules lie closer than normal to the epidermis.

PHYSICAL LESIONS

There are single or multiple 1-to-3-mm yellow umbilicated papules with overlying telangiectasias that appear on the face. The forehead, cheeks, and nose are the most common locations. It can rarely present on the areola.

DIFFERENTIAL DIAGNOSIS

Most commonly mistaken for basal cell carcinoma.

LABORATORY EXAMINATION

None is indicated. Biopsy if considering basal cell carcinoma.

COURSE

Benign, but do not regress or resolve without therapy.

KEY CONSULTATIVE QUESTIONS

Any history of the lesion bleeding.

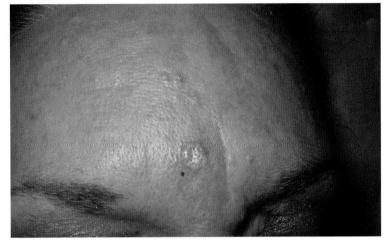

Figure 15.1 *Large sebaceous hyperplasia on the forehead*

MANAGEMENT

There is no medical indication to treat sebaceous hyperplasia. Still, some individuals are significantly bothered by its appearance and request removal, particularly in the circumstance of multiple lesions. Treatments include oral, destructive, laser, and photodynamic therapies. Each has its side effects and risk of recurrence.

TREATMENTS

All patients should be informed before any treatment modality that improvement is variable and in the future new lesions may arise requiring follow-up treatments.

■ Destructive Modalities

- "Light" cryotherapy and electrosurgery are quick, inexpensive means of treating sebaceous hyperplasia.

■ Laser Therapy

- The 1,450-nm diode laser has been studied in 10 patients for the treatment of sebaceous hyperplasia (Figs. 15.2 and 15.3).
  - Each patient was treated 1 to 5 times.
  - Fluences of 16 to 17 J/cm^2 were employed, with cooling durations of 40 to 50 ms.
  - After two to three treatments with the diode laser, 84% of lesions decreased in size greater than 50%, and 70% decreased greater than 75%. Patient and physician satisfaction was high.
  - Side effects included one case of an atrophic scar and one case of hyperpigmentation.
- Pulsed dye laser (PDL) (585 nm) has been shown to improve sebaceous hyperplasia.
  - Successful treatment has been shown with three-stacked 5-mm pulses at fluences of 7 and 7.5 J/cm^2.
  - Most lesions respond after one treatment with flattening, shrinking, or resolution.
  - Seven percent of lesions recurred completely.
  - One study showed clearance in two patients treated with the PDL at 585 nm, 6.5 to 8 J/cm^2, and a pulse width of 300 to 450 seconds. Two to three treatments were performed.
- Erbium:YAG or CO$_2$ laser ablation can also improve sebaceous hyperplasia.
- Laser-assisted photodynamic therapy with topical 20% 5-aminolevulinic acid and PDL irradiation (595 nm), blue light or intense pulse light; 1 to 4 treatments are needed with variable improvement and future recurrence achieved more effective improvement of sebaceous hyperplasia than PDL alone.

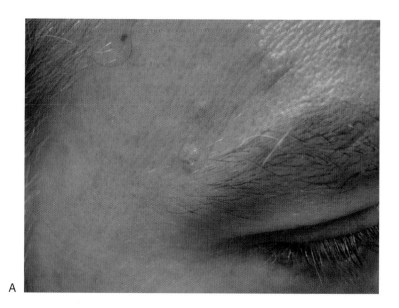

A

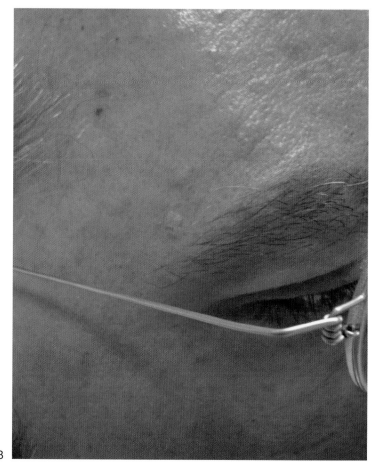

B

Figure 15.2 (A) *Patient with sebaceous hyperplasia on the right temple and forehead.* **(B)** *Improvement 1 month after treatment with 1,450-nm diode laser (Smoothbeam, Candela Corp., Wayland, MA) utilizing a 6-mm spot with a fluence of 14 J/cm^2 and a pulse duration of 35 ms*

– Treatments were performed at 1-to-6-week intervals.

– Both therapies showed greater improvement than no therapy at all. There were no long-term results.

– Side effects were limited to mild temporary redness, edema, and crusting.

PITFALLS TO AVOID/OUTCOME EXPECTATIONS/COMPLICATIONS/ MANAGEMENT

• Patients should be informed that complete resolution is difficult and not always permanent.

• Destructive modalities such as cryotherapy and electrodesiccation can produce pigmentary changes and even scarring if done too aggressively. Recurrences are common.

• Local excision leaves a scar.

• Oral therapy with isotretinoin is clearly an alternative treatment and is not as efficacious as other modalities and carries with it the risk of significant side effects such as teratogenicity, dry skin and mucous membranes, high triglycerides and cholesterol, diffuse skeletal hyperostosis, liver function abnormalities, reduced night vision, pseudotumor cerebri, leukopenia, possible depression, and suicidal ideation. Topical tretinoin can produce skin irritation.

• Laser therapy must be used with caution, especially in dark skin phototypes, given the risk of hyperpigmentation.

• There can be scarring, redness, edema, and crusting, as shown in Figure 15.3. Recurrence is not uncommon.

BIBLIOGRAPHY

Aghassi D, Gonzalez E, Anderson RR, Rajadhyaksha M, Gonzalez S. Elucidating the pulsed-dye laser treatment of sebaceous hyperplasia in vivo with real-time confocal scanning laser microscopy. *J Am Acad Dermatol.* 2000; 43(1 pt 1):49-53.

Alster TS, Tanzi EL. Photodynamic therapy with topical aminolevulinic acid and pulsed dye laser irradiation for sebaceous hyperplasia. *J Drugs Dermatol.* 2003;2(5): 501-504.

Kim SK, Do JE, Kang HY, Lee ES, Kim YC. Combination of topical 5-aminolevulinic acid-photodynamic therapy with carbon dioxide laser for sebaceous hyperplasia. *J Am Acad Dermatol.* 2007;56(3):523-524.

Richey DF. Aminolevulinic acid photodynamic therapy for sebaceous gland hyperplasia. *Dermatol Clin.* 2007;25(1): 59-65. Review.

Schonermark MP, Schmidt C, Raulin C. Treatment of sebaceous gland hyperplasia with the pulsed dye laser. *Lasers Surg Med.* 1997;21(4):313-316.

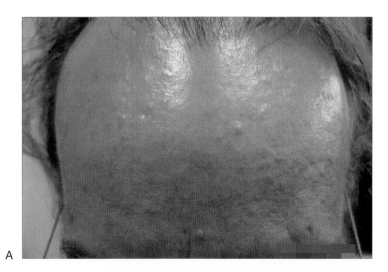

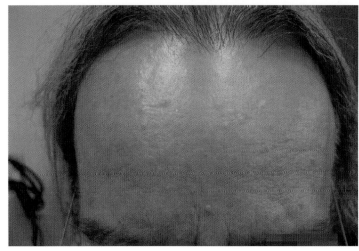

Figure 15.3 (A) *Sebaceous hyperplasia—before.* **(B)** *Improvement one month after treatment with 1450 nm diode laser 14.5 J/cm², 35 ms cooling, single pulse per lesion*

SECTION THREE

Disorders of Eccrine Glands

CHAPTER 16 Hyperhidrosis

Hyperhidrosis is the secretion of excessive amounts of sweat from the eccrine sweat glands at rest and at normal room temperature. It produces both physical and social discomfort. The most commonly affected areas are the axillae, palms, and plantar feet. It can present in a bilateral or symmetric fashion. The most common cause of hyperhidrosis is idiopathic.

EPIDEMIOLOGY

Incidence: no good epidemiologic studies of prevalence.

Age: palmoplantar: birth; axillary: puberty.

Race: no racial predilection.

Sex: equal.

Precipitating factors: idiopathic, emotional, central nervous system injury/disease, drug, surgical injury are the most common causes. In most cases, there is a family history.

PATHOGENESIS

Eccrine glands are primarily innervated by sympathetic fibers that are cholinergic rather than adrenergic in neural response.

PHYSICAL FINDINGS

- Palmoplantar: excessive sweat and sweat droplets producing a moist appearance and clammy feel
- Axillary: staining of shirts in the underarm area

DIFFERENTIAL DIAGNOSIS

Clinical appearance does not suggest other disorders.

LABORATORY EXAMINATION

Starch-iodine or ninhydrin test are useful in defining areas of sweating (Fig. 16.1).

DERMATOPATHOLOGY

No characteristic findings. Biopsy plays no role in management.

COURSE

Does not remit spontaneously; may improve slightly with age.

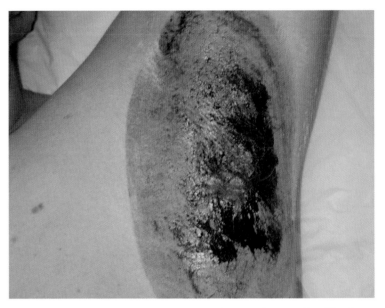

Figure 16.1 *An example of the starch-iodine test in the left axilla. Note the prominent dark blue-black discoloration at sites of hyperhidrosis*

KEY CONSULTATIVE QUESTIONS

- Medication history
- Past treatments and response
- Assess for systemic abnormality
- Recent surgery

MANAGEMENT

The goal of the treatment is to substantially decrease sweat production to improve physical and social discomfort, not complete elimination. There are multiple treatments for hyperhidrosis (Fig. 16.2). Botulinum toxin A is a very effective treatment providing temporary reduction in sweating. Topical and oral medications are only modestly effective. Surgical therapy, including liposuction, is more effective than topical therapy.

Compensatory hyperhidrosis secondary to sympathectomy limits its use at present except as a final therapeutic modality.

TOPICAL MEDICATIONS

- Aluminum chloride hexahydrate.

  - Application of 10% to 30% aluminum chloride hexahydrate solution in ethanol with or without occlusion to unshaven skin for 6 to 8 hours nightly for 3 to 4 days can be beneficial but is complicated by local irritation. Retreatment once or twice weekly for maintenance is recommended. Treated skin should be washed the following morning.

  - In the axillae, it is applied at night to unshaven skin and washed off in the morning.

  - Frequency of application diminishes with improvement.

- Tap water iontophoresis can be effective.

  - The procedure requires continual application for 15 to 20 minutes 2 to 3 times per week.

  - Blistering and burning have been reported as side effects.

  - Contraindications include pregnancy, cardiac pace makers, and metal implants.

ORAL MEDICATIONS

Oral anticholinergics including bornaprine, glycopyrronium bromide, propantheline, and methanthaline bromide are of limited efficacy. They produce dose-related anticholinergic side effects.

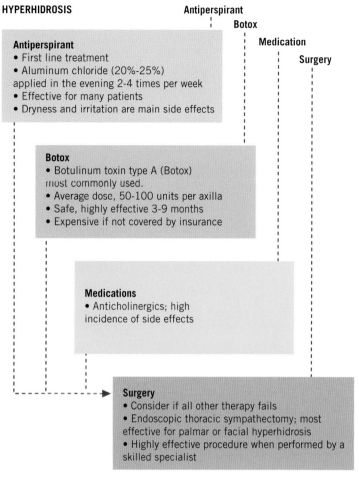

Figure 16.2 *Hyperhidrosis treatment diagram*

SURGERY

Surgical procedures include the following:

- Endoscopic or classic sympathectomy is usually reserved as a final therapeutic option for palmar hyperhidrosis. Surgery provides long-lasting control. General anesthesia is required. Side effects include bleeding, scar formation, infection, reaction to anesthesia, compensatory hyperhidrosis, gustatory sweating, pneumothorax, and Horner's syndrome.
- Selective gland removal is reserved for axillary hyperhidrosis.
- Liposuction for axillary hyperhidrosis involves subdermal liposuction. The liposuction cannula is held with the bevel side up at the subdermal level for suctioning of this region.

BOTULINUM TOXIN A

Botulinum toxin A provides temporary effective treatment for this condition. It is a bacterial toxin that decreases sweating by irreversibly blocking acetylcholine release from cholinergic presynaptic vesicles (Fig. 16.3).

■ Anesthesia

- Topical anesthetic cream and/or ice generally can provide sufficient anesthetic effect.
- Still, nerve blocks should be considered prior to plantar and palmar treatments to minimize the associated pain.
  - Plantar: sural and posterior tibial nerves
  - Palmar: ulnar and median nerves

■ Treatment

- A starch-iodine test performed prior to treatment can help delineate the areas to be injected. Iodine is placed on the affected area, followed by the application of cornstarch producing a prominent dark blue-black discoloration. The starch-iodine paste should be washed off prior to Botox injections.
- Effective Botox dilutions vary. A Botox A (100 U/vial) dilution of 2.0 U/0.1 cc is effective.
- Injections are performed at 1 to 2 cm intervals intradermally throughout the affected area (Figs. 16.4, 16.5 and 16.6). Two units should be injected per site.
- A total dose ranging from 50 to 100 U/axilla, palm, or sole can be injected, for a total dose of 100 to 200 U for both treatment sites. A decreased dose can be used for localized hyperhidrosis.
- Temporary hand and finger muscle weakness may be a complication of palmar botulinum toxin A injections, especially with increasing dosages. Patients should use

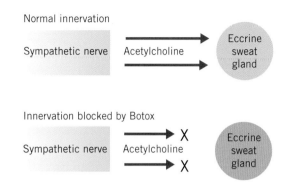

Figure 16.3 *Mechanism of action of Botox in hyperhidrosis. Blocking acetylcholine release from cholinergic presynaptic vesicles*

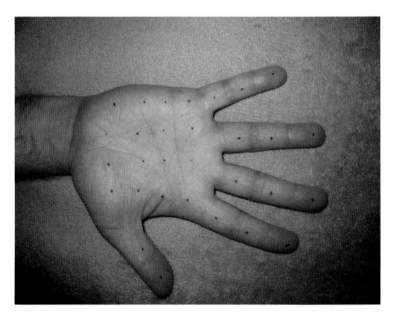

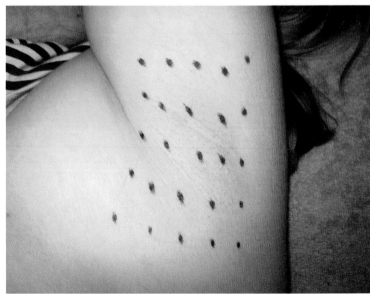

Figure 16.4 *Appropriate injection sites of botulinum toxin A for treatment of* **(A)** *palmar hyperhidrosis and* **(B)** *axillary hyperhidrosis. Each injection should be approximately 1 to 2 cm apart*

caution when holding cups and other objects supported by the thenar muscle while the weakness is present. This weakness generally dissipates within 3 to 4 weeks.

- Decreased sweating is observed within 1 to 2 weeks. Benefits generally are noted between 3 and 9 months.
- Side effects may include local muscle weakness for palmar injections, bruising, antibody resistance, and rarely an anaphylactic reaction.
- The efficacy of botulinum toxin injections is not affected by laser hair removal in the same area of treatment.

■ Medications

- Anticholinergics; high incidence of side effects

PITFALLS TO AVOID

- Temporary hand and finger muscle weakness may be a complication of palmar injections of botulinum toxin A, especially with increasing dosages.
- Botox injections are contraindicated in patients with underlying neuromuscular conditions as well as in pregnant and lactating patients.
- Decreased doses should be considered for patients on angiotensin-converting enzyme (ACE) inhibitors, which can potentiate Botox effects.
- It is important to counsel that the benefits of Botox are temporary and require repeat treatments.
- None of the therapies is universally efficacious. The patient must be aware that the treatment endpoint is a reduction in sweating and not complete elimination.
- Treatment side effects may be considerable depending on the treatment chosen, and must be reviewed at depth with the patient prior to any treatment initiation.

BIBLIOGRAPHY

Campanati A, Lagalla G, Penna L, Gesuita R, Offidani A. Local neural block at the wrist for treatment of palmar hyperhidrosis with botulinum toxin: Technical improvements. *J Am Acad Dermatol.* 2004;51(3):345-348.

Glaser DA. Treatment of axillary hyperhidrosis by chemodenervation of sweat glands using botulinum toxin type A. *J Drugs Dermatol.* 2004;3(6):627-631.

Goh CL. Aluminum chloride hexahydrate versus palmar hyperhidrosis. *Int J Dermatol.* 1990;29:368-370.

Gregoriou S, Rigopoulos D, Makris M, et al. Effects of botulinum toxin-a therapy for palmar hyperhidrosis in plantar sweat production. *Dermatol Surg.* 2010;36(4): 496-498.

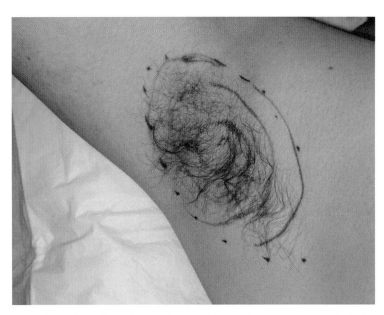

Figure 16.5 *Injection sites marked on right axilla of a male prior to botulinum toxin A injection*

Hamm H. The place of botulinum toxin type A in the treatment of focal hyperhidrosis. *Br J Dermatol.* 2004;151(6):1115-1122.

Heckmann M, Ceballos-Bauman AO, Plewig G. Botulinum toxin A for axillary hyperhidrosis (excessive sweating). *N Engl J Med.* 2001;344:488-493.

Herbst F, Plas EG, Fuggo R, Fritsch A. Endoscopic thoracic sympathectomy for primary hyperhidrosis of the upper limbs: A critical analysis and long-term results in 480 operations. *Ann Surg.* 1994;220:86-90.

Lowe N, Campanati A, Bodokh I, et al. The use of topical glycopyrrolate in the treatment of hyperhidrosis. *Clin Exp Dermatol.* 1998;23:204-205.

Paul A, Kranz G, Schindl A, Kranz GS, Auff E, Sycha T. Diode laser hair removal does not interfere with botulinum toxin A treatment against axillary hyperhidrosis. *Lasers Surg Med.* 2010;42(3):211-214.

Reinauer S, Nuesser A, Schauf G, Holzle E. Iontophoresis with alternating current and direct current offset (A/C iontophoresis): A new approach for treatment of hyperhidrosis. *Br J Dermatol.* 1993;129:166-169.

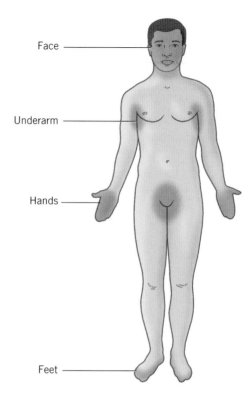

Figure 16.6 *The sites of hyperhidrosis*

SECTION FOUR

Disorders of Hair Follicles

CHAPTER 17 | Hirsutism

Hirsutism represents a male pattern overgrowth of terminal and vellus hairs in women. Far from being solely a cosmetic concern, hirsutism can be an important manifestation of an underlying endocrine disorder arising from increased androgenic activity. Often, it results from an overproduction of adrenal and ovarian hormones and may accompany other signs of virilization. Its appearance produces social anxiety, distress, and ostracism in affected patients. It also merits an appropriate medical workup. By contrast, hypertrichosis features fine hairs in androgen-sensitive as well as androgen-insensitive areas. Normal racial and ethnic variations may cause confusion with these disorders.

EPIDEMIOLOGY

Incidence: common.

Age: usually postpubertal but age of onset can vary in the setting of medication, tumor, or endocrine abnormality.

Race: racial and cultural factors affect the perception of what constitutes abnormal hair growth. Skin type affects treatment options as well.

Sex: female.

Precipitating factors: hirsutism is caused by a host of endocrine abnormalities. Adrenal causes include Cushing's disease, ectopic adrenocorticotropic hormone (ACTH) production, primary androgen-producing neoplasms, and congenital adrenal hyperplasia. Ovarian causes can be related to polycystic ovarian syndrome and primary tumors among other causes. Finally, medications such as oral contraceptive pills, anabolic steroids, and androgens may cause hirsutism.

PHYSICAL EXAMINATION

There is an overgrowth of hair in androgen-sensitive hair follicles. Common sites include the beard area of the face, chin, preauricular face, linea alba, periareolar area, and chest. Depending on the severity of the condition, other signs of virilization such as increased muscle mass, deep voice, male pattern hair loss, and clitoral enlargement may be present.

DIFFERENTIAL DIAGNOSIS

While both hirsutism and hypertrichosis feature hair overgrowth, these conditions can be differentiated by the location and quality of the hair growth. Hirsutism is characterized by terminal hair overgrowth in androgen-dependent areas, while hypertrichosis features fine hairs

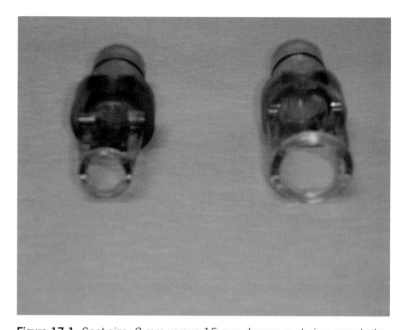

Figure 17.1 *Spot size, 8 mm versus 15 mm. Larger spot sizes penetrate deeper and allow quicker treatments*

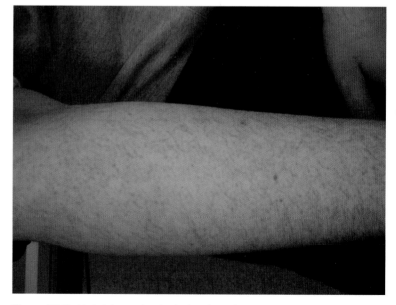

Figure 17.2 *Hair trimmed prior to treatment*

in androgen-sensitive as well as androgen-insensitive areas. Normal racial and ethnic variations may cause confusion with these disorders.

LABORATORY TESTS

The laboratory workup should be guided by the patient's clinical findings as well as by a detailed patient history. Testing can help establish if there is an adrenal or ovarian source of the hair growth. Ovarian, adrenal, and pituitary tumors should be ruled out in cases of rapid onset by an endocrinologist and/or a gynecologist. Total testosterone levels, dehydroepiandrosterone sulfate levels, urinary free cortisol levels, dexamethasone suppression test, prolactin levels, ACTH stimulation, luteinizing hormone/follicle-stimulating hormone (LH/FSH) ratio, 17-hydroxy progesterone levels, and pelvic ultrasound may all present important components of a thorough endocrinologic workup.

COURSE

Course is dependent on the etiology of the hirsutism.

KEY CONSULTATIVE QUESTIONS

- Menstrual history—regular or irregular
- Medication history
- Onset and progression of symptoms
- Family history of inflammatory cystic acne and hair loss
- History of endocrine abnormalities

MANAGEMENT

The primary goal of the treatment is to determine the underlying cause of hirsutism and treat. After determining the cause and ensuring appropriate medical therapy, the goal can transition to reversing the abnormal hair growth. There are multiple means by which temporary and permanent hair removal can be achieved.

■ Consultation with Endocrinology

In cases of hirsutism, the first priority is to uncover the source of the aberrant hair growth. Numerous laboratory investigations, as detailed above, may be required. Consultation and referral to an endocrinologist is strongly recommended as part of such a workup.

■ Nonlaser Therapies

There are several temporary means to conceal hair overgrowth. They include makeup, bleaches, and hydrogen peroxide. Shaving also can temporarily hide hair growth.

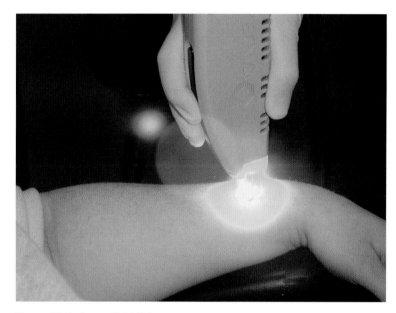

Figure 17.3 *Laser light firing*

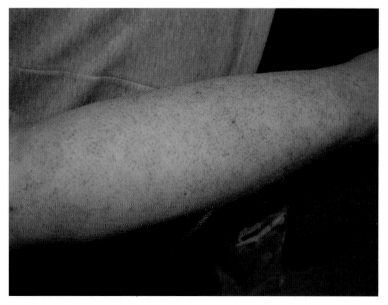

Figure 17.4 *Characteristic posttreatment perifollicular erythema*

Hair removal can be achieved with depilation, epilation, laser therapy, electrolysis, and topical eflornithine.

Depilation

Depilation is the process of removing part of the hair shaft. Its effects are temporary. There are chemical and mechanical methods of depilation. Chemical depilatories, such as thioglycolate salts and sulfides of alkali metals, dissolve hair shafts. They can produce localized irritation at the site of treatment. Mechanical depilation can be quite crude including shaving of hair as well as rubbing hair with a pumice stone.

Epilation

Epilation is the process of removing the entire hair shaft. It provides more longevity than depilation but is not permanent. It includes waxing, plucking, threading, and electrical devices that remove the hair shaft. Each of these options is relatively inexpensive but can produce pain and irritation as side effects. Plucking can result in localized infection, ingrown hairs, and even scarring. Each of these treatments can be used in combination with topical eflornithine on the face of women.

Topical eflornithine (Vaniqa)

Topical eflornithine twice daily has been approved by the U.S. Food and Drug Administration (FDA) for temporary hair removal on the face of women. It should only be used on the face and not on other parts of the body. It decreases the rate of hair growth by inhibiting ornithine decarboxylase. It should be used in conjunction with other hair removal methods, such as shaving, waxing, or plucking. Patients should use the medications for 8 weeks to judge its efficacy. If there is no improvement after 8 weeks, the medication should be discontinued. If the medication works, it should be continued. Discontinuation of treatment results in a resumption of hair growth. Side effects include local irritation. It should not be used during pregnancy.

■ Electrolysis

- Removal can be permanent.

- Electrolysis uses direct electrical current to destroy the dermal papilla of the hair follicle. A fine needle placed directly into the hair follicle delivers the electrical current to the follicle's base without producing scarring. The site of treatment is shaved several days prior to therapy and topical anesthetic cream can be used 1 hour prior to the procedure to reduce pain. Side effects include scar, hypo-/hyperpigmentation, and infection. It is most appropriate for small areas of treatment.

- Need for multiple treatments for limited treatment zone.

- Greater risk of side effects, painful.

- Not practical for large areas of the body.

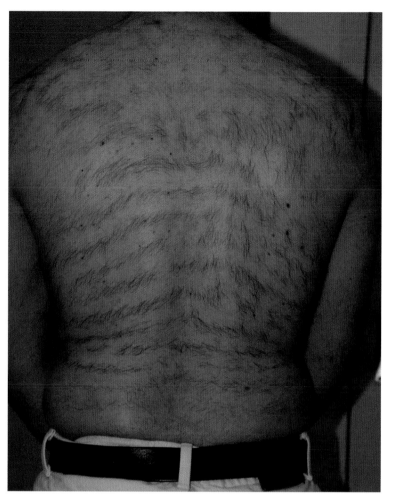

Figure 17.5 *Bizarre growth of back hair on a male due to poor technique*

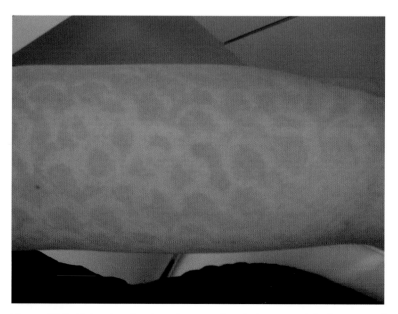

Figure 17.6 *Extensive dyschromia secondary to inappropriate fluence and pulse duration*

Laser hair removal

Lasers are the treatment of choice for permanent reduction of unwanted, pigmented terminal hair follicles. Laser hair removal is quick, relatively nonpainful, especially compared to electrolysis. Furthermore, it can cover a far more extensive area of affected skin with less pain in less (ie, improper spacing and overlap) time. An average of five to seven treatments are needed for greater than 50% reduction.

Mechanism of action

Lasers are based on the selective photothermolysis. The light is absorbed by the pigment in hair follicles. Therefore, if hair follicles have no pigment (ie, blond or gray hair), lasers do not work. Lasers work best on thicker hair follicles.

Patient Consultation

- Hair color.
- Skin type—all skin types can benefit from laser hair removal.
- Past medical history.
- Medications.
- Past treatments.
- Emphasize the need for five to seven treatments on an average to remove the majority of unwanted hair.
- Improvement is variable.
- Low risk of no improvement or increased hair (especially in females of Mediterranean heritage).
- Risk of hyper- or hypopigmentation that may last months; rarely permanent.
- Scarring is rare.
- Likelihood of at least some pain; the amount of pain associated with the procedure is a reflection of the caliber and density of hair in the treated region.
- Ideal candidate has dark course hair and light skin phototype.
- Average candidate—fine/light brown hair
- Poor candidate—blond/gray hair should not be treated with a 810-nm diode laser with current lasers. Additionally, patients with unrealistic expectations or medical contraindications should not be treated.

Patient Consultation Prior to Treatment

- Sun avoidance is crucial. If a patient is tanned, the procedure should be postponed until the tan completely fades. If the procedure is performed on tanned skin, the risk of dyschromia is markedly increased.

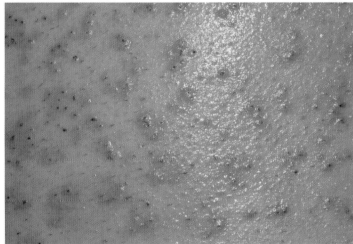

Figure 17.7 (A) *Appearance of skin prior to laser hair removal.* **(B)** *Hair on lateral cheeks*

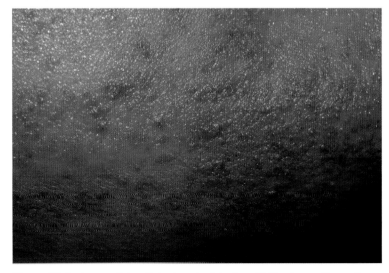

Figure 17.8 *Appropriate clinical endpoint of perifollicular erythema in this 24-year-old female with type VI skin and polycystic ovarian syndrome treated with the long-pulsed 1,064-nm Nd:YAG laser*

- Shave hair prior to arriving in the office. Alternatively, the hair can be trimmed in the office with a moustache trimmer. This will focus the majority of energy to the pigmented hair follicles in the skin.

- A topical anesthetic cream can be applied 1 hour prior to therapy to decrease the pain during the procedure. It is important to advise the patient to apply topical anesthetic over a limited surface of the skin to avoid any risk of lidocaine toxicity.

- Hair waxing should not be performed 2 to 3 weeks before treatment.

- If there is a history of recurrent herpes simplex virus, prophylaxis should be provided before laser hair removal on face.

- Pregnancy: there are no clear studies demonstrating safety or risk. It is important to educate pregnant patients desiring hair removal as to this uncertainty. Most physicians will not treat patients while pregnant. If treatment is pursued, it is recommended to treat only limited areas during third trimester after medical clearance from an obstetrician.

■ Just Prior to Treatment

- Written consent
- Photography
- Trim hair

■ Laser Hair Removal Technique (Figs. 17.1–17.8) (Table 17.1)

Key concepts for optimal results are as follows:

- For skin types I to III, use relatively high energy with a shorter pulse duration for optimal results.

TABLE 17.1 ■ Laser Hair Removal Technique

Laser type	Safest skin type	Wavelength (nm)	Pulse duration	Energy (J/cm^2)	Comments
Ruby	I–III	694	1–20 ms	10–40 J/cm^2	First laser used for hair removal; slower to use
Alexandrite	I–III	755	Skin types I–III 3 ms; skin types III and IV 10–20 ms	Skin types I–III 20–25 J/cm^2; skin type IV 15–20 J/cm^2	3 ms and 10–20 ms pulse duration demonstrate equal efficacy
Diode	I–V	810	3–100 ms	30–40 J/cm^2	Longer pulse duration for treatment of skin types IV and V
Nd:YAG	I–VI	1064	Skin types I–III 10–20 ms; skin types IV–VI 25–100 ms	Skin types I–III 30–50 J/cm^2; skin types III–VI 25–35 J/cm^2	Safest device for removing hair in skin types IV–VI
Intense pulsed light—noncoherent light	I–IV	550–1200	1.5–3.5 ms	25–50 J/cm^2	Most variable results

LASER SAFETY

Hazard: ocular

Dangers

Cornea, retina, or lens can be damaged

Damage can occur from direct exposure or reflected beams, i.e. patient jewelry, watches

Q-switched lasers are most hazardous, can cause blindness

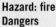

Enhance Safety

Baseline eye exam

Laser goggle optical density (OD) should be equal to or greater than 7 (check goggles)

Inspect goggles for visible damage or degradation of the filter media

Always check that appropriate goggles for wavelength are used

Remove, ebonize or cover any reflective surfaces in laser room, i.e. mirrors, metallic garbage cans

Remove patient jewelry, watches

Hazard: fire

Dangers

All lasers can potentially cause fire hazards

Most commonly seen with CO_2 lasers

Damage can occur from direct exposure or reflected beams

Enhance Safety

Remove, ebonize, or cover any reflective surfaces in laser room, i.e. mirrors, metallic garbage cans

Avoid alcohol or ensure that it is fully vaporized prior to start of treatment

Drape treatment site with wet gauze or towels

Remove all flammable items, i.e. dry gauze, towels, drapes

Coat exposed hair with water-based jelly

Decrease FiO_2 to 40% when treating near endotracheal tubes

Hazard: plume, splatter, infection

Dangers

Intact virions and viral DNA such as HPV may be present in the plume of CO_2 lasers

Tissue particles can splatter and aerosolize with Q-switched lasers

Enhance Safety

Use mask

Smoke evacuator

Hazard: electrocution

Dangers

Even with power off, can cause shock/electrocution

Enhance Safety

Only qualified laser technicians should open lasers

Check for water spills, hose ruptures or condensations

Hazard: general

Dangers

Anticipate dangers

Enhance Safety

Always immediately put laser on standby mode when not treating patient

Ensure proper sign is on the door of laser room

Educate staff members as to laser safety

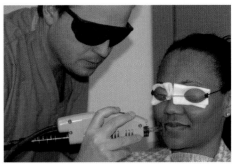

A

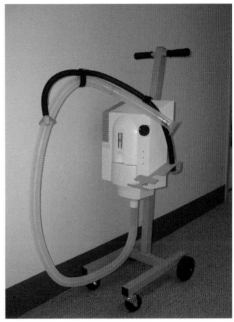

B

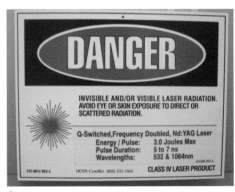

C

Figure 17.9 *Laser safety. It is important to emphasize that lasers present special safety concerns for physicians, staff, and patients. Among the risks are ocular injury, fire, electrocution, and dissemination of infectious disease. No lasers should be operated in the absence of a detailed knowledge of laser safety issues between the physician and the staff. Educating staff members is an essential component of safe laser practices. Periodic laser safety training is required by many hospitals and remains good practice for private physician offices as well.* **(A)** *Patient and all personnel are wearing protective eyewear. Note gauze is moist to reduce the risk of fire.* **(B)** *Smoke evacuator.* **(C)** *Safety sign placed outside appropriate laser room to ensure proper warning of laser use*

- Skin types IV to VI must use longer pulse and longer wavelength such as a 1064-nm YAG.

- If uncertain as to treatment parameters, perform test sites with variable fluencies and pulse durations.

- All machines utilize cooling of epidermal skin via cryogen, contact cooling, or gel.

- Optimal cooling settings must be utilized to lower the risk of dyschromia.

- Use larger spot sizes for deeper penetration and more rapid treatment of larger areas.

- Safety goggles for patient and medical team.

- Use the largest spot size possible for target region.

- Overlap laser pulses 10% over the entire treatment region.

■ Posttreatment Instructions to Patient

- Expect redness for up to several hours after treatment.

- If redness or pain persists for more than 12 hours, call the office. If there are any cutaneous changes in the skin the day after the procedure or beyond, the patient must be told to contact the treating physician.

- Once redness fades, patient may continue to wear makeup.

- Avoid sun for 48 hours; no tanning.

- Hair removal is not entirely immediate. Some hair will fall out 1 to 3 days after treatment.

- Do not worry if some hair persists after treatment.

- Call the office if discoloration develops in the treated sites.

- Call the office with questions or concerns.

PITFALLS TO AVOID/COMPLICATIONS/ MANAGEMENT (Figs. 17.5–17.6)

- There is no effective mechanism for laser removal of light or blond hair.

- Excessive fluencies or incorrect pulse duration may produce epidermal damage and dyschromia. These effects are typically temporary but can be permanent. If there is any doubt regarding laser parameters, perform a test site.

- Skin types IV to VI require longer pulse durations and lower fluencies.

- Coincident tattoos and lentigines may experience lightening. Patients should be informed of this possibility.

- Always keep contact cooling against the skin to avoid burning.

- Overlap (10%) in the treated zone. Do not leave "gaps" that can create bizarre hair growth patterns as hair regrows.

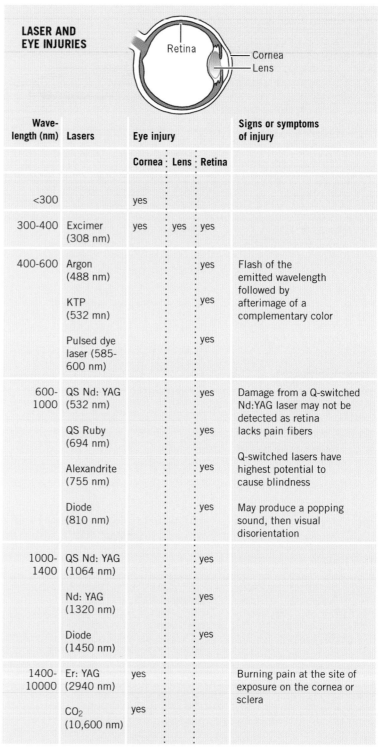

Wave-length (nm)	Lasers	Eye injury			Signs or symptoms of injury
		Cornea	Lens	Retina	
<300		yes			
300-400	Excimer (308 nm)	yes	yes	yes	
400-600	Argon (488 nm)			yes	Flash of the emitted wavelength followed by afterimage of a complementary color
	KTP (532 mn)			yes	
	Pulsed dye laser (585-600 nm)			yes	
600-1000	QS Nd: YAG (532 nm)			yes	Damage from a Q-switched Nd:YAG laser may not be detected as retina lacks pain fibers
	QS Ruby (694 nm)			yes	
	Alexandrite (755 nm)			yes	Q-switched lasers have highest potential to cause blindness
	Diode (810 nm)			yes	May produce a popping sound, then visual disorientation
1000-1400	QS Nd: YAG (1064 nm)			yes	
	Nd: YAG (1320 nm)			yes	
	Diode (1450 nm)			yes	
1400-10000	Er: YAG (2940 nm)	yes			Burning pain at the site of exposure on the cornea or sclera
	CO$_2$ (10,600 nm)	yes			

Figure 17.10 *Lasers and eye injuries (http://www.eyesafety.4ursafety.com/laser-eye-safety.html)*

• For Nd:YAG lasers, patients may experience pain even after topical anesthesia.

BIBLIOGRAPHY

Azziz R. The evaluation and management of hirsutism. *Obstet Gynecol.* 2003;101(5 pt 1):995-1007.

Battle EF, Hobbs LM. Laser-assisted hair removal for darker skin types. *Dermatol Ther.* 2004;17(2):177-183.

Bouzari N, Tabatabai H, Abbasi Z, Firooz A, Dowlati Y. Laser hair removal: Comparison of long-pulsed Nd:YAG, long-pulsed alexandrite, and long-pulsed diode lasers. *Dermatol Surg.* 2004;30(4 pt 1):498-502.

Goldberg DJ. Laser hair removal. *Dermatol Clin.* 2002;20(3):561-567.

Tanzi EL, Alster TS. Long-pulsed 1064-nm Nd:YAG laser-assisted hair removal in all skin types. *Dermatol Surg.* 2004;30(1):13-17.

CHAPTER 18 | Pseudofolliculitis

Pseudofolliculitis is a common, chronic inflammatory disorder that presents with inflammatory papules and pustules in the beard distribution of males, particularly those with darker skin phototypes and tightly coiled hair. Nonetheless, pseudofolliculitis can present in any skin that is regularly shaved and in all skin phototypes. In females it is most commonly seen in the axillary and pubic areas. It tends to present in a more mild form in lighter skin phototypes.

EPIDEMIOLOGY

Incidence: over 50% of African American males

Age: begins with shaving or plucking

Race: more common in beard distribution of males with darker skin phototypes

Sex: male > females

Precipitating factors: shaving in any region of the body

PATHOGENESIS

This disorder is induced by shaving. Shaving sharpens curled hair. Sharpened, tightly curled hairs pierce into the skin adjacent to the hair follicle and invade into the dermis producing an inflammatory reaction. It can also follow hair plucking, especially in females with hirsutism.

DERMATOPATHOLOGY

Hair penetration results in epidermal invagination with associated microabscess, mixed inflammatory infiltrate, and foreign body giant reaction at the tip of the invading hair. Dermal fibrosis may be observed.

PHYSICAL LESIONS

Most commonly, it presents with follicular papules, pustules, and postinflammatory hyperpigmentation in the beard area and anterolateral neck of males and underarms and bikini areas of females. Papules can develop into cysts. Scar formation may be observed. The upper cutaneous lip is typically spared.

DIFFERENTIAL DIAGNOSIS

Acne vulgaris, folliculitis.

LABORATORY EXAMINATION

None.

COURSE

Begins with shaving or plucking and continues until cessation or modification in the hair removal technique.

MANAGEMENT

The goal of the treatment is to prevent the formation of the papules, pustules, scarring, and postinflammatory hyperpigmentation associated with this disorder. There are multiple treatment options available to accomplish this goal. Cessation of shaving or plucking is the most successful treatment but it is impractical and undesirable for many patients. Laser therapy is highly effective with high patient satisfaction.

TREATMENT

■ Shaving Cessation

The most simple, inexpensive, and effective treatment for pseudofolliculitis is the cessation of shaving. Many patients will find this option undesirable or impractical.

■ Modification of Shaving Technique

A proper shaving technique may prevent or significantly decrease the risk of pseudofolliculitis. Among these practices are lifting, not plucking ingrown hairs, thoroughly

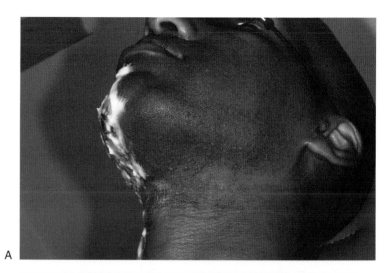

A

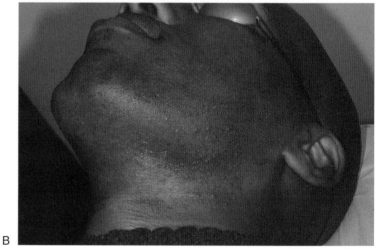

B

Figure 18.1 (A) *A young male with type VI skin phototype and pseudofolliculitis barbae prior to treatment.* **(B)** *Same patient 3 months later after several treatments with long-pulsed 1,064-nm Nd:YAG laser. (Courtesy of E. Victor Ross, MD)*

wetting the area prior to applying shaving cream, using a sharp razor, shaving in the direction of the hair growth, and avoiding shaving in more than one direction in the same area. The Bump Fighter Razor prevents the shaved hair from being cut too short. Additionally, cutting the hair twice daily with hair clippers prevents hairs from piercing into the skin.

▪ Topical Treatment

Topical antibiotics are effective in treating the inflammation and occasional impetiginization associated with this condition. Topical tretinoin, benzoyl peroxide, and glycolic acids can be helpful adjuncts.

▪ Laser Hair Removal (Figs. 18.1 and 18.2)

- Laser hair removal is a safe, highly effective treatment modality for short and long-term improvement.
- Skin types I to III
  - The long-pulsed alexandrite laser (755 nm), diode laser (810 nm), intense pulse light (590–100 nm), and long-pulsed Nd:YAG (1064 nm) laser have the appropriate wavelengths to selectively target the chromophore melanin found in the hair bulb.
  - Multiple treatments (average of 5–10) every 4 to 8 weeks achieve an average of 50% to 75% permanent reduction of follicular papules/pustules.
- Skin types IV to VI
  - The long-pulsed 1,064-nm Nd:YAG laser is the treatment of choice in skin phototypes IV to VI. It is safe and effective. Long pulse durations are necessary for epidermal protection. Pulse durations of 30 to 100 ms are generally recommended. Optimal fluences range from 20 to 40 J/cm^2. Treatment is performed with nonoverlapping pulses utilizing cooling to the epidermis via cryogen, contact cooling, or gel.
  - Newer generation diode lasers with longer pulse durations up to 400 ms can also be utilized with caution in darker skin types.
  - Typically, 5 to 10 treatments spaced every 4 to 8 weeks are needed for 50% to 75% permanent reduction.

PITFALLS TO AVOID/OUTCOME EXPECTATIONS/COMPLICATIONS/ MANAGEMENT

- Tanned patients should not be treated with laser hair removal. Once the tan/inflammation subsides, hair removal can begin.
- Do not pluck or wax hair prior to or during the course of laser hair removal.

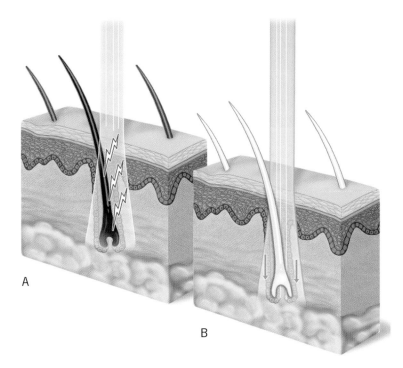

Figure 18.2 *Pseudofolliculitis—laser therapy: pigmented versus unpigmented hair follicle*

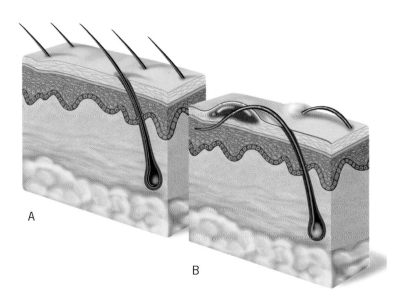

Figure 18.3 *Etiology of pseudofolliculitis*

- Patients with unpigmented hair (blond, gray, red) will not benefit from laser hair removal and should not be treated.

- There is the risk of transient and long-term hyperpigmentation and hypopigmentation. Transient erythema, scabbing, and risk of scar formation also exist.

- A majority of patients will see 75% improvement. A small minority will see little or no improvement.

- Future maintenance treatments may be needed.

- A small minority of patients will experience a paradoxical increase in hair growth, particularly females of Mediterranean descent.

- Treatment may not benefit preexisting hyperpigmentation and will not improve scars.

- It is important to inform patients that side effects are often delayed in skin phototypes IV to VI and may not be observed for 1 to 2 weeks after treatment. Test spot is advised for these patients (Figs. 18.3 and 18.4).

BIBLIOGRAPHY

Battle EF Jr, Hobbs LM. Laser-assisted hair removal for darker skin types. *Dermatol Ther.* 2004;17(2):177-183.

Bridgeman-Shah S. The medical and surgical therapy of pseudofolliculitis barbae. *Dermatol Ther.* 2004;17(2): 158-163.

Haedersdal M, Wulf HC. Evidence-based review of hair removal using lasers and light sources. *J Eur Acad Dermatol Venereol.* 2006;20(1):9-20.

Kontoes P, Vlachos S, Konstantinos M, Anastasia L, Myrto S. Hair induction after laser-assisted hair removal and its treatment. *J Am Acad Dermatol.* 2006;54(1):64-67.

Ross EV, Cooke LM, Timko AL, Overstreet KA, Graham BS, Barnette DJ. Treatment of pseudofolliculitis barbae in skin types IV, V, and VI with a long-pulsed neodymium: Yttrium aluminum garnet laser. *J Am Acad Dermatol.* 2002;47(2):888-893.

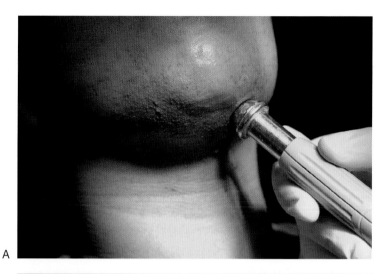

A

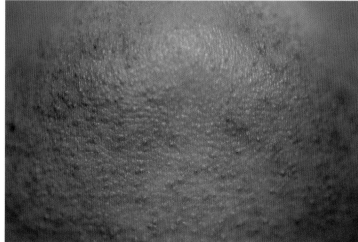

B

Figure 18.4 (A) *Test spot treatment under chin and on cheek is advised for darker skin phototypes before treating pseudofolliculitis.* **(B)** *Two weeks after test spot treatment, some hair removal is achieved with no pigmentary changes*

CHAPTER 19 | Male Pattern Hair Loss

Male pattern hair loss classically presents with bitemporal hair loss that progresses to the loss of hair on the vertex, frontal, and temporal scalp. Parietal and occipital hairs are usually unaffected. It is a nonscarring form of alopecia that occurs in genetically susceptible males. The gradual *involuntary* loss of hair does change the natural frame hair provides around our face. The gradual loss of hair resulting in an involuntary change in appearance creates varying degree of emotional and psychological stress. Many men seek treatment for male pattern hair loss because of unhappiness with its cosmetic appearance and association with aging.

EPIDEMIOLOGY

Incidence: 30% of males older than 30 years; more than half of males older than 50 years.

Age: begins after puberty.

Precipitating factors: polygenetic inherited predisposition. No diagnostic tests exist to determine the etiology and natural progression.

PATHOGENESIS

The precise pathophysiology remains unknown. This process is believed to result from both a polygenetic inherited susceptibility as well as androgenic stimulation. The most important androgen in this process is dihydrotestosterone.

There is a diminution in the size of affected terminal follicles that regress to become vellus follicles that eventually disappear. There is an increase in telogen hairs and a decrease in anagen hairs.

PHYSICAL EXAMINATION AND NATURAL PROGRESSION

Typically, frontal and temporal hair loss/thinning is present first. This begins in puberty and progresses over decades. The rate and extent of hair loss varies from individual to individual. Some progress to complete baldness in early 20s and others gradually thin over decades.

DIFFERENTIAL DIAGNOSIS

In males, the pattern of hair loss is characteristic suggesting no other diagnoses.

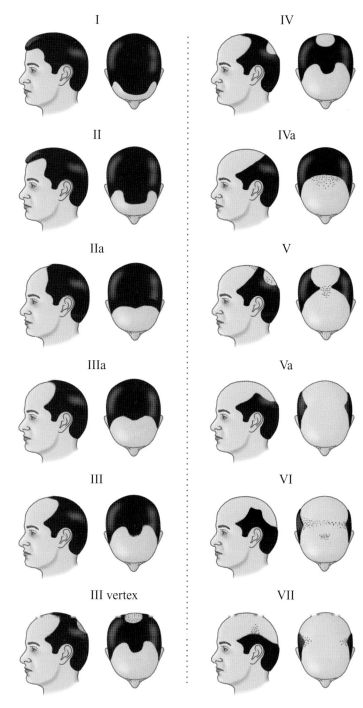

Figure 19.1 *Norwood classification of the natural progression of male pattern hair loss*

TABLE 19.1 ■ **Minoxidil and Finasteride—The Only Two FDA-Approved Medications for Male Pattern Hair Loss**

	Finasteride	Minoxidil
Mechanism of action	5-α reductase type II inhibitor blocking the conversion of testosterone to dihydrotestosterone	Unknown
Key to success	Emphasize maintenance over regrowth of hair and compliance for at least 6–8 months to see benefit	Emphasize maintenance over regrowth of hair and compliance 6–8 months to see benefit
Side effects	2% of men experience sexual dysfunction. Reversible within days if discontinued No allergic reactions, blood monitoring or drug interactions. Pre menopause of females should never handle or take medication. Women may have some benefit	Dryness and pruritus of the scalp. Rare allergic reaction
Clinical onset of action	6–8 months	6–8 months
Dose	1 mg qd with or without food	Two to four drops one to two times daily to frontal and vertex of scalp
Candidate selection		
Norwood II–IV	Highly effective	Highly effective
Norwood IV–VII	Somewhat effective	Somewhat effective

LABORATORY EXAMINATION

In males, no laboratory workup is typically required.

MEDICAL THERAPY

■ Key Consultative Questions

- Age of onset
- Rate of hair loss
- Past medical history
- Medications used to date and success of therapy
- Patient expectation of any medical or surgical therapy

■ FDA-Approved Medical Therapy (Table 19.1)

Minoxidil and finasteride are the only two medications for male pattern hair loss approved by the U.S. Food & Drug Administration (FDA).

HAIR TRANSPLANTATION

■ Definition

All patients should expect consistently natural appearing transplanted hair. Based on the theory of donor dominance, hair follicles maintain their genetic destiny wherever they grow on our scalp. Hair transplanted from the posterior scalp will grow for as long as it was genetically programmed to grow. For the vast majority of men, transplanted hair will grow for decades.

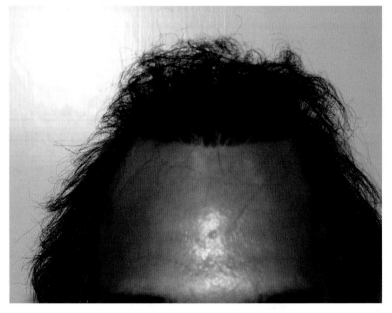

Figure 19.2 *Unnatural "pluggy" hairline using 10 to 25 hair grafts. Should never happen in twenty-first century*

Hair naturally grows in 1 to 4 hair follicular bundles. Contemporary hair transplantation utilizes a large number of 1 to 4 hair follicular groupings. The result is consistently natural appearing transplanted hair for men and women.

THE CONSULT

■ Key Questions

- How long have you noticed hair loss?
- Rate of hair loss?
- Which medications, whether prescription or alternative, have been tried and for how long?
- Expectations?

■ Physical Examination

- Norwood stage (Fig. 19.1)
- Donor density
- Caliber of hair follicles
  - Ideal candidate: high donor density, thick caliber hair follicle, realistic expectation (Figs. 19.3 and 19.4)
  - Poor candidate: poor donor density, below average hair caliber, unrealistic expectations

■ Key Points to Emphasize Before Hair Transplantation

- Net perceived density from a hair transplant = the number of hair follicles transplanted–ongoing hair loss.
- Fine hair follicles will create thin natural coverage, and thick caliber follicles will create more perceived density.
- Ongoing hair loss will affect the cosmetic appearance of a transplant.
- Visible donor scar or scars if hair is shaved or closely cropped in posterior scalp.
- Limited donor supply!

Key to success: physician and patient have similar expectations of what the procedure will and will not achieve over the short (1–3 years) and long term (10–20 years).

■ Medication and Transplantation

Medication to maintain existing hair will maximize the density from a transplant but medications should always remain elective. Hairline design and distribution of recipient sites should always assume ongoing hair loss.

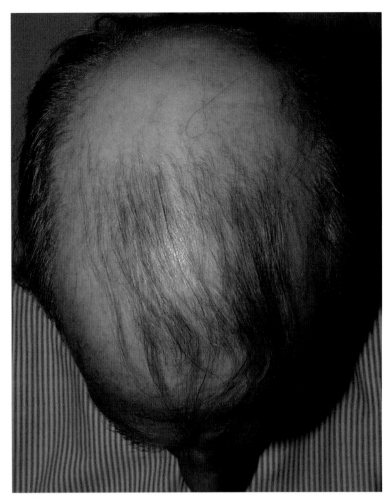

Figure 19.3 *Realistic expectations using 1 to 4 hair grafts. Before Norwood V*

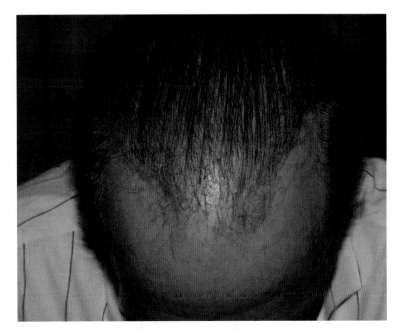

Figure 19.4 *Realistic expectations using 1 to 4 hair grafts. After 1,100 1 to 4 hair grafts*

SURGICAL PROCEDURE

■ Preoperative Instructions

- No specific blood tests
- Medical clearance if appropriate
- Photographs
- Informed written consent sent to the patient for review at least 1 week before the procedure

■ Day of Procedure

- Written consent with postoperative instructions reviewed
- Introduce hair transplant team
- Review procedure and goals with patient

■ Donor Region—Only Limiting Factor in Hair Transplantation (Figs. 19.5 and 19.10)

Anesthesia in donor region

- 1% Lidocaine with 1:200,000 epinephrine
- 30 to 60 cc saline

  Saline in donor region provides

  - anesthesia
  - hemostasis
  - less transection of hair follicles
  - less likely to transect the occipital arteries

Donor harvesting techniques (Tables 19.2 and 19.3)

- Elliptical strip harvesting: >95% of patients
- Follicular unit extraction: <5% of patients (Fig. 19.11)

Elliptical strip harvesting

- Use skin hooks to retract when removing donor ellipse to minimize transaction of hair follicles (Fig. 19.12)

TABLE 19.2 ■ Advantages and Disadvantages of Follicular Unit Extraction (FUE)

Advantage	Disadvantage
–No linear donor scar	–More time consuming
–Often minimally visible scarring in trimmed donor region; advantage for patients with short hairstyle	–More FUE sessions to equal density from ellipse
–Can be used for patients with extensive scarring in posterior scalp from multiple previous surgeries	–Greater transection of hair follicles with potential decreased yield

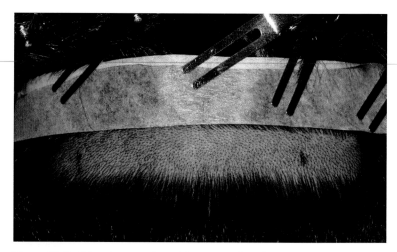

Figure 19.5 *Trim donor region with moustache trimmer, and tape hair up so donor suture will not be visible in the postoperative period*

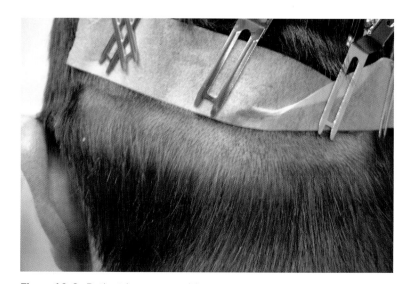

Figure 19.6 *Patient in prone position*

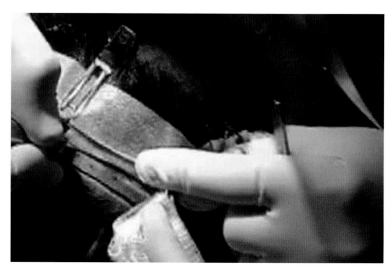

Figure 19.7 *Donor strip should not be more than 1 cm wide. Strips >1 cm have an increased risk of creating a hypertrophic scar*

TABLE 19.3 ■ Donor Harvesting Techniques: Elliptical Strip Harvesting Versus Follicular Unit Extraction

	Ellipse	Follicular unit extraction
Minimal transection of donor hair	Yes	No
Number of 1–4 grafts safely harvested per procedure	1,500–2,000	200–500
Time to harvest donor hair	15–20 min	1–2 h
Visible donor scar with hair length >1 cm	No	No
Visible donor scar with hair length <0.5 cm	Yes	Likely not
Overall percentage of cases used	>95%	<5%

- Undermining donor region rarely necessary
- Double layer of sutures rarely necessary
- Sutures or staples to close in single layer
- Sutures or staples out in 7 to 10 days

Keys to success in donor harvesting of ellipse

- Donor strip width <1 cm
- After lidocaine, add saline to donor region to provide hemostasis, anesthesia, and reduce transection of hair follicles
- Skin hooks to retract tissue while removing ellipse
- Do not rush!

■ Follicular unit extraction

Definition: removal of follicular groupings from the posterior scalp using 1-mm punches.

Excellent treatment option for patients' very short donor hair that do want a visible donor scar and for patients with severely depleted donor regions from multiple previous hair transplants.

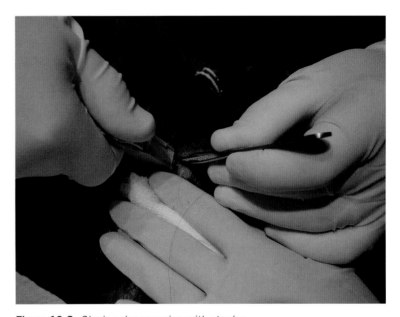

Figure 19.8 *Closing donor region with staples*

■ Graft creation

All grafts should mimic the natural 1 to 4 follicular bundles that naturally occur on the scalp.

Keys to success in creating 1 to 4 hair grafts

- Good ergonomics and instruments. Prep blades and #10 blades are often used to separate follicular groupings from the donor ellipse. Magnification can aid the process in separating follicular groupings from the donor ellipse.
- Do not allow grafts to dry. They must always be in chilled saline.
- Well-trained staff of three to four surgical assistants.

Staff training

- Enthusiasm/interest in procedure
- Patience; 6 to 12 months for an assistant to learn to create 200 to 300 grafts per hour

■ Anesthesia in Recipient Region

- Field block and local infiltration with 1% lidocaine with 1:200,000 epinephrine and 0.25% Marcaine with 1:200,000 epinephrine.

- Supraorbital and supratrochlear block is optional.

- Superficial infiltration in dermis, not subcutaneous tissue, will create good hemostasis.

■ Hairline Design

Definition: a hairline is an irregular, ill-defined transition zone from skin to increasing density of terminal pigmented hair follicles.

- Always consider the frontal, temporal, and posterior hairlines.

- The frontal and posterior hairlines should be irregular and in the same plain. This means generally avoiding transplanting the vertex, particularly in younger patients. The reason is the ever-expanding balding spot in the vertex.

  – When designing a frontal temporal hairline, always assume progression of hair loss to Norwood stage V.

  – Frontal hairline at least 9 cm above glabella.

  – Be conservative.

■ Recipient Site Creation (Fig. 19.18)

Commonly used needles to create recipient sites are

- #19 or #20 gauge needle

  – Magnification to reduce transaction of existing pigmented terminal hair

- SP 88 to 90 gauge needle

- 0.5- to 1.0-mm cag needle

Key points

- Distribute recipient sites randomly and closely together and in a distribution that will appear natural if all hair is lost in the frontal two-thirds of the scalp

- Avoid trauma to existing hair follicles

  – Magnification in recipient sites

  – Follow the natural 15- to 30-degree angle of hair follicles in the frontal two-thirds of the scalp

- Excellent hemostasis using 1:100,000 epinephrine

- 10 to 30 sites/cm^2 depending on the amount of existing hair and area (cm^2) to distribute grafts

■ Graft Placement (Fig. 19.19)

Two or three surgical assistants place the grafts into recipient sites using microvascular forceps.

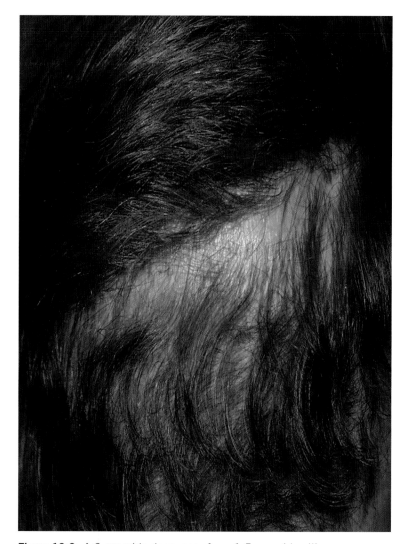

Figure 19.9 *A 2-cm-wide donor scar from 1.5-cm-wide ellipse*

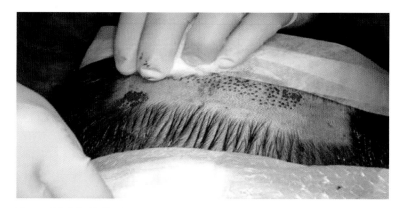

Figure 19.10 *Follicular unit extraction using 1-mm sites*

Keys to success

- Handle grafts in perifollicular tissue—never crush hair follicles
- Keep all grafts in chilled saline—never allow a graft to desiccate
- Staff training
- Excellent hemostasis using 1:100,000 epinephrine
- Patience

■ Postoperative Period

- Overnight dressing to protect grafts.
- Oral steroids 40 mg qd for 3 to 4 days to reduce frontal edema.
- Tylenol #3, one tablet q 4 to 6 hours for 1 day PRN. There should be no discomfort morning after surgery.
- Shower in morning after surgery. Avoid trauma to transplanted zone.
  - Perifollicular hemorrhagic crusting remains 5 to 8 days
  - The vast majority of patients return to work 2 to 3 days after the procedure
- Normal activities immediately. No heavy exercise for 5 to 7 days.
- Topical antibiotic to donor wound for 7 to 10 days.
- Sutures or staples removed 7 to 10 days after surgery.

■ Common Post Hair Transplant Side Effects

- Frontal edema lasting 3 to 4 days postoperatively
- Pruritus in donor and/or recipient zone
- Transitory folliculitis
- Telogen effluvium in patients with diffuse thinning

■ Rare Side Effects

- Hypertrophic scarring in donor region in ellipses less than 1 cm
- Persistent numbness or discomfort in donor or recipient zone
- Cystic nodules
- Poor quality growth of transplanted hair
- Infection

■ Postsurgical Period after Sutures/Staples Removed

- Resume full sports 1 week after surgery
- Dye hair 2 weeks after surgery

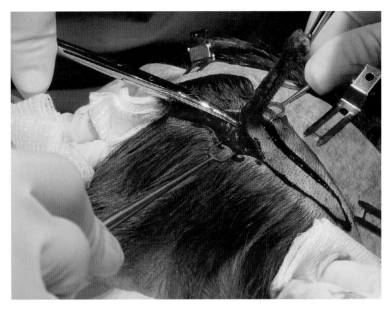

Figure 19.11 *Skin hooks to aid in removal of donor ellipse*

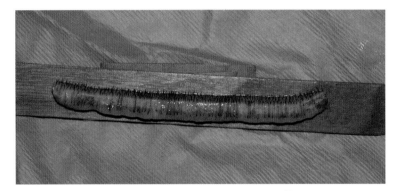

Figure 19.12 *Donor ellipse with natural follicular bundles*

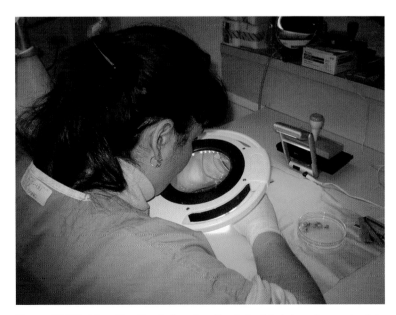

Figure 19.13 *Magnification helps visualize 1 to 4 hair bundles and minimize transection when separating with surgical prep blades*

TABLE 19.4 ■ **Treatment Options for Corrective Hair Transplant Surgery**

Treatment option	Advantage	Disadvantage
Adding 1–3 hair grafts between existing large 10–25 hair "plugs"	Dramatically soften hairline and add further density to existing "plugs"	Donor region may be depleted
Excision of grafts	Patient requesting "I would rather just be bald" Status quo ante	Patient not psychologically able to go through another hair transplant procedure Potential visible erythematous scar for weeks to months Permanent scar and/or dyschromia
Laser hair removal	Noninvasive	40–80% improvement after—five to seven does not work on bland hair
Combination	Reduce "pluggy" grafts Majority of patients utilize a combination of the above for optimal results	As above

- Initial followup 8 to 12 months after surgery
- Full cosmetic result 9 to 15 months after surgery

■ Corrective Hair Transplant Surgery (Table 19.4)

For the majority of men, corrective hair transplant surgery is cosmetically and emotionally mandatory, not elective.

Consult

Key question: what is your chief concern and goal for possible corrective surgery?

BIBLIOGRAPHY

Avram MR. Polarized light-emitting diode magnification for optimal recipient site creation during hair transplant. *Dermatol Surg.* 2005;31(9 pt 1):1124-1127. Discussion 1127.

Epstein JS. The treatment of female pattern hair loss and other applications of surgical hair restoration in women. *Facial Plast Surg Clin North Am.* 2004;12(2):241-247.

Harris JA. Follicular unit transplantation: Dissecting and planting techniques. *Facial Plast Surg Clin North Am.* 2004;12(2):225-232.

Leavitt M, Perez-Meza D, Rao NA, et al. Effects of finasteride (1 mg) on hair transplant. *Dermatol Surg.* 2005;31(10):1268-1276. Discussion 1276.

Limmer BL. Elliptical donor stereoscopically assisted micrografting as an approach to further refinement in hair transplantation. *J Dermatol Surg Oncol.* 1994;20(12): 789-793.

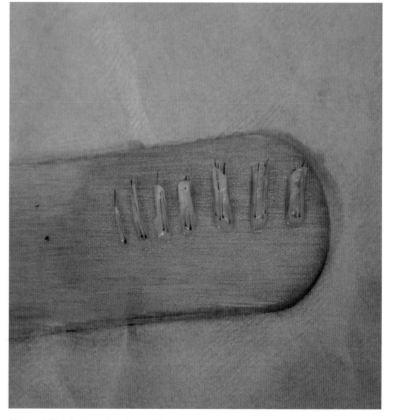

Figure 19.14 *1 to 4 hair grafts*

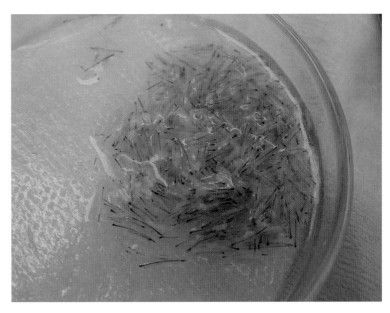

Figure 19.15 *1 to 4 hair grafts in chilled saline*

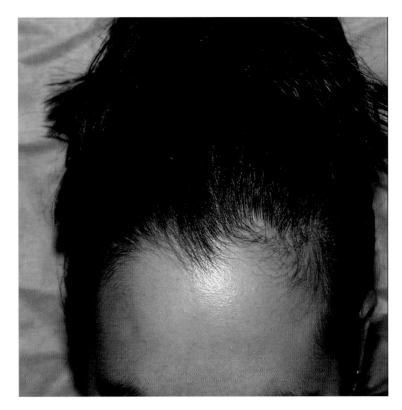

Figure 19.16 *Natural irregular frontal hairline*

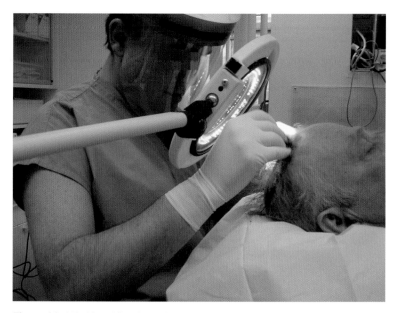

Figure 19.17 *Magnification with polarized light to create recipient sites*

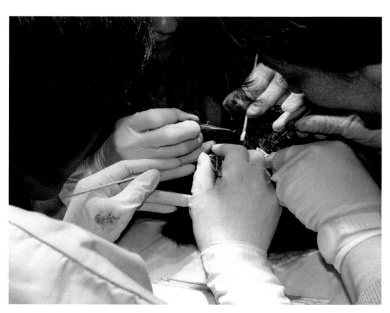

Figure 19.18 *Placing 1 to 4 hair grafts with microvascular forceps*

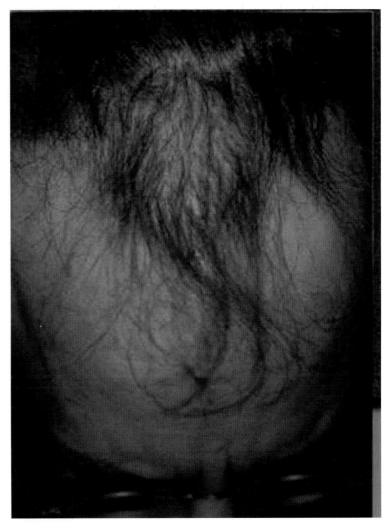

Figure 19.19 *Preoperative Norwood III*

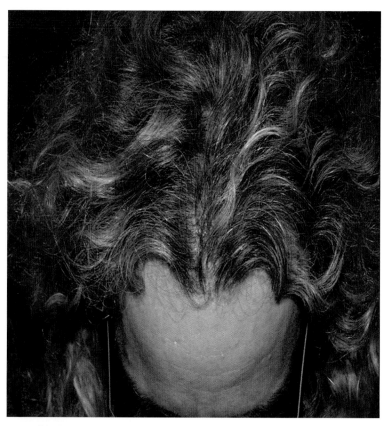

Figure 19.20 *After 2,400 1 to 4 hair grafts*

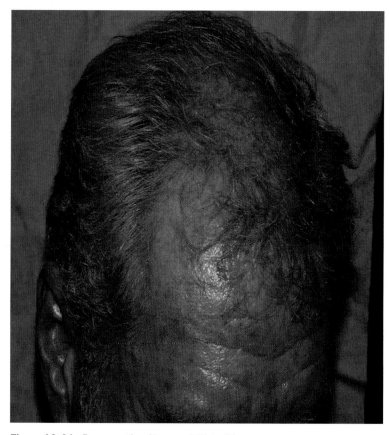

Figure 19.21 *Preoperative Norwood III to IV*

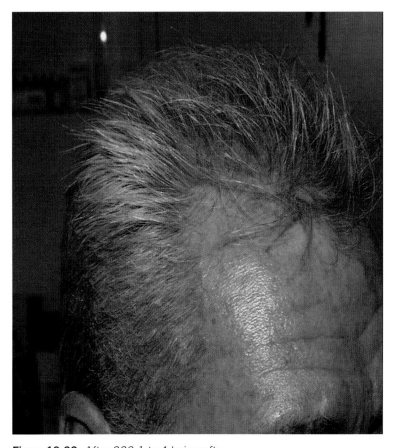

Figure 19.22 *After 900 1 to 4 hair grafts*

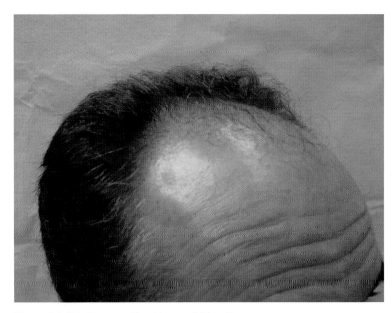

Figure 19.23 *Preoperative Norwood IV to V*

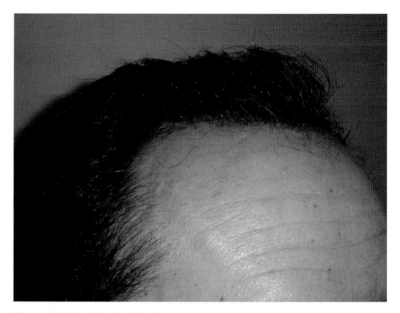

Figure 19.24 *After 2,030 1 to 4 hair grafts*

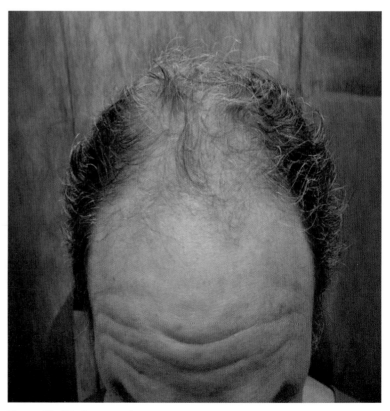

Figure 19.25 *Preoperative Norwood IV to V*

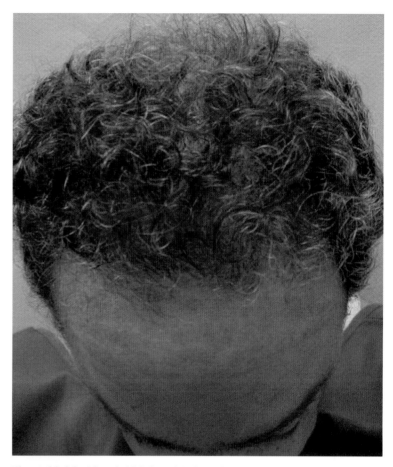

Figure 19.26 *After 1,000 1 to 4 hair grafts*

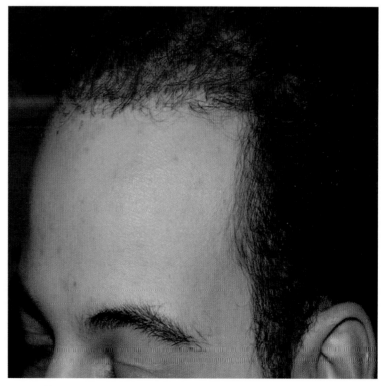

Figure 19.27 *Straight "pluggy" frontal hairline*

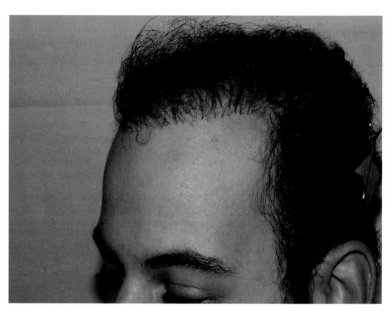

Figure 19.28 *After 650 1 to 3 hair grafts. Note improvement. Not completely natural hairline*

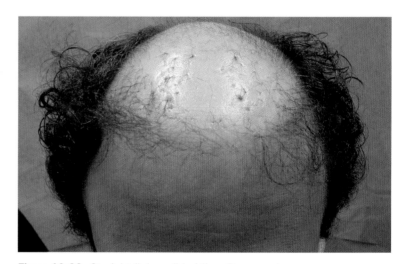

Figure 19.29 *Straight "pluggy" hairline. Depressed scars*

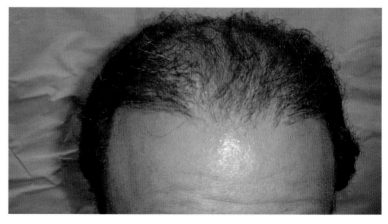

Figure 19.30 *After 1,000 1 to 3 grafts*

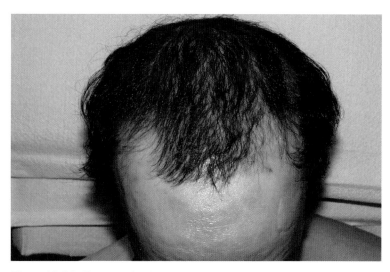

Figure 19.31 *Preoperative Norwood IV to V*

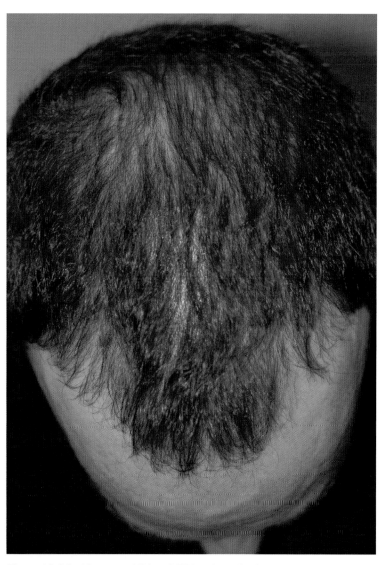

Figure 19.32 *After an additional 700 hair grafts (second surgery)*

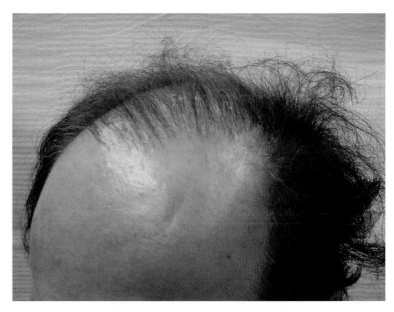

Figure 19.33 *Straight "pluggy" hairline*

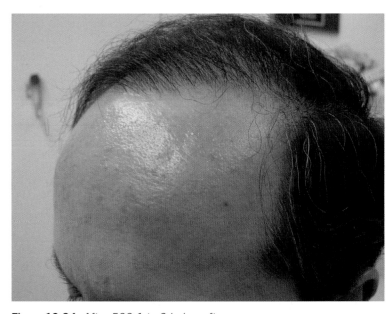

Figure 19.34 *After 500 1 to 3 hair grafts*

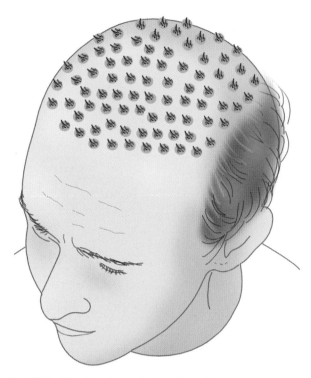

Illustration 19.1 *Obsolete 4-mm "pluggy" grafts*

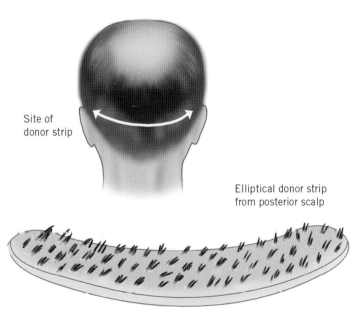

Site of
donor strip

Elliptical donor strip
from posterior scalp

Illustration 19.2 *Elliptical donor strip from posterior scalp*

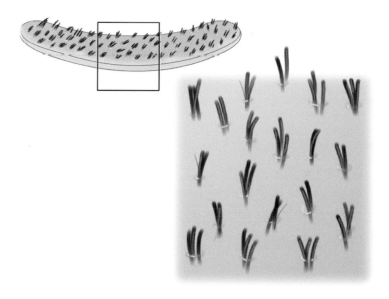

Illustration 19.3 *1 to 3 hair follicular groupings within donor strip*

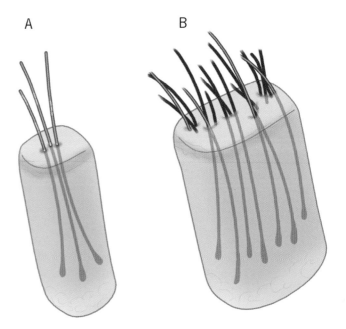

Illustration 19.4 *Versus 10 to 20 hair "pluggy" graft. Natural 1 to 3 follicular groupings*

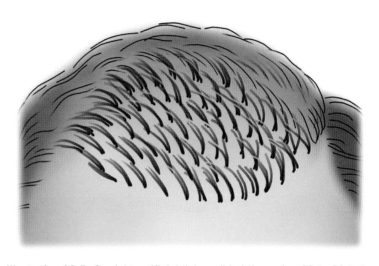

Illustration 19.5 *Straight artificial "pluggy" hairline using 10 to 20 hair grafts*

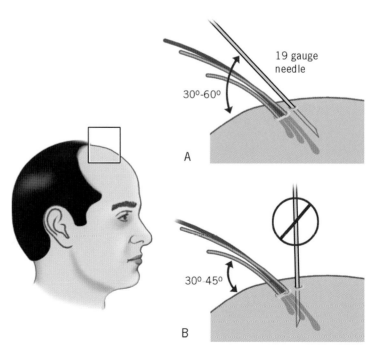

Illustration 19.6 *Recipient sites created at 15- to 45-degree angles not 90 degrees*

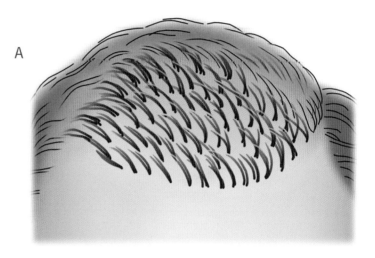

A

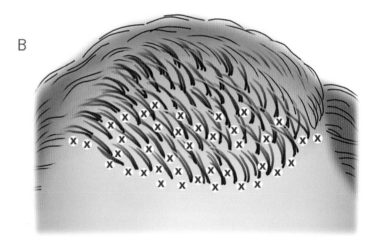

B

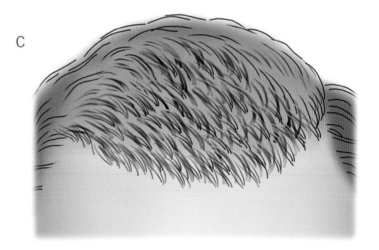

C

Illustration 19.7 *Corrective hair transplant adding 1 to 3 hair grafts between and in front of "pluggy" grafts*

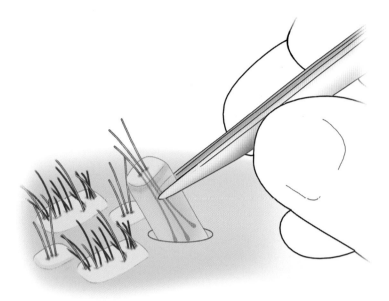

Illustration 19.8 *Adding 1 to 3 hair grafts between large "pluggy" grafts to improve cosmetic appearance*

CHAPTER 20 | Female Pattern Hair Loss

Female pattern hair loss presents with a diffuse thinning of the mid-scalp with a characteristic maintenance of the frontal hairline. It may also present with the typical bitemporal hair recession seen in male pattern hair loss. Parietal and occipital hairs are usually unaffected. Female pattern hair loss is particularly problematic for women for whom hair loss produces greater social and self-esteem difficulties than for men with male pattern hair loss (Figs. 20.1 and 20.2).

EPIDEMIOLOGY

Incidence: nearly 30% of females older than 30 years.

Age: begins in second and in third decade.

Race: none reported in females.

Precipitating factors: polygenetic inherited predisposition is present. It is not one parent's fault!

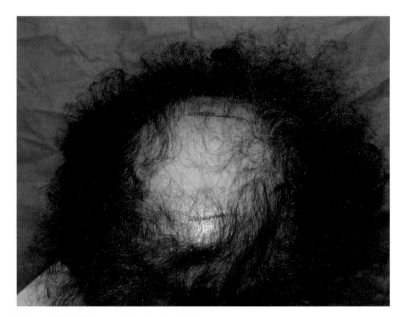

Figure 20.1 *Preoperative Ludwig III*

PATHOGENESIS

There is a diminution in the size of affected terminal follicles that regress to become vellus follicles that eventually disappear. There is an increase in telogen hairs and a decrease in anagen hairs. Hormones play a role but the exact pathophysiology is uncertain.

COURSE

Begins in twenties and progresses over decades. The rate and extent of hair loss varies.

KEY CONSULTATIVE QUESTIONS

• Duration of hair loss

• Menstrual history

• Medication history

• Nutrition, dieting, weight loss

• Hair care—bleaching, braiding

• Family history of hair loss

• History of major unexpected emotional or physical stress

• Medical history, that is, thyroid disease, iron deficiency

PHYSICAL EXAMINATION

Nonscarring alopecia—no erythema, scale, atrophy in skin with female pattern hair loss

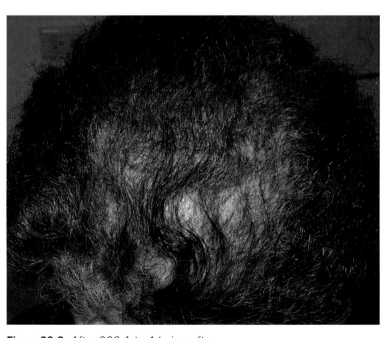

Figure 20.2 *After 900 1 to 4 hair grafts*

DIFFERENTIAL DIAGNOSIS OF FEMALE PATTERN HAIR LOSS

- Telogen effluvium
- Poor hair styling—chemicals, excessive dying
- Iron deficiency, thyroid disease, chronic medical disease, polycystic or other endocrine imbalance
- Medication-related hair loss
- Poor nutrition, weight loss
- Trichotillomania
- Diffuse alopecia areata—rare

KEY QUESTIONS TO DISTINGUISH DIFFERENTIAL DIAGNOSIS

- How long has your hair loss persisted?
- Changes in diet or weight loss over past 6 to 12 months?
- Any new prescription, over-the-counter (OTC) medications, or supplements?
- Any major surgery or unusual emotional stress?
- Any change in hair care? Chemicals to hair?

KEY POINTS

- Patients may have a combination of etiologies.
- If there is any questioning after history and physical examination, scalp biopsy is indicated.
- Thyroid function tests, iron studies, antinuclear antibody (ANA), rapid plasma reagin (RPR).
- Referral to gynecologist and/or endocrinologist if appropriate on history and/or examination.

MEDICAL THERAPY

Topical minoxidil (2% and 5% solution) are the only medications for female pattern hair loss approved by the U.S. Food and Drug Administration (FDA) (Table 20.1). The mechanism of action is unknown. It is safe for long-term application.

TABLE 20.1 ■ **Minoxidil**

Mechanism of action	Unknown
Onset of action	6–8 months
Side effects	Dryness, pruritus, "greasy hair"
Use with pregnancy or breast-feeding	No
5% versus 2%	5% slightly more effective but more "greasy" slight increased risk of hirsutism

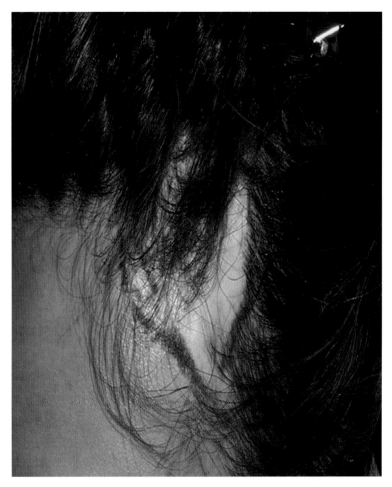

Figure 20.3 *Preoperative temporal scar—chief complaint: "I cannot wear my hair back"*

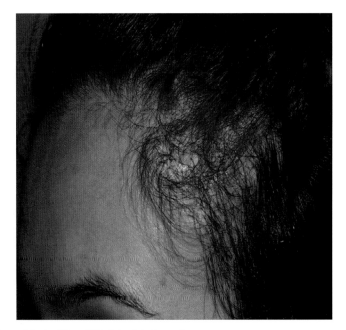

Figure 20.4 *After 650 1 to 3 hair grafts*

Minoxidil 5% foam is only approved for men but often is used by women. The reason is due to minoxidil in small percentage of women, inducing unwanted pigmented terminal hairs. The medication-induced hirsutism is reversible if the medication is discontinued.

Many women who do get minoxidil-induced hirsutism also get excellent growth of hair on their scalp and opt to continue the medication and use lasers to remove the unwanted hair on the face.

The foam creates much less irritation on the scalp making it much easier to be compliant than the solution.

KEYS TO SUCCESS

- Compliance: must use for 6 to 8 months to produce the desired effect.
- Emphasize maintenance over regrowth of hair. Minoxidil stops hair loss in the majority of patients and grows back pigmented terminal hair in a minority of patients.

NON-FDA APPROVED MEDICATIONS

- Finasteride, a type II 5-α reductase inhibitor, is contraindicated in women of childbearing age. Studies demonstrate some efficacy in postmenopausal females.
- Oral androgen receptor antagonists such as spironolactone and cyproterone acetate are other alternatives with limited proof of efficacy in both premenopausal and postmenopausal females. They are contraindicated in pregnant patients, given the risk of producing sexual defects in a male fetus. They should, therefore, be discontinued months prior to a planned pregnancy.

SURGICAL

■ Consultation

Chief complaint: "see through" frontal hairline, "limited styling options," "fear of windy days."

■ Key Questions

- How long has hair loss persisted on?
- Medical workup to date
- Medication used to treat hair loss and for how long
- Patient's chief cosmetic concern
- Patient's goal for hair transplantation

PHYSICAL EXAMINATION

- Donor density

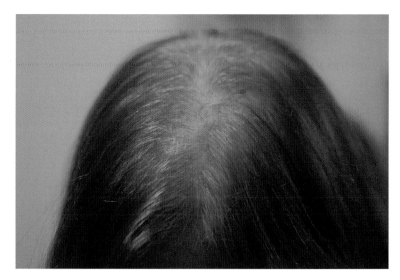

Figure 20.5 *Preoperative Ludwig I to II*

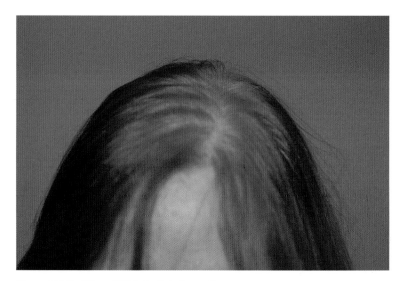

Figure 20.6 *After 600 1 to 3 hair grafts*

- Caliber of hair loss
- Extent of hair loss

KEY POINTS

- Emphasize unpredictable donor density. The transplanted hair will grow for as long as it was genetically programmed to grow.
- Increased risk of postsurgical telogen effluvium.
- Ongoing hair loss will affect perceived density of hair transplant.

SURGICAL APPROACH: FEMALE VERSUS MALE HAIR TRANSPLANTATION (Table 20.2)

Hair transplantation for men and women utilize the same donor harvesting techniques, graft creation, instruments, anesthesia, and pre- and postsurgery course.

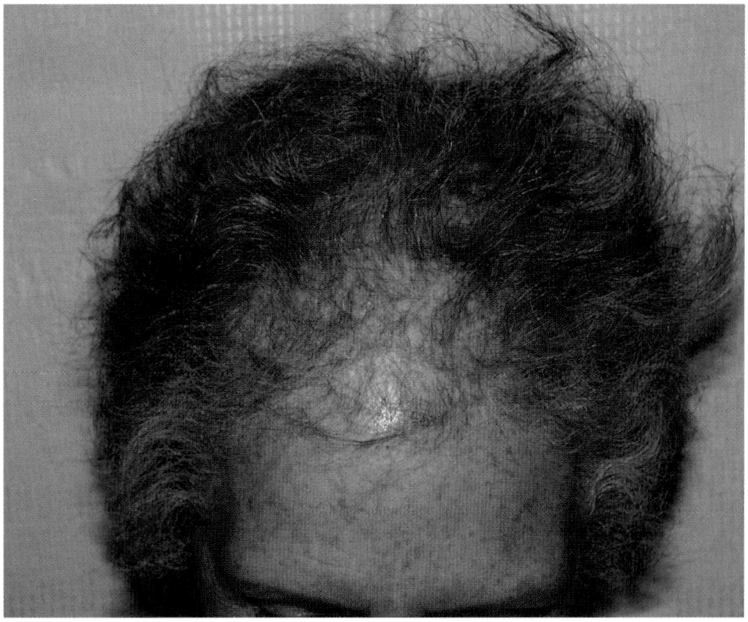

Figure 20.7 *Preoperative Ludwig I to II.*

FEMALE SURGICAL PLANNING

Transplant frontal one-third of scalp only! This will address chief complaint and reduce the risk of telogen effluvium.

- Chief complaint: "see through" frontal hairline
- Stable frontal, temporal, and posterior hairlines
- Diffuse thinning—no bald spots
- Risk of telogen effluvium
  - Unpredictable long-term growth of hair from the donor region

TABLE 20.2 ■ Surgical Approach: Female Versus Male Hair Transplantation

	Male	Female
Donor density	More predictable	Less predictable long term
Hairline design	Unstable and receding frontal temporal and posterior hair-line	
	Need to design hair transplant for long-term natural cosmetic appearance (>10 years)	Stable hairlines. Major cosmetic advantage over men for surgical planning
Caliber of hair	Variable between individuals	Variable between individuals
Medication use with hair transplantation	If existing hair remains, medication will add density by limiting further hair loss	All women should use minoxidil to help maintain existing hair and decrease risk of postsurgery telogen effluvium
	Medication always remains elective	
	Need to design hair transplant assuming ongoing hair loss and receding hairlines	Density = number of hair follicles transplanted—ongoing hair loss
Expectations	Key to success	Key to success

■ Preoperative Instructions

- β-Human chorionic gonadotropin (B-HCG) in appropriate patient
- Consent
- Photos
- Medical clearance if appropriate
- Ok to dye hair up until day before procedure
- Procedure
- Introduce staff
- Review surgical plan
- Review postsurgical care, anesthesia, instruments, donor harvesting, graft creation, grafts placement are the same as for men

■ Postoperative Instructions

- Overnight dressing to protect grafts as they heal.
- Resume regular activities. Light exercise 2 to 3 days after surgery. Full exercise when staples/sutures removed 7 to 10 days postoperatively.
- If any discomfort or pain, take Tylenol #3 with food q 4 to 6 hours. Fifty percent of patients take no pain medication and the other 50% take one or two tablets. If a patient has any discomfort or pain after the day of surgery, they should contact their physician.
- Prednisone 40 mg qd for 3 to 4 days to prevent frontal edema. If a patient cannot or will not take prednisone, ice forehead for 10 minutes every 30 minutes over the dressing for the first afternoon/evening of surgery to reduce but not eliminate edema. Edema begins 24 hours after surgery, peaks 72 hours postsurgery, and disappears 5 to 6 days postsurgery. Rare periorbital ecchymoses.
- The morning after surgery the dressing is removed. All patients are encouraged to shower to help reduce postsurgery hemorrhagic crusting. Patients should NOT pick or rub scabs; this may permanently damage transplanted hair.
- After shower, blow dry with warm not hot air on low power.
- Apply topical antibiotic or Aquaphor to donor region twice daily for 7 days.
- Resume minoxidil 48 to 72 hours post surgery.

■ Postoperative Period

- Continue minoxidil one to two times daily.
- Telogen effluvium may begin 2 to 3 weeks after surgery and continue for 2 to 3 months.

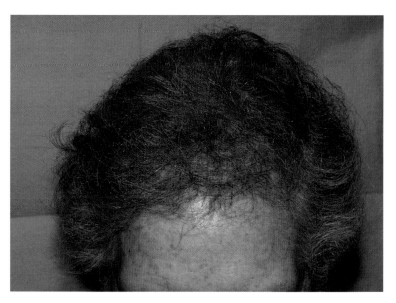

Figure 20.8 *After 750 1 to 3 hair grafts.*

- If telogen effluvium occurs, hair density will decrease but will rarely be cosmetically noticeable.
- Can dye hair 2 weeks after surgery.
- Initial followup 9 to 12 months after surgery and then every 3 months until 15 months when final density from the procedure will appear.

KEYS TO SUCCESS WITH FEMALE HAIR TRANSPLANTATION

- Emphasize ongoing hair loss will affect long-term density of hair transplant. The net perceived density of the hair transplant = number of hair follicles transplanted—ongoing hair loss.
- Patients with thick caliber hair will appear to have more hair than a patient with an equal number of fine hair follicles. The same effect will occur with a hair transplant.
- Discuss the risk of postsurgical telogen effluvium.
- Minoxidil will help reduce not eliminate the risk of telogen effluvium and help slow or stop ongoing hair loss for the majority of patients.
- Unpredictable future loss of donor hair. Transplanted hair will grow for as long as it was genetically programmed.
- Limit the majority of transplanted grafts to frontal one-third of scalp for maximum cosmetic impact.
- Well-trained staff.

HAIR TRANSPLANTATION TO CORRECT ALTERED TEMPORAL HAIRLINE FROM LIFTING PROCEDURE

After female pattern hair loss, transplanting to correct scars left from lifting procedures such as facelifts and browlifts are the most common reasons for hair transplantation in women.

CHIEF COMPLAINT (Figs. 20.3 AND 20.4)

"I cannot wear my hair up or back."

CONSULT (Figs. 20.5–20.8)

■ Key Points

- After hair loss following a lift, wait at least 12 months before considering surgery.
- The loss may be a telogen effluvium and the hair may grow back on its own.

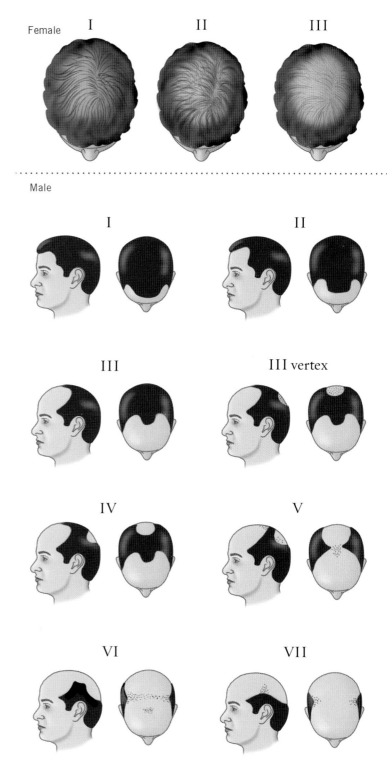

Illustration 20.1 *Female versus male pattern hair loss*

- Hair growth in scar tissue is unpredictable. The majority of patients have excellent growth but a small minority do not.

- Emphasize greater risk of frontal and potentially periorbital edema. It is not medically concerning, but may impact postoperative cosmetic appearance of the patient.

■ Procedure

Preoperative, intraoperative, and postoperative medication, technique, and wound care are the same for male and female hair transplantation. When creating recipient sites, follow the natural direction of hair growth in the temporal region.

■ Keys to Success

- Wait at least 12 months after loss before considering surgery.

- Follow the natural angle of hair in the temporal region, that is, 15-degree angle pointing down toward the neck.

- With appropriate patient selection, there is high patient satisfaction.

BIBLIOGRAPHY

Avram MR. Accurately communicating the extent of a hair transplant procedure. A proposal of a follicular-based classification scheme. *Dermatol Surg.* 1997;23(9):817-818.

Avram MR. Polarized light-emitting diode magnification for optimal recipient site creation during hair transplant. *Dermatol Surg.* 2005;31(9 pt 1):1124-1127. Discussion 1127.

Avram MR, Cole JP, Gandelman M, et al. The potential role of minoxidil in the hair transplantation setting. *Dermatol Surg.* 2002;28(10):894-900. Discussion 900.

Epstein JS. The treatment of female pattern hair loss and other applications of surgical hair restoration in women. *Facial Plast Surg Clin North Am.* 2004;12(2):241-247.

Harris JA. Follicular unit transplantation: Dissecting and planting techniques. *Facial Plast Surg Clin North Am.* 2004;12(2):225-232.

Leavitt M, Perez-Meza D, Rao NA, Barusco M, Kaufman KD, Ziering C. Effects of finasteride (1 mg) on hair transplant. *Dermatol Surg.* 2005;31(10):1268-1276. Discussion 1276.

Limmer BL. Elliptical donor stereoscopically assisted micrografting as an approach to further refinement in hair transplantation. *J Dermatol Surg Oncol.* 1994;20(12):789-793.

CHAPTER 21 Low Level Light Therapy (LLLT) and Hair Loss

Low level light laser therapy (LLLT) has been used to treat a variety of medical disorders from ulcers to musculoskeletal disorders. In 2007, a low level light device was approved by the U.S. Food and Drug Administration (FDA) to treat male pattern hair loss (Fig. 21.1; Hairmax, Boca Raton, Florida). The laser comb is a handheld device that was approved as a device which has a different standard for FDA approval than a medication. The device is sold over the counter without physician prescription or physician monitoring. There are various other manufacturers of light therapy devices that are sold to physicians' offices that are not handheld, such as the Sunetics device (Figs. 21.2 and 21.3; Sunetics International, Las Vegas NV).

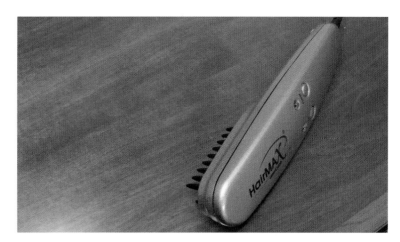

Figure 21.1 *Hand held LLLT device (hairmax lasecomb Boca Raton, Florida)*

MECHANISM OF ACTION—UNKNOWN

• Candidate selection—all skin types. All hair colors. Most effective at earlier stages of hair loss. FDA approved for male pattern hair loss. Many physicians believe it may have a role in treating female pattern hair loss.

APPROPRIATE USE

• The manufacturer recommends slowly combing the device throughout the affected areas of hair more than 10 minutes three times weekly (Fig. 21.4).

• There are no published studies comparing different frequency and time of use of the device.

PEARLS OF WISDOM

• All patients with hair loss should be evaluated by a dermatologist to establish a diagnosis before considering any medical therapy.

• Minoxidil for men and women and finasteride for men remain the medical treatment of choice for male and female pattern hair loss.

• LLLT appears to be safe but long-term independent studies confirming efficacy over placebo have not been done.

• Corporate-funded studies have demonstrated some efficacy in the treatment of male pattern hair loss.

• LLLT should be considered after clear medical failure with minoxidil and/or finasteride.

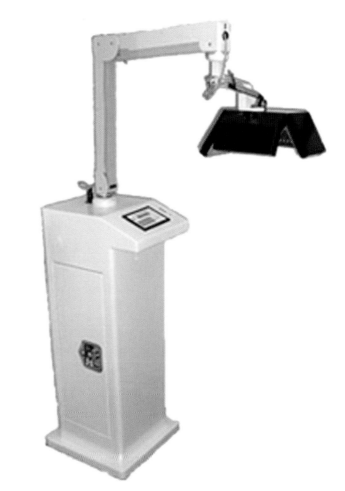

Figure 21.2 *Office based LLLT device (Sunnetics, las Vegas, Nevada)*

BIBLIOGRAPHY

Avram MR, Leonard RT Jr, Epstein ES, Williams JL, Bauman AJ. The current role of laser/light sources in the treatment of male and female pattern hair loss. *J Cosmet Laser Ther.* 2007;9(1):27-28. Review.

Avram MR, Rogers NE. Hair transplantation for men. *J Cosmet Laser Ther.* 2008;10(3):154-160. Review.

Avram MR, Rogers NE. The use of low-level light for hair growth: Part I. *J Cosmet Laser Ther.* 2009;11(2):110-117.

Hodson DS. Current and future trends in home laser devices. *Semin Cutan Med Surg.* 2008;27(4):292-300.

Leavitt M, Charles G, Heyman E, Michaels D. HairMax LaserComb laser phototherapy device in the treatment of male androgenetic alopecia: A randomized, double-blind, sham device-controlled, multicentre trial. *Clin Drug Investig.* 2009;29(5):283-292.

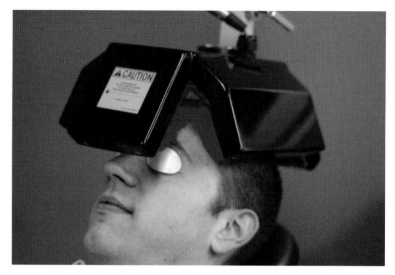

Figure 21.3 *Patient undergoing LLLT treatment for male pattern hair loss in a physician office*

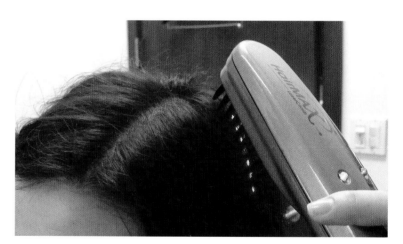

Figure 21.4 *Patient performing home LLLT treatment*

SECTION FIVE

Disorders of Pigmentation

CHAPTER 22 | Café Au Lait Macule

Café au lait macules (CALMs) are benign well-demarcated, light brown macules that typically present in early childhood. The pigmentation is typically uniform. Lesions may be multiple or isolated. They grow in proportion to the growth of the child. They are present in as many as 20% of the population and, rarely, can be associated with a host of genodermatoses.

EPIDEMIOLOGY

Incidence: 10% to 20% of the population

Age: birth and early childhood

Race: more common in African Americans than Caucasians

Sex: none

Precipitating factors: most commonly these are benign, isolated findings in healthy children. Multiple CALMs can be associated with genodermatoses such as neurofibromatosis, tuberous sclerosis, Bloom syndrome, McCune–Albright syndrome, Russell–Silver syndrome, Watson syndrome, and Westerhof syndrome

PATHOGENESIS

Unknown.

PATHOLOGY

Increased melanin in basal keratinocytes. Clinically darker lesions contain more melanocytes than lighter ones.

PHYSICAL LESIONS

Lesions are well demarcated, uniformly pigmented macules that vary in color from hues of tan to light brown to brown. They can present anywhere on the body but spare mucous membranes. Their size can range from a few millimeters to over 20 cm.

DIFFERENTIAL DIAGNOSIS

Postinflammatory hyperpigmentation, Becker's nevus, melasma, lentigines, ephelides, berloque dermatitis, and congenital nevus.

LABORATORY EXAMINATION

Biopsy is not indicated. Additional laboratory workup may be appropriate in the event of suspicion of an underlying systemic disorder.

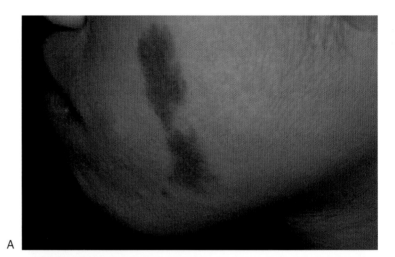

A

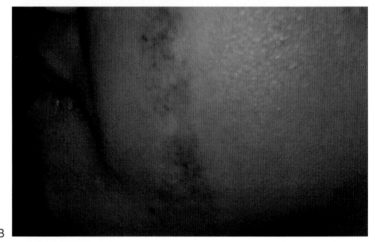

B

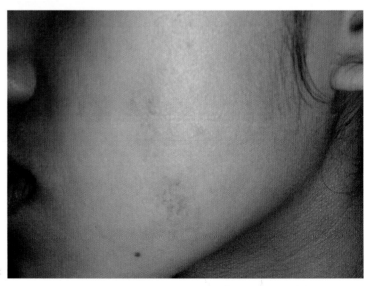

C

Figure 22.1 **(A)** *Café au lait macule on left cheek of a 17-year-old female prior to treatment.* **(B)** *Erythema and lightening of café au lait macule after one treatment with 694-nm Q-switched ruby laser.* **(C)** *Significant clearing after four treatments with Q-switched ruby laser*

COURSE

They grow in proportion to the growth of the child. Once a child has fully grown, CALMs do not change in size or color. There is no increased risk of malignant transformation.

KEY CONSULTATIVE QUESTIONS

- Time of onset
- Failure to meet milestones
- Photosensitivity
- Intellectual impairment
- History of multiple fractures
- Central nervous system disorders or tumors
- Poor growth
- Scoliosis
- Ophthalmologic impairment

MANAGEMENT

CALMs do not require treatment unless their appearance is disfiguring or distressing to the patient or parents. Multiple lesions may suggest an underlying systemic disorder. If there is any indication of underlying systemic abnormalities in the setting of multiple CALMs, referral to appropriate pediatric specialists is indicated. Laser therapy is often employed as a treatment. CALMs tend to be more difficult to treat than other benign pigmented lesions such as ephelides and lentigines. They require multiple treatments and complete resolution can be challenging. Recurrence is common. Cryotherapy and surgical excision are alternatives to laser therapy but carry the risk of pigmentary alterations, poor cosmesis, pain, and scarring.

LASER TREATMENT (Figs. 22.1–22.3)

Prior to treatment, a test site should be performed to assess for efficacy and hyperpigmentation. CALMs respond variably to multiple modalities of laser therapy.

- Q-switched lasers including the frequency-doubled Q-switched Nd:YAG (532 nm), Q-switched ruby (694 nm), and the Q-switched alexandrite (755 nm) are employed for selective pigment removal.

  It is important to note that treatment with Q-switched lasers is not cookbook. Energy settings vary from laser to laser. They also vary before and after maintenance. Thus, treatment should be based on achieving epidermal whitening after treatment. Without epidermal whitening, the treatment is unlikely to be effective.

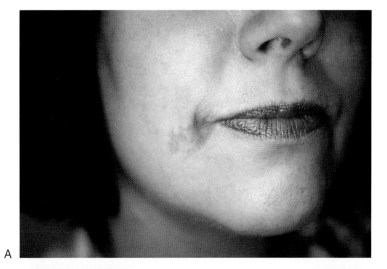

A

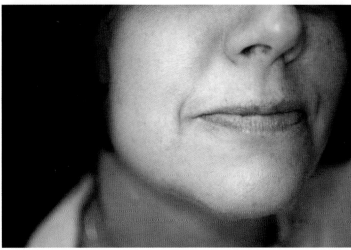

B

Figure 22.2 (A) *Café au lait macule adjoining right lateral commissure of lips.* **(B)** *Near clearance after three treatments with a 755-nm Q-switched alexandrite laser*

However, it is important to note that overly aggressive treatments produce pigmentary changes such as hypo- and hyperpigmentation.

– In one study, Q-switched ruby and frequency-doubled Q-switched Nd:YAG treatments, each at 6 J/cm^2, produced variable responses including

  ○ Significant lightening, which was most frequently observed

  ○ Clearance with recurrence

  ○ Darkening

– Q-switched lasers have a decreased risk of textural change versus other laser therapies, but still carry the risk of hyperpigmentation.

– Results are variable with approximately 50% of lesions showing a response.

– While full resolution can be obtained with the Q-switched lasers, there are frequent recurrences. Frustratingly, recurrences may occur 6 months to 1 year after treatment. Sometimes lightening, rather than full resolution, is the best obtainable result. All of these lasers produce equivalent results in the treatment of CALMs.

TOPICAL TREATMENT

CALMs are not responsive to topical bleaching creams.

PITFALLS TO AVOID/OUTCOME EXPECTATIONS/COMPLICATIONS/ MANAGEMENT

• Unfortunately, despite their superficial nature, CALMs can be difficult to treat completely.

• The key clinical finding is epidermal whitening after Q-switched laser treatment.

• Lightening, rather than full clearance, is often the best result, even after multiple treatments.

• There is a high risk of recurrence of CALMs up to 1 year after treatment.

• Studies indicate a risk for hyper- and hypopigmentation associated with the Q-switched lasers, especially in darker skin phototypes.

• Treating above the therapeutic threshold may result in prolonged healing and increased risk of pigmentary changes.

• Patients with darker skin types should be treated cautiously and conservatively, given the lower therapeutic threshold.

• Laser treatment of tanned patients should be avoided.

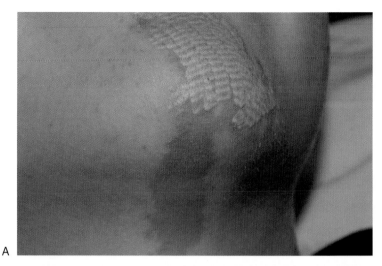

A

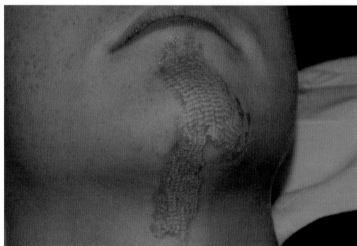

B

Figure 22.3 **(A)** *Treatment of café au lait macule on the chin of a young man with a 532-nm frequency-doubled Q-switched Nd:YAG laser.* **(B)** *Completion of treatment of café au lait macule with the appropriate clinical endpoint of tissue whitening and erythema*

BIBLIOGRAPHY

Alora MB, Arndt KA. Treatment of a cafe-au-lait macule with the erbium:YAG laser. *J Am Acad Dermatol.* 2001;45(4):566-568.

Grossman MC, Anderson RR, Farinelli W, Flotte TJ, Grevelink JM. Treatment of café au lait macules with lasers: A clinicopathologic correlation. *Arch Dermatol.* 1995;131:1416-1420.

Kim JS, Kim MJ, Cho SB. Treatment of segmental café au lait macules using 1064-nm Q-switched Nd:YAG laser with low pulse energy. *Clin Exp Dermatol.* 2009;34(7): 222-223.

Levy JL, Mordon S, Pizzi-Anselme M. Treatment of individual cafe au lait macules with the Q-switched Nd:YAG: A clinicopathologic correlation. *Cutan Laser Ther.* 1999; 1(4):217-223.

CHAPTER 23 | Ephelides

Ephelides, more commonly known as freckles, are benign, small, well-demarcated, brown macules found on the sun-exposed skin of blond, light brown, and red-haired individuals. They present in early childhood and decrease in older age. They can be distinguished from lentigines in that they darken in times of high sun exposure and fade during periods of limited sun exposure.

EPIDEMIOLOGY

Incidence: very common, particularly in fair-skinned patients

Age: early childhood

Race: more common in Caucasians, but also seen in Asians

Sex: equal

Precipitating factors: individuals with light hair and complexion such as blonds and redheads

PATHOGENESIS

The brown pigmentation associated with ephelides results from increased production of melanin in sun-exposed areas of the skin.

PATHOLOGY

Keratinocytes display an increase in melanin especially in the basal layer, but there is no substantial increase in the number of melanocytes in ephelides.

PHYSICAL LESIONS

Ephelides are well-demarcated light brown to dark brown macules of several millimeters diameter that present in sun-exposed areas of the skin.

DIFFERENTIAL DIAGNOSIS

The differential diagnosis includes other benign lesions such as lentigines and junctional nevi.

LABORATORY EXAMINATION

None.

COURSE

They present in early childhood. They darken in periods of high sun exposure and lighten during periods of limited sun exposure.

KEY CONSULTATIVE QUESTIONS

• Sun exposure.

MANAGEMENT

There is no medical indication to treat ephelides. The cosmetic appearance, however, may displease some individuals. Sun avoidance and sunscreens protect against darkening of ephelides. Bleaching creams, such as hydroquinone, and topical retinoids can produce lightening. Cryotherapy and laser treatment are also effective. Recurrence is frequent, particularly with sun exposure.

TREATMENTS

■ Topical Treatment

Topical bleaching creams may provide some lightening. Multiple formulations are available differing in their product contents and strengths.

• Hydroquinone (2–4%) creams have traditionally been employed.
  – Twice daily application of the cream to the ephelides over 3 months is generally necessary to achieve significant, if not complete, improvement.
  – Side effects include irritation, pruritus, peeling, and dryness of the treated areas.

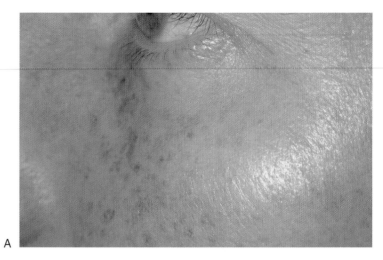

A

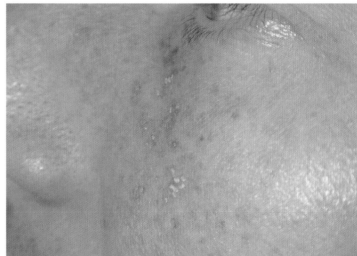

B

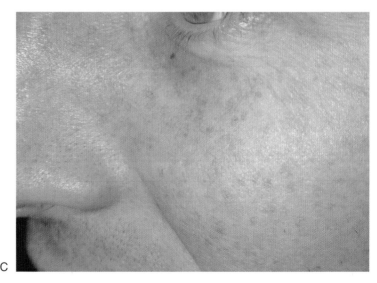

C

Figure 23.1 (A) *A 38-year-old male from Southern California with extensive ephelides.* **(B)** *Same patient with posttreatment whitening immediately after frequency-doubled Q-switched Nd:YAG (532 nm) laser therapy.* **(C)** *Significant improvement 2 weeks after single treatment with frequency-doubled Q-switched Nd:YAG (532 nm) laser utilizing a fluence of 1.5 J/cm² and a 2.0 mm spot size*

- – If erythema and irritation occur, exercise caution to avoid hyperpigmentation, especially in darker skin phototypes.

- – Patients must discontinue the treatment if any lightening of nonlesional skin is observed.

- – Bleaching creams are contraindicated in pregnant and lactating women.

- – Prolonged treatment may produce skin discoloration known as pseudo-ochronosis.

- Retinoids

  - – Retinoids have been added in products such as Solage (2% mequinol and 0.01% tretinoin) and Triluma (0.01% fluocinolone acetonide, 4% hydroquinone, and 0.05% tretinoin) to provide an exfoliative benefit.

  - – Application of Triluma must be limited in duration due to the possibility of side effects with repeated corticosteroid usage such as skin atrophy and acne.

- Azelaic acid (20%) cream is unpredictably effective for ephelides and lentigines.

- Kojic acid (1–2.5%) cream.

■ Chemical Peels

Chemical peels can be helpful in reducing the appearance of ephelides. Superficial depth peels, medium depth peels, and deeper peels are all effective. A careful evaluation of skin type, however, is essential prior to treatment. As the depth of the peel increases, the chance for improvement, along with adverse side effects, increases.

- Over-the-counter α-hydroxy acid peels are a beneficial adjunct to physician-strength chemical peels. The continual exfoliation achieved from consistent use of the peels will result in mild lightening.

- Glycolic acid peels (35–70%) are administered every 2 to 3 weeks utilizing increasing strengths as tolerated. Lightening of ephelides may be observed after four to six peels. Strict photoprotection is stressed. Salicylic acid peels (20–30%) are also effective. They can be used safely in all skin types.

- Jessner peels (resorcinol, lactic acid, and salicylic acid) are administered every 6 to 8 weeks.

  - – Strict photoprotection for 2 to 3 months is advised.

  - – Multiple treatments are recommended.

  - – Contraindicated in pregnant and lactating women.

- Combination Jessner/10% trichloroacetic (TCA) peels may also be employed in a similar fashion as the Jessner peel.

  - – The Jessner peel results in exfoliation allowing for greater penetration of the TCA peel.

  - – Multiple peels are generally needed. Contraindicated in pregnant and lactating women.

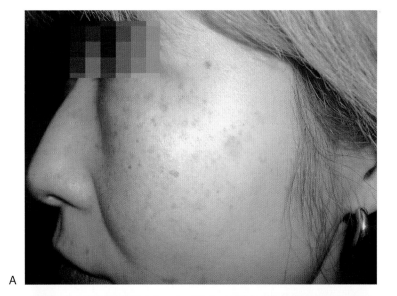

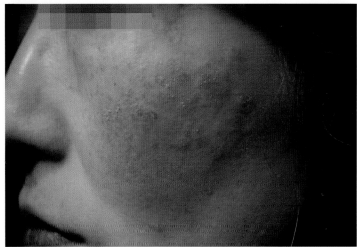

Figure 23.2 **(A)** *A 40-year-old Japanese female with ephelides and lentigines prior to 694-nm Q-switched ruby laser treatment.* **(B)** *Immediate tissue whitening and erythema after treatment*

• Caution to avoid pigmentary changes, especially in darker skin types.

• A test site can be considered.

■ Cryotherapy

Cryotherapy can produce lightening of freckling.

• Has a risk of hypo- or hyperpigmentation at and around treated sites, especially in darker skin phototypes and tanned patients.

• Recurrence is common.

■ Laser Therapy (Figs. 23.1 and 23.2)

Laser and light source therapy can be effective in treating ephelides.

• Intense pulsed light, frequency-doubled Q-switched Nd:YAG (532 nm), Q-switched alexandrite (755 nm), Q-switched ruby (694 nm), Q-switched Nd:YAG (1064 nm), pulsed dye (595 nm), fractional resurfacing, and KTP lasers (532 nm) are all effective.

• With Q-switched lasers:

  – Perform a test spot on darker skin types.

  – Treatment endpoint for Q-switched lasers is immediate tissue whitening. For the Q-switched Nd:YAG (1064 nm), small pinpoint bleeding may be seen.

  – A 7-to-10-day healing time can be expected for crusting to resolve with Q-switched lasers.

• One study used the frequency-doubled Nd:YAG (532 nm) to treat ephelides in 20 patients with type IV skin. Eighty percent of patients showed better than 50% improvement. Recurrence was common. Hypopigmentation, textural changes, and hyperpigmentation all resolved within 2 to 6 months after final treatment.

• In another study, 197 Asians were treated with the Q-switched alexandrite (755 nm) at 7.0 J/cm^2, with a pulse width of 100 ns at 8-week intervals. Clinical followup after an average of 1.5 treatment sessions showed a 76% decrease in the number of ephelides. No scarring, textural changes, or pigmentary changes were noted.

• The Q-switched ruby (694 nm) and alexandrite lasers (755 nm) are also effective.

  – If the clinical endpoint of immediate whitening is achieved, the ephelides should clear with one treatment.

• Q-switched lasers are most effective for darker lesions.

• Fractional resurfacing (Fraxel Laser; Reliant technologies, San Diego, CA) is also effective (Fig. 23.3).

  – Treatment is generally performed at superficial depths compared to treatments of rhytides and acne scars.

  – High treatment densities are most effective.

  – Mild-to-moderate erythema, resembling a sunburn reaction, is observed. Postprocedure swelling is also common.

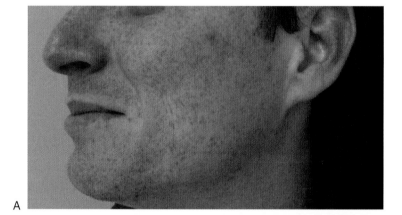

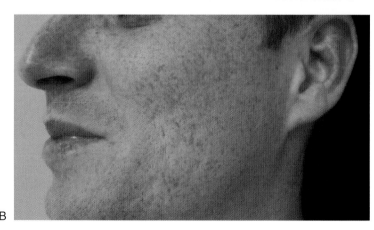

Figure 23.3 (A) *Young male with ephelides on his left cheek at baseline.* **(B)** *Improvement of ephelides after several nonablative fractional resurfacing treatments.*

– The erythema resolves in 3 to 5 days and can be covered with makeup within a day of the treatment.

– Long-term data are currently lacking.

• Intense pulse light is also effective.

– The clinical endpoint is darkening of the lentigines.

• Caution should be employed when treating patients with darker skin types to avoid hyperpigmentation that may persist for months.

• Recurrence of freckling after treatment, however, is common.

• Sunscreen and sun avoidance are mandatory adjuncts to laser therapy.

PITFALLS TO AVOID/COMPLICATIONS/ MANAGEMENT

• Laser treatment of ephelides is frequently successful but often transient.

• Patients should be informed that recurrence is highly likely, especially with sun exposure.

• Daily strict photoprotection with a sunscreen with UVA/UVB protection and/or a physical block such as titanium dioxide or zinc oxide are stressed as well as sun avoidance.

• If bleaching creams produce erythema, caution is advised as erythema can produce irritation and hyperpigmentation.

• Patients should be counseled regarding the possibility of postinflammatory pigmentation changes after treatment. Laser removal of ephelides may also produce an unattractive, spotty hypopigmentation, especially in darken skin phototypes.

BIBLIOGRAPHY

Jang KA, Chung EC, Choi JH, Sung KJ, Moon KC, Koh JK. Successful removal of freckles in Asian skin with a Q-switched alexandrite laser. *Dermatol Surg*. 2000;26(3): 231-234.

Mishima Y, Ohyama Y, Shibata T, et al. Inhibitory action of kojic acid on melanogenesis and its therapeutic effect for various human hyperpigmentation disorders. *Skin Res*. 1994;36(2):134-150.

Nakagawa M, Kawai K. Contact allergy to kojic acid in skin care products. *Contact Dermatitis*. 1995;31(1):9-13.

Ngujen QH, Bui TP. Azelaic acid: Pharmacokinetic and pharmacodynamic properties and its therapeutic role in hyperpigmentary disorders and acne. *Int J Dermatol*. 1995;34(2):75-84.

Rashid T, Hussain I, Haider M, Haroon TS. Laser therapy of freckles and lentigines with quasi-continuous, frequency-doubled, Nd:YAG (532 nm) laser in Fitzpatrick skin type IV: A 24-month follow-up. *J Cosmet Laser Ther*. 2002;4(3-4):81-85.

CHAPTER 24 | Lentigines

There are two major types of lentigines: lentigo simplex and solar lentigos. They are benign lesions. Although both are clinically identical, they appear in entirely different clinical settings. Lentigo simplex typically first present in childhood as multiple well-demarcated, brown or black macules that can appear on any part of the skin or mucous membranes. They are clinically indistinguishable from junctional nevi. There is no association with sun exposure in this type of lentigo. In contrast, solar lentigos, more commonly known as "liver spots," are well-defined, brown macules that appear on sun-exposed skin of adults. They increase in number with age. They most often appear on the dorsal hands, shoulders, and face of lightly pigmented and red-haired patients.

EPIDEMIOLOGY

Incidence: very common, particularly in fair-skinned patients

Age: bimodal distribution in childhood and in sun-damaged skin of adults

Race: more common in Caucasians

Sex: equal

Precipitating factors: sun exposure is closely related to solar lentigines. Multiple lentigines are associated with a few genodermatoses including LEOPARD syndrome, LAMB syndrome, and Peutz–Jeghers syndrome

PATHOGENESIS

Unknown.

PATHOLOGY

There is a uniform elongation of the rete ridges of the epidermis along with increased melanin in melanocytes and basal keratinocytes. In addition, there are an increased number of melanocytes in the basal cell layer. Melanophages are present in the papillary dermis.

PHYSICAL LESIONS

Well-defined brown macules. Lentigo simplex macules tend to be evenly distributed and small, measuring only a few millimeters. Solar lentigos have a predilection for the sun-exposed areas of the dorsal hands and face. They can be larger than lentigo simplex.

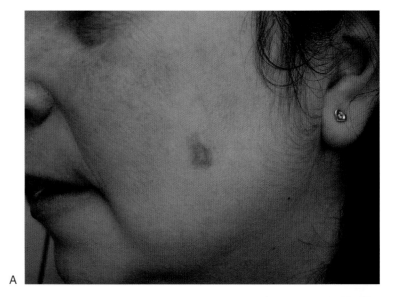

A

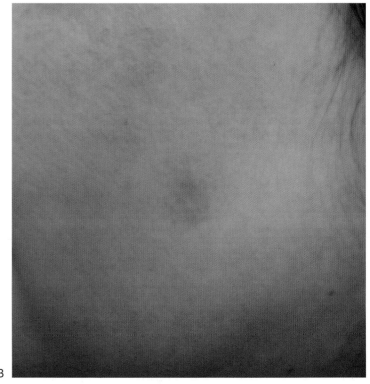

B

Figure 24.1 **(A)** *Lentigo on left cheek of a female.* **(B)** *Significant improvement after one treatment with a 532-nm Q-switched Nd:YAG laser at a fluence of 1.0 J/cm^2 and a 2-mm spot size*

DIFFERENTIAL DIAGNOSIS

Seborrheic keratosis, junctional nevi, ephelides, lentigo maligna, melanoma may all mimic lentigines.

TABLE 24.1 ■ Solar Lentigo Versus Ephelid

	Solar lentigo	Ephelid
Presents in childhood	No	Yes
Permanent	Yes	No
Decreases with age	No	Yes
High recurrence after treatment	Yes	Yes
Increase in melanin	Yes	Yes
Increase in melanocytes	Yes	No

LABORATORY EXAMINATION

Biopsy is indicated if there is suspicion of a lentigo maligna or melanoma. Medical workup is appropriate if there is suspicion for a genodermatosis.

COURSE

There is a bimodal distribution for lentigines. They appear in childhood and in sun-exposed adults.

KEY CONSULTATIVE QUESTIONS

- Has there been any change in the color or size of the lesion?
- Does the lesion bleed?
- Sun exposure
- Sunscreen use

MANAGEMENT

There is no medical indication to treat lentigines. The cosmetic appearance, however, displeases many due to the perception that lentigines are associated with aging. Cryotherapy and laser treatment are the mainstays of treatment. Laser therapy is more effective than one-time application of cryotherapy. Cryotherapy, however, is an effective and less expensive option for the patient. Chemical peels, topical tretinoin, local dermabrasion, and topical bleaching agents represent other treatment options.

TOPICAL MEDICATIONS

- Bleaching creams such as 4% hydroquinone can lighten lesions over a period of several months. A topical combination of hydroquinone, steroid, and retinoid, ie, Triluma (4% hydroquinone, 0.05% tretinoin, 0.01%

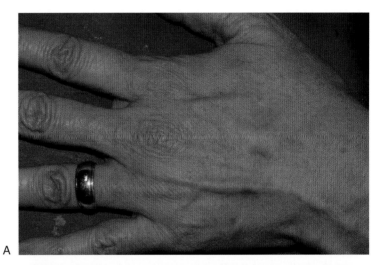
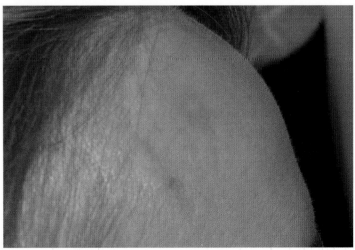

Figure 24.2 *Two examples of chrysiasis, a rare but well-described complication of Q-switched laser therapy in patients with a history of ingesting gold salts. In both of these patients, the characteristic dark-blue pigmentation was produced after Q-switched laser treatments of lentigines on the* **(A)** *dorsal hand and* **(B)** *forehead, respectively*

fluocinolone acetonide) can be used as well. However, bleaching creams are often not completely effective.

- Topical tretinoin can produce lightening, but not usually clearance of lesions. It may also, in combination with sun avoidance and sunscreen use, prevent the development of lentigines.

- Retreatment is often necessary.

- If any of these topical medications produce significant inflammation or irritation, it is important to discontinue their use to avoid postinflammatory hyperpigmentation. In addition, pseudo-ochronosis may occur with continuous, long-term use of topical hydroquinone.

- Bleaching creams are relatively contraindicated in pregnant and lactating women.

CRYOTHERAPY

- This is a cheap, swift, and effective means for treating lentigines.

- Application of cryotherapy can be accomplished with a small cotton-tip applicator or with a cryotherapy gun.

- It is often less effective than one-time treatment with a Q-switched laser.

   There is a significant risk of hypopigmentation with cryotherapy if it is applied excessively, or on a tanned patient.

CHEMICAL PEELS

Superficial depth peels, medium depth peels, and deeper peels are all effective for lentigines. A careful evaluation of skin type, however, is essential to avoid pigmentary complications. As the depth of the peel increases, the chance of improvement, along with adverse side effects, increases.

LASER AND LIGHT SOURCE TREATMENT

Multiple different therapies are effective for treating lentigines. In general, darker lentigines fare best with Q-switched lasers. Where there are numerous, fainter lentigines, intense pulsed light sources and, to a lesser extent, nonablative fractional resurfacing lasers are very effective.

- Intense pulsed light, frequency-doubled Q-switched Nd:YAG laser (532 nm) (Fig. 24.1), Q-switched alexandrite laser (755 nm) (Fig. 24.2), Q-switched ruby laser (694 nm), Q-switched Nd:YAG laser (1064 nm), pulsed dye laser with pigmented lesion window (595 nm), and fractional resurfacing lasers are all effective.

- With Q-switched lasers:

   – Perform a test spot on darker skin types.

   – Treatment endpoint for Q-switched lasers is immediate tissue whitening. For the Q-switched Nd:YAG (1064 nm), small pinpoint bleeding may be seen.

- A 7-to-10-day healing time can be expected for crusting to resolve after Q-switched laser treatment.

- Legs respond more slowly than the face and hands.

- Caution should be taken while treating lower legs as they often hyperpigment. Hyperpigmentation may persist for months.

- The frequency-doubled Q-switched Nd:YAG (532 nm) laser has been shown to improve lentigines safely and effectively.

  - In one study, 37 patients were treated once with a fluence of 2 to 5 J/cm^2, a 2.0-mm spot size, and a 10-ns pulse width.

  - Higher fluences provided best results with 60% of patients showing 75% or better clearances.

  - Minor, transient hypopigmentation, hyperpigmentation, and erythema were noted in a few patients.

  - Has been shown to produce better clearing than 35% TCA peel.

  - Has been shown to treat lentigines more effectively than cryotherapy.

- The Q-switched ruby (694 nm) laser is also very effective.

  - In one treatment, substantial clearing occurred at fluences of 4.5 and/or 7.5 J/cm^2 and a pulse width of 40 ns.

  - If the clinical endpoint of immediate whitening is achieved, the lentigo should clear with one treatment.

- Fractional resurfacing can also be effective.

  - Treatment is generally performed at superficial depths and lower energies compared to treatments of rhytides and acne scars.

  - High treatment densities are most effective. Typically, requires multiple treatments.

  - Mild-to-moderate erythema, resembling a sunburn reaction, is observed. Postprocedure swelling is also common.

  - The erythema resolves in 3 to 5 days and can be covered with makeup within a day of the treatment.

  - Long-term data are currently lacking.

- Intense pulse light is also effective.

  - Seventy-four percent clearance of lentigines in 18 patients with one treatment.

  - The clinical endpoint is darkening of the lentigines.

PITFALLS TO AVOID/COMPLICATIONS/ MANAGEMENT/OUTCOME EXPECTATIONS

- Q-switched laser and light source treatment for lentigines is frequently successful. Nonablative fractional resurfacing is the least effective of this group.

- Patients should be counseled regarding the possibility of postinflammatory pigmentation changes after treatment, especially on the lower legs.

- Recurrence after treatment is not uncommon.

- Biopsy any lesion that demonstrates any clinical atypia prior to treating with laser or cryotherapy. Laser therapy of a malignant lesion such as a lentigo maligna or melanoma may mask its clinical appearance and thus cause a delay in diagnosis.

Avoid using Q-switched lasers in patients with any prior history of gold intake. Chrysiasis, presenting as blue-gray circular macules on the skin, can occur after Q-switched laser treatment of solar lentigines in these patients (Fig. 24.2).

BIBLIOGRAPHY

Bjerring P, Christiansen K. Intense pulsed light source for treatment of small melanocytic nevi and solar lentigines. *J Cutan Laser Ther.* 2000;2:177-181.

Galeckas KJ, Ross EV, Uebelhoer NS. A pulsed dye laser with a 10-mm beam diameter and a pigmented lesion window for purpura-free photorejuvenation. *Dermatol Surg.* 2008;34(3):308-313.

Geist DE, Phillips TJ. Development of chrysiasis after Q-switched ruby laser treatment of solar lentigines. *Am Acad Dermatol.* 2006;55(Suppl 2):S59-S60.

Kilmer SL. Laser eradication of pigmented lesions and tattoos. *Dermatol Clin.* 2002;20(1):37-53.

Kilmer SL, Wheeland RG, Goldberg DJ, Anderson RR. Treatment of epidermal pigmented lesions with the frequency-doubled Q-switched Nd:YAG laser. A controlled, single-impact, dose-response, multicenter trial. *Arch Dermatol.* 1994;130(12):1515-1519.

Li YT, Yang KC. Comparison of the frequency-doubled Q-switched Nd:YAG laser and 35% trichloroacetic acid for the treatment of face lentigines. *Dermatol Surg.* 1999;25(3):202-204.

Sadighha A, Saatee S, Muhaghegh-Zahed G. Efficacy and adverse effects of Q-switched ruby laser on solar lentigines: A prospective study of 91 patients with Fitzpatrick skin type II, III, and IV. *Dermatol Surg.* 2008;34(11):1465-1468.

Stern RS, Dover JS, Levin JA, Arndt KA. Laser therapy versus cryotherapy of lentigines: A comparative trial. *J Am Acad Dermatol.* 1994;30(6):985-987.

Taylor CR, Anderson RR. Treatment of benign pigmented epidermal lesions by Q-switched ruby laser. *Int J Dermatol.* 1993;32(12):908-912.

Todd MM, Rallis TM, Gerwels JW, Hata TR. A comparison of 3 lasers and liquid nitrogen in the treatment of solar lentigines: A randomized, controlled, comparative trial. *Arch Dermatol.* 2000;136(7):841-846.

CHAPTER 25 | Melasma

Melasma is an acquired brown macular hyperpigmentation usually of the face. It is far more common in females than in males. It usually presents bilaterally and symmetrically on the face, but extensor forearms may also be involved. There are believed to be three histologic variants of melasma: epidermal, dermal, and mixed dermal and epidermal. Epidermal melasma responds best to therapy. All forms have a high rate of recurrence, making this a frustrating condition to treat. Sun exposure, pregnancy, and oral contraceptive pills are all associated with its presentation and recurrence (Fig. 25.1).

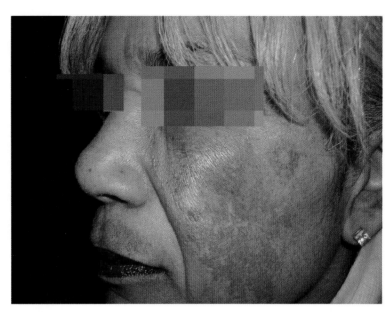

Figure 25.1 *Female with extensive melasma recalcitrant to multiple topical regimens for several years*

EPIDEMIOLOGY

Incidence: common

Age: young females

Race: Central and South American, Middle Eastern, Indian, East Asian females are most frequently affected

Sex: females > males (9:1)

Precipitating factors: pregnancy, oral contraceptive pills, sun exposure, hormone replacement therapy

PATHOGENESIS

Unknown.

DERMATOPATHOLOGY

In epidermal melasma, there is increased melanin deposition in the epidermis, particularly in the basal and suprabasal layers. In dermal melasma, there are perivascular melanin-containing macrophages in the superficial and middermis. Mixed-type melasma exhibits features of each of the above findings.

PHYSICAL LESIONS

Patients present with well-demarcated light brown to dark brown symmetric macular hyperpigmentation. In approximately two-thirds of patients it appears on the central face including the forehead, nose, upper cutaneous lip, and chin. It presents less frequently on the malar areas and jawline. More rarely, it appears on the dorsal forearms. Dermal melasma has more of a blue-gray hue. Mixed-type melasma has a brown-gray coloration.

DIFFERENTIAL DIAGNOSIS

Postinflammatory hyperpigmentation, exogenous ochronosis, drug-induced/photo-hyperpigmentation, nevus of Ota, erythema dyschromicum perstans.

LABORATORY EXAMINATION

Wood's lamp examination accentuates the increased epidermal pigmentation in melasma but does not highlight its dermal component.

COURSE

The pigmentation presents over a period of weeks. It occurs most commonly in summertime, with high estrogen states, during pregnancy, and prior to menstruation. It may fade completely months after delivery or after discontinuation of oral contraceptive pills. It may reappear in subsequent pregnancies and/or sun exposure.

KEY CONSULTATIVE QUESTIONS

- Medication history
- Pregnancy
- Sun exposure
- Time of onset
- Previous treatments

MANAGEMENT

There is no medical indication to treat melasma. Nevertheless, many patients understandably are distressed by its appearance and desire treatment. The goal of the treatment is to lighten or remove the pigmentation. Treating melasma can be quite frustrating. Prior to initiating therapy, it is essential for the physician to explain melasma and its treatment in detail to the patient. While there are many treatments for melasma, it should be stressed that many are often only partially effective. Recurrences are very common.

It is also important to determine which form of melasma is being treated, that is, epidermal versus mixed-type versus dermal melasma (Fig. 25.2). There are multiple topical and laser therapies available (Fig. 25.3). Treatment is frustrating and often ineffective. There is a high rate of recurrence. Dermal and mixed-type melasma are least responsive to therapy. In all melasma patients, strict sun avoidance is crucial with a sunscreen with UVA/UVB protection and/or a physical block such as titanium dioxide or zinc oxide during and after any treatment regimen.

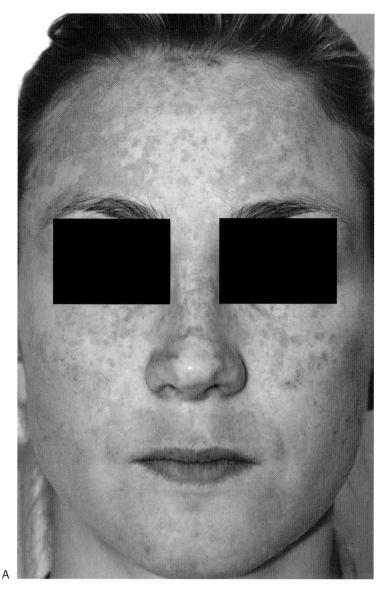

A

Figure 25.2 (A) *A female patient with therapy-resistant melasma. (Courtesy of Howard Conn)*

TOPICAL TREATMENT (Table 25.1)

There are a host of topical treatments for melasma.

- Numerous formulations containing bleaching agents such as 4% hydroquinone are effective treatments to lighten or resolve pigmentation. They are most effective if used over a period of weeks to a few months. If the skin becomes significantly irritated from treatment, discontinue its use to avoid postinflammatory hyperpigmentation. Prolonged usage of hydroquinone can result in a characteristic skin discoloration known as pseudo-ochronosis.

- Retinoids such as topical 0.1% tretinoin applied once daily for 40 weeks has been shown to be effective, but less effective than hydroquinone.

- Combination therapy of 0.05% tretinoin, 4% hydroquinone, and 0.01% fluocinolone acetonide, that is, Triluma, produces favorable clinical results for melasma and postinflammatory hyperpigmentation with decreased irritation. Treatment duration is limited by side effects of prolonged topical steroid use including skin atrophy and acne.

- Azelaic acid has also been shown to produce improvement.

CHEMICAL PEELS

Chemical peels are often effective for melasma.

- In one study, there was no difference in results when comparing Jessner's solution versus 70% glycolic acid peels after performing three peels 1 month apart on each side of the face.

- Glycolic acid peels performed every 3 weeks in combination with daily sunscreen and a combination

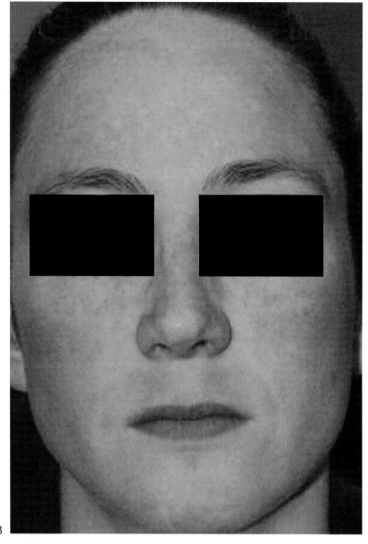

B

Figure 25.2 (B) (*Continued*) *Marked resolution in the melasma after four treatment sessions with Fraxel laser. (Courtesy of Howard Conn)*

TABLE 25.1 ■ Treatment of Pigmented Lesions on the Face

	Retinoid/hydroquinone	Glycolic acid peels	Q-switched laser	Ablative resurfacing	Fractional resurfacing
Melasma	Variable improvement	Multiple light peels in conjunction with sunscreen and topical retinoid/ hydroquinone	No	Yes; but careful patient selection and long postlaser recovery	Yes in skin types I–III; caution skin type IV
Postinflammatory hyperpigmentation	Yes; weeks to months to see clinical improvement	Variable improvement	No	No	No
Lentigo	Minimal/moderate improvement after months of use	Minimal/moderate change with three to four peels	Yes; one to two treatments are highly successful	Yes; post-inflammatory erythema chief obstacle	Mild/moderate
Nevus of Ota	None	None	Yes; multiple treatments result in improvement	No	No

glycolic acid/hydroquinone cream has been shown to be effective.

- Serial superficial chemical peels such as salicylic acid and glycolic acid peels are the safest peels in darker skin phototypes.

Caution is required for darker skin phototypes to avoid hyperpigmentation.

LASERS

■ Q-Switched Lasers

Q-switched laser treatment for melasma is not recommended given its high incidence of postinflammatory hyperpigmentation. Additionally, it is not dramatically effective except in some cases of superficial melasma.

■ Ablative Laser

In cases refractory to topical creams and chemical peels, erbium:YAG laser produced significant, temporary improvement in 10 patients in one study but was complicated by subsequent postinflammatory hyperpigmentation in all 10 patients.

■ Non-Ablative Fractional Resurfacing

Non-Ablative Fractional resurfacing can be successful for some cases of melasma, especially epidermal types (Fig. 25.2).

- Long-term data are lacking.
- Treatment is generally performed at superficial depth relative to treatments for rhytides and acne scars.
- Treatment is generally performed at higher densities.

It is most successful in patients with lighter skin phototypes, such as skin types I and II. Improvement is less predictable in skin type III, but is often achieved.

Skin phototypes IV and V often do not respond favorably to fractional resurfacing. Postinflammatory hyperpigmentation is a high risk.

- Pre- and posttreatment use of hydroquinone and longer intervals between treatments may reduce postinflammatory hyperpigmentation in darker skin phototypes.

PITFALLS TO AVOID/ COMPLICATIONS/MANAGEMENT/ OUTCOME EXPECTATIONS

- All forms of melasma are difficult and frustrating to treat. Recurrence is common.
- Dermal melasma is particularly difficult.
- Patients should be apprised of the recalcitrant nature of this condition in some cases.

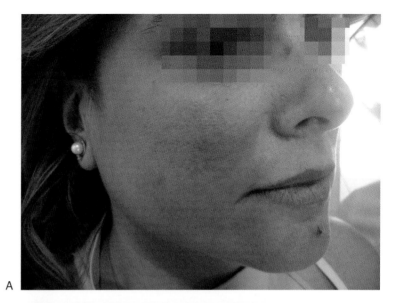

A

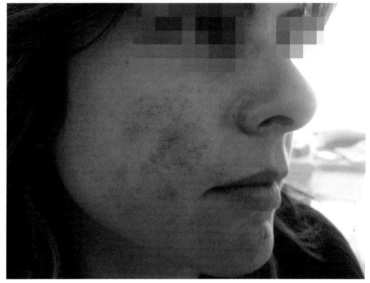

B

Figure 25.3 (A) *Young female with melasma.* **(B)** *Characteristic darkening of melasma 1-day post intense pulsed light treatment*

• Postpartum state and discontinuance of oral contraceptive pills are frequently successful therapies.

• Some treatments worsen its appearance.

• Strict sun avoidance is crucial with a sunscreen with UVA/UVB protection and/or a physical block such as titanium dioxide or zinc oxide during and after any treatment regimen.

BIBLIOGRAPHY

Finkel LJ, Ditre CM, Hamilton TA, Ellis CN, Voorhees JJ. Topical tretinoin (retinoic acid) improves melasma. A vehicle-controlled, clinical trial. *Br J Dermatol.* 1993;129: 415-421.

Grimes PE. Management of hyperpigmentation in darker racial ethnic groups. *Semin Cutan Med Surg.* 2009; 28(2):77-85.

Lawrence N, Cox SE, Brody HJ. Treatment of melasma with Jessner's solution versus glycolic acid: A comparison of clinical efficacy and evaluation of the predictive ability of Wood's light examination. *J Am Acad Dermatol.* 1997;36:589-593.

Lee HS, Won CH, Lee DH, et al. Treatment of melasma in Asian skin using a fractional 1,550 nm laser: An open clinical study. *Dermatol Surg.* 2009;35(10):1499-1504.

Manaloto RM, Alser TM. Erbium:YAG laser resurfacing for refractory melasma. *Dermatol Surg.* 1999;25:121-123.

Rokhsar CK, Fitzpatrick RE. The treatment of melasma with fractional photothermolysis: A pilot study. *Dermatol Surg.* 2005;31 (12):1645-1650.

Torok HM, Jones T, Rich P, Smith S, Tschen E. Hydroquinone 4%, tretinoin 0.05%, fluocinolone acetonide 0.01%: A safe and efficacious 12-month treatment for melasma. *Cutis.* 2005;75(1):57-62.

Verallo-Rowell VM, Veralo V, Graupe K, Lopez-Villafuerte L, Garcia Lopez M. Double-blind comparison of azeleic acid and hydroquinone in the treatment of melasma. *Acta Derm Venereol.* 1989;143:58-61.

Victor FC, Gelber J, Rao B. Melasma: A review. *J Cutan Med Surg.* 2004;8(2):97-102.

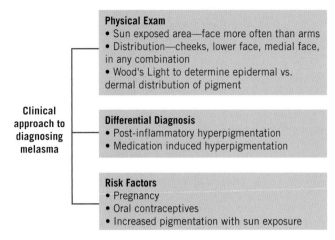

Figure 25.4 *Clinical approach to diagnosing melasma*

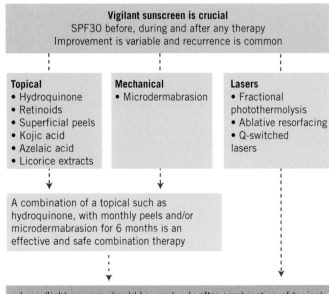

Figure 25.5 *Melasma treatment protocol*

CHAPTER 26 | Nevus of Ota

Nevus of Ota, also known as nevus fuscoceruleus ophthalmomaxillaris, represents a benign partially confluent macular brown-blue pigmentation of the skin and mucous membranes in the distribution of the first and second branches of the trigeminal nerve. It may be unilateral or bilateral. The ipsilateral sclera is frequently involved.

EPIDEMIOLOGY

Incidence: 0.4% to 0.8% of Japanese dermatology patients

Age: bimodal distribution at birth and puberty

Race: more common in Asians and blacks than whites

Sex: more females than males seek treatment for this condition; unknown if there is a sex predilection

Precipitating factors: sporadic, not an inherited disorder

PATHOGENESIS

Hyperpigmentation arises as a result of dermal melanocytes that have not migrated to the epidermis.

PATHOLOGY

Heavily pigmented, elongated, dendritic melanocytes are located among the reticular dermal collagen. Most typically, these melanocytes are found in the upper one-third of the reticular dermis but are also seen in the papillary dermis in some lesions.

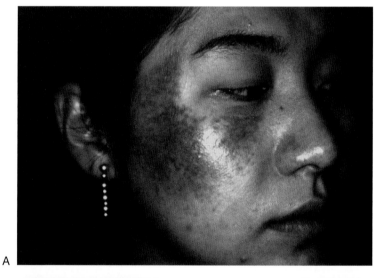

A

PHYSICAL LESIONS

It presents as confluent or partially confluent brown-blue patches in the distribution of the first and second branches of the trigeminal nerve. Gray, black, and purple coloration may be present in some lesions as well. It can be unilateral or bilateral. The magnitude of involvement can vary from local periocular involvement to much of the side of the face. Approximately two-thirds of patients feature ipsilateral scleral involvement.

DIFFERENTIAL DIAGNOSIS

Melasma, café au lait macule, Hori's macule blue nevus, bruising, ochronosis, argyria, photodermatoses, fixed drug eruption, and other medication-related eruptions should be considered in the proper clinical setting.

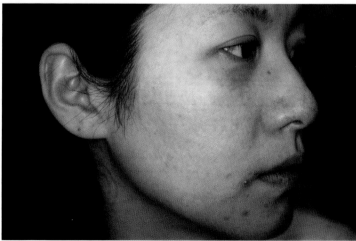

B

Figure 26.1 (A) *Nevus of Ota prior to treatment with Q-switched ruby laser.* **(B)** *Significant clearance after serial treatments with Q-switched ruby laser*

LABORATORY EXAMINATION

Biopsy may be indicated if the diagnosis is in question or to exclude the rare case of melanoma arising in this lesion.

COURSE

There is a bimodal distribution for nevus of Ota, birth and puberty. It remains relatively similar in appearance after initial presentation.

KEY CONSULTATIVE QUESTIONS

- Onset of eruption
- Medication history

MANAGEMENT

There is no medical indication to treat nevus of Ota. Cosmetic appearance, however, is distressing to patients. While cryotherapy and topical bleaching treatments have been utilized, the treatment of choice is Q-switched laser treatment.

TOPICAL TREATMENT

Makeup can camouflage or assist in camouflaging nevus of Ota. Topical medications are less effective than laser.

TREATMENT

- Numerous studies have shown that nevus of Ota is amenable to successful resolution with Q-switched laser therapies including the Q-switched ruby (694 nm), the alexandrite (755 nm), and the Nd:YAG (1,064 nm) lasers (Figs. 26.2 and 26.3).
- Test spot can be performed prior to treatment.
- The Q-switched ruby laser has been shown to be effective at producing 75% or greater clearance at fluences of 5 to 7 J/cm^2, 4-mm spot size, and a 30-ns pulse width at 3-to-4-month treatment intervals.
  - In a study of 46 children and 107 adults with nevus of Ota, treatments were more successful in children than in adults.
  - The mean number of treatment sessions to achieve significant clearing or better was 3.5 for the younger age group and 5.9 for the older age group.
  - Additionally, complications were lower in the children than adults, that is, 4.8% as compared to 22.4%.
  - One retrospective study examined 101 patients 1 year after treatment with Q-switched ruby laser and

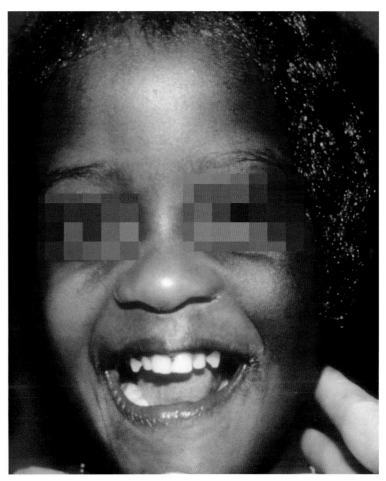

Figure 26.2 *Nevus of Ota. Periorbital blue-gray pigmentation with scleral involvement (Kay K, Jen R, Richard J, et al eds. Color Atlas & Synopsis of Pediatric Dermatology. McGraw-Hill, Inc.; 2002)*

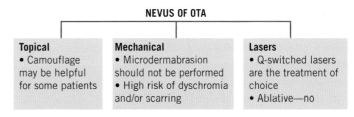

Figure 26.3 *Treatment of nevus of Ota algorithm*

found that 16.8% displayed hypopigmentation and 5.9% showed hyperpigmentation. One patient who had complete resolution developed recurrence.

- The Q-switched alexandrite laser is also effective for the treatment of nevus of Ota. Dermal whitening is the key clinical endpoint when treating nevus of Ota with Q-switched lasers.

  - One group reported the successful treatment of nevus of Ota with fractional photothermolysis. Nonetheless, Q-switched laser is the treatment of choice.

■ Topical

- Camouflage may be helpful for some patients.

■ Mechanical

- Microdermabrasion should not be performed.
- High risk of dyschromia and/or scarring.

■ Lasers

- Q-switched lasers are the treatment of choice.
- Ablative—no.
- Multiple treatments with Q-switched lasers are needed.
- Improvement moderate to dramatic after multiple treatments.
- Q-switched laser treatment of lesions that arise in infancy may respond better to laser therapy than later in life.
- If a Q-switched YAG laser is used, a combination of 532 nm/1,064 nm may result in better clinical improvement than 1,064 nm alone.

  - One study treated 13 patients at fluences ranging between 6 and 8 J/cm^2 at 8-week intervals. The mean number of treatments was approximately seven. Seven patients achieved 75% or better lightening, three patients achieved between 51% and 75% improvement, one achieved between 25% and 50% improvement, and another achieved less than 25% improvement.

  - Two patients experienced transient hyperpigmentation; one experienced transient hypopigmentation.

- The Q-switched Nd:YAG (1,064 nm) laser has also proven to be effective.

  - Slightly less effective than other Q-switched lasers.

  - It is safer for use in dark skin types.

  - Less risk of hypopigmentation.

PITFALLS TO AVOID/OUTCOME EXPECTATIONS/COMPLICATIONS/ MANAGEMENT

- Laser treatment for nevus of Ota is frequently successful.
- Given the high proportion of patients with dark skin phototypes, there is the risk of hypo- and hyperpigmentation.
- The risk of such an adverse reaction should be discussed with the patient prior to therapy.
- Additionally, a test site can be treated before performing full treatment of any lesion.
- Q-switched laser treatment can be associated with transient hyperpigmentation.
- Recurrence after treatment is infrequent.

BIBLIOGRAPHY

Chan HH, Leung RS, Ying SY, et al. A retrospective analysis of complications in the treatment of nevus of Ota with the Q-switched alexandrite and Q-switched Nd:YAG lasers. *Dermatol Surg.* 2000;26(11):1000-1006.

Chan HH, Ying SY, Ho WS, Kono T, King WW. An in vivo trial comparing the clinical efficacy and complications of Q-switched 755 nm alexandrite and Q-switched 1064 nm Nd:YAG lasers in the treatment of nevus of Ota. *Dermatol Surg.* 2000;26(10):919-922.

Kono T, Chan HH, Ercocen AR, et al. Use of Q-switched ruby laser in the treatment of nevus of Ota in different age groups. *Lasers Surg Med.* 2003;32(5):391-395.

Kono T, Nozaki M, Chan HH, Mikashima Y. A retrospective study looking at the long-term complications of Q-switched ruby laser in the treatment of nevus of Ota. *Lasers Surg Med.* 2001;29(2):156-159.

Kouba DJ, Fincher EF, Moy RL. Nevus of Ota successfully treated by fractional photothermolysis using a fractionated 1440-nm Nd:YAG laser. *Arch Dermatol.* 2008; 144(2):156-158.

Radmanesh M. Naevus of Ota treatment with cryotherapy. *J Dermatol Treat.* 2001;12(4):205-209.

CHAPTER 27 | Postinflammatory hyperpigmentation

Postinflammatory hyperpigmentation (PIH) is a common sequela of inflammatory dermatoses or injury to the skin. It occurs most commonly in darker skin types. Depending on the etiology of the hyperpigmentation, pigment may be deposited in the dermis or epidermis with important implications for treating the pigment changes. It is a common sequela of laser treatment, particularly in darker skin phototypes (Fig. 27.1).

EPIDEMIOLOGY

Incidence: common, especially in darker skin types

Age: all ages

Race: more common in darker skin types

Sex: none

Precipitating factors: any inflammatory disorder or injury to the skin can produce hyperpigmentation. It may also result from laser therapy, dermabrasion, cryotherapy, or chemical peels. It presents more exuberantly and with a greater duration in darker skin phototypes

PATHOGENESIS

Unknown.

DERMATOPATHOLOGY

Basal cell layer pigmentation and dermal melanophages are seen.

PHYSICAL LESIONS

In epidermal PIH, patients display indistinct tan to dark brown macules at sites of previous skin inflammation. In dermal PIH, there is more of a brown-gray hue.

DIFFERENTIAL DIAGNOSIS

Mastocytosis, macular amyloidosis, minocin hyperpigmentation, exogenous ochronosis, melasma, and erythema dyschromicum perstans.

LABORATORY EXAMINATION

None.

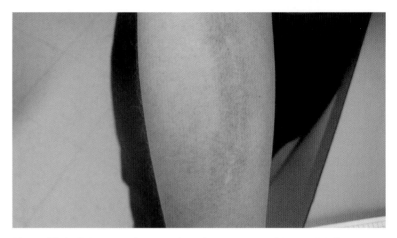

Figure 27.1 *PIH seen after a series of treatments with nonablative fractional resurfacing for a scar. The PIH resolved on its own within 3 weeks*

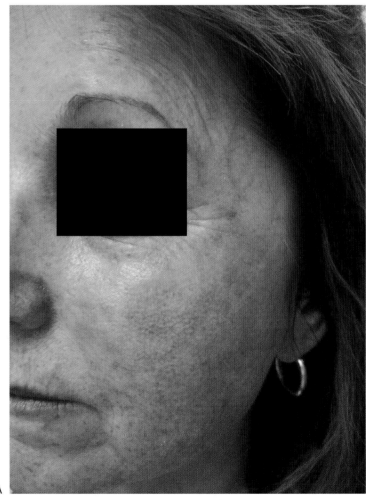

A

Figure 27.2 (A) *Pseudo-ochronosis seen after years of hydroquinone treatment.*

COURSE

PIH does not worsen in the absence of further insult or inflammation at the affected site. PIH usually resolves over a period of a few months. In the case of dermal hyperpigmentation, there may not be improvement.

KEY CONSULTATIVE QUESTIONS

• Sun exposure, sunscreen use

• Time of onset

• Recent rashes, injury, or treatment of skin

• Medication use

MANAGEMENT

While there is no medical indication to treat PIH, many patients are as bothered by PIH as they are by the processes that produced it initially. Furthermore, PIH can endure far longer than the original eruption. There are multiple treatments including topical, laser, and chemical peels (Table 27.1). It is essential to first determine the cause of the hyperpigmentation. Culprits range from hemosiderin to pigment to vascular. Without determining the etiology correctly, treatment will, at best, provide no improvement, or worsen the PIH. Frequently, the safest and most effective treatment is time. Attempted treatment of PIH, especially in darker skin phototypes, can often worsen and prolong hyperpigmentation. Normally, epidermal PIH will resolve on its own over a period of months.

Therapeutic options include topical retinoids, bleaching creams, chemical peels (including glycolic acid peels,

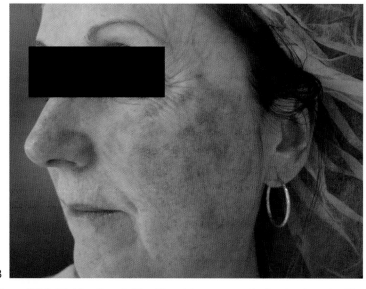

B

Figure 27.2 (B) (*Continued*) *Significant improvement after treatment with Q-switched laser*

TABLE 27.1 ■ Post-inflammatory Hyperpigmentation treatment

Therapeutic options	Retinoid/ hydroquinone	Peels/ microdermabrasion	Q-switched laser	Ablative lasers	Fractional resurfacing
Post-inflammatory hyperpigmentation	Needs to be used for weeks to months for improvement	20-70% glycolic acid peels, jessner peels, combination jessner TCA/peels and Salicilyc acid peels and/or microdermabrasion may help improve more quickly	No	No	No
	Face/upper body improves more quickly than lower half of the body	Risk of paradoxically making postinflammatory changes *worse* if too much inflammation is created			

Jessner peels, combination Jessner/TCA peels, and salicylic acid peels), and fractional laser treatment. There is a risk of paradoxically making post-inflammatory changes *worse* if too much inflammation is created.

SUNPROTECTION

Sunblocks and sunscreens used daily are crucial to prevent worsening, as is sun avoidance. Without their use, other therapies will not be effective. If a patient does not avoid sun exposure, PIH will worsen. Sun avoidance includes avoiding peak sun hours, wearing a hat out doors to protect the face from sun exposure and an awareness that UVA rays penetrates through windows while driving, while at work and while at home.

TOPICAL TREATMENTS

There are a host of topical treatments for PIH that produce mild improvement and may expedite resolution.

- Hydroquinone formulations, particularly with sunscreens
  - Hydroquinone (2%–4%) creams are effective, first-line treatment.
  - Prolonged usage of hydroquinone can result in a characteristic skin discoloration known as pseudo-ochronosis (Fig. 27.2).
  - Bleaching creams are contraindicated in pregnant and lactating women.
- Retinoids
  - Solage (2% mequinol and 0.01% tretinoin) and Triluma (0.01% fluocinolone acetonide, 4% hydroquinone, and 0.05% tretinoin) provide an exfoliative benefit.
  - Triluma should not be used indefinitely due to its corticosteroid content and risk for atrophy.
- Azelaic acid (20%) cream applied twice daily provides slow lightening of pigmentation.
- Kojic acid (1%–2.5%) cream.
  - The exact concentration of kojic acid needed for effective results is unknown.
- If any of these topicals produces significant inflammation or irritation, it is important to discontinue its use to avoid worsening of PIH.

CHEMICAL PEELS

Chemical peels are an effective treatment option for the reduction of PIH.

- Over-the-counter α-hydroxy acid peels are a beneficial adjunct to physician-strength chemical peels. The continual exfoliation achieved from consistent use of the peels may result in mild lightening.

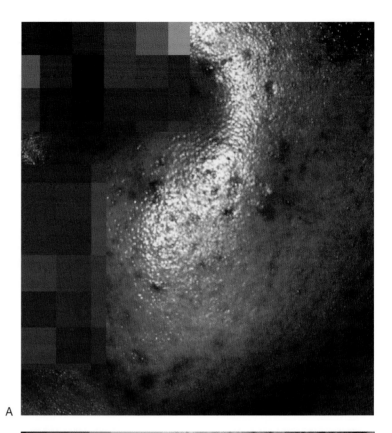

A

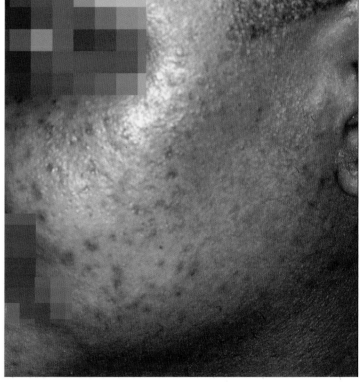

B

Figure 27.3 (A) *Hyperpigmentation on left side of face before treatment.* **(B)** *Improvement after a series of salicylic acid peels and topical application of 4% hydroquinone (Courtesy of Pearl E. Grimes, MD)*

- Glycolic acid peels (20%–70%) are administered every 2 to 3 weeks utilizing increasing strengths as tolerated.
  - The treatment endpoint is mild confluent erythema.
  - Treated areas must be fully neutralized with sodium bicarbonate or water at the completion of the peel.
  - Lightening of superficial PIH may be observed after four to six peels.
  - Strict photoprotection for 1 month is essential and must be stressed.
- Jessner peels (resorcinol, lactic acid, and salicylic acid) are administered every 6 to 8 weeks.
  - Treatment endpoint is a light whitening of the skin.
  - Strict photoprotection for 2 to 3 months is advised.
  - Multiple treatments are recommended.
  - Contraindicated in pregnant and lactating women.
- Combination Jessner/10% trichloroacetic (TCA) peels may also be employed in a similar fashion as the Jessner peel. The Jessner peel results in exfoliation allowing for greater penetration of the TCA peel.
  - Multiple peels are generally needed.
  - Contraindicated in pregnant and lactating women.
  - Deeper peels are rarely employed given the risk of PIH exacerbation with healing.
- Caution must be used in treating skin phototypes III to VI, particularly with medium depth peels. Salicylic acid peels are safest for dark skin phototypes (Fig. 27.3).

LASERS

Traditionally, laser treatment for PIH does not produce reliable improvement and is not first-line therapy. In fact, laser therapy may exacerbate PIH. In general, it is not recommended.

Fractional photothermolysis (FP) can, however, provide improvement of PIH (Fig. 27.4). This is especially true for patients with lighter skin phototypes. In darker skin types, PIH often worsens. It should not be recommended as a first-line therapy. Rather, bleaching creams and chemical peels provide more consistent, reproducible results.

Typically, FP treatments should be directed toward superficial skin depth and avoid higher treatment densities.

PITFALLS TO AVOID/COMPLICATIONS/ MANAGEMENT/OUTCOME EXPECTATIONS

- It is important to reassure patients that PIH will resolve on its own with time, except if it is a dermal process.
- Laser treatment is unreliable and may produce worsening. It is usually not recommended.

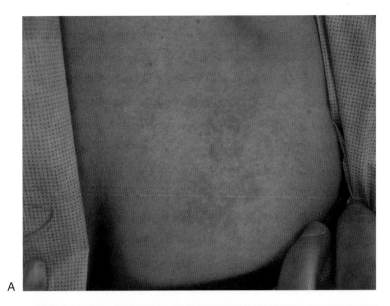

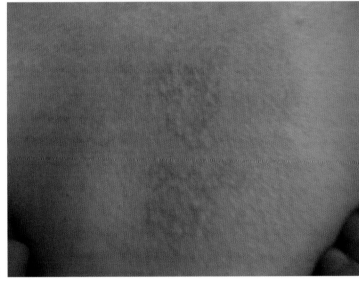

Figure 27.4 (A) *Hyperpigmentation after a series of Q-switched laser tattoo treatments.* **(B)** *Improvement of PIH after two nonablative fractional resurfacing treatments utilizing superficial depth and lower treatment densities*

- It is important to discontinue any topical medications that produce inflammation or irritation to avoid worsening PIH.
- Chemical peels are likely to only lighten and not fully eliminate the PIH. Caution should be taken in darker skin phototypes.
- It is better and safer to utilize serial superficial peels rather than a single deeper peel to minimize the risk of PIH.
- PIH may not improve despite serial chemical peel use. PIH resulting from hemosiderin (ie, leg vein treatments) will not respond to lasers, peels, and bleaching creams. In fact, treatment will likely worsen the PIH.

BIBLIOGRAPHY

Kilmer SL. Laser eradication of pigmented lesions and tattoos. *Dermatol. Clin.* 2002;20(1):37-53.

Mishima Y, Ohyama Y, Shibata T, et al. Inhibitory action of kojic acid on melanogenesis and its therapeutic effect for various human hyperpigmentation disorders. *Skin Res.* 1994;36(2):134-150.

Nakagawa M, Kawai K. Contact allergy to kojic acid in skin care products. *Contact Dermatitis.* 1995;31(1):9-13.

Ngujen QH, Bui TP. Azelaic acid: Pharmacokinetic and pharmacodynamic properties and its therapeutic role in hyperpigmentary disorders and acne. *Int J Dermatol.* 1995;34(2):75-84.

CHAPTER 28 | Vitiligo

Vitiligo is an acquired idiopathic condition that produces symmetric depigmented patches of the skin. It is particularly distressing and clinically apparent in patients with darker skin phototypes.

EPIDEMIOLOGY

Incidence: approximately 2% of the world population

Age: can present at any age but most commonly presents in the second to fourth decade

Race: equal

Sex: equal

Precipitating factors: inheritance, trauma, illness, emotional states

PATHOGENESIS

Unknown.

DERMATOPATHOLOGY

There are no melanocytes in basal cell layer.

PHYSICAL LESIONS

Patients display well-demarcated, symmetric, depigmented, chalk-white macules. Common locations include elbows, knees, sacral area, penis, perioral areas, and neck. Hair may also lose pigmentation (Figs. 28.1 and 28.2).

DIFFERENTIAL DIAGNOSIS

Chemical leukoderma, postinflammatory hypopigmentation, nevus depigmentosus, nevus anemicus, pityriasis alba, lupus erythematosus, leprosy, and genodermatoses.

LABORATORY EXAMINATION

Wood's lamp examination is helpful in making the diagnosis. In cases of uncertainty, biopsy should be performed of both lesional and nonlesional skin in order to determine if there is an absence of melanocytes in the affected skin. Check thyroid-stimulating hormone (TSH) for hypothyroidism.

COURSE

Vitiligo can pursue a variable course. After an initial rapid presentation, it tends to stabilize. Typically, it is a chronic

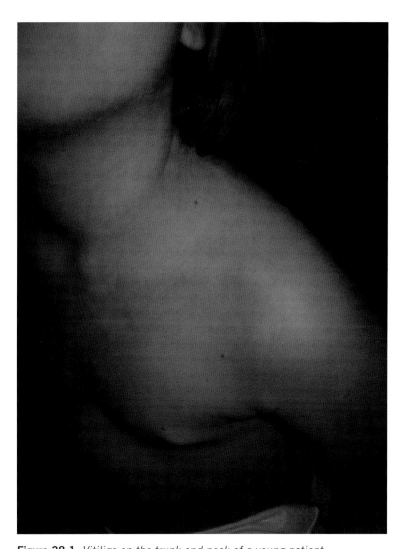

Figure 28.1 *Vitiligo on the trunk and neck of a young patient*

disease with periods of partial repigmentation but not resolution. It may improve in the summertime. In some cases, depigmentation becomes extensive.

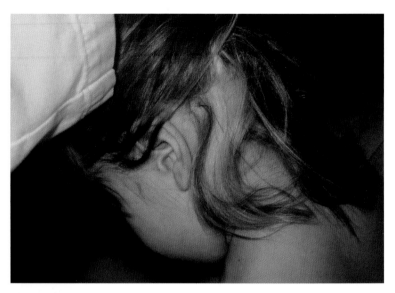

Figure 28.2 *White forelock in the same patient*

KEY CONSULTATIVE QUESTIONS

- Age of patient
- Time of onset
- Family history
- Occupation
- Chemical exposures

MANAGEMENT

There are multiple treatment modalities for vitiligo. Unfortunately, treatment is frustrating and often ineffective. Patients understandably are distressed by the appearance of vitiligo and desire treatment. In extensive cases, it produces a striking appearance, particularly for patients with darker skin phototypes.

PREVENTION

Sunscreens and sun avoidance protect vitiliginous skin from burning and are an important component of therapy. Further, tanning unaffected skin will accentuate the contrast between normal and vitiliginous skin, worsening the cosmetic appearance of the disease.

TOPICAL TREATMENT

There are a host of topical treatments for vitiligo. They include

- Corticosteroids
  - Topical
  - Intralesional
- Calcineurin inhibitors: tacrolimus, pimecrolimus
- Monobenzylether of hydroquinone
  - Produces permanent depigmentation
  - Twice daily over 1-year period
  - Permanent depigmentation is produced in less than 50% of patients
  - Poor or no depigmentation in nearly half of patients
  - Caution prior to pursuing this permanent treatment
  - Side effects include contact dermatitis, erythema, and pruritus
  - Heightened risk of sunburn after this permanent treatment
- Camouflaging makeup and self-tanning agents to hide depigmented macules

PHOTOTHERAPY

Phototherapy is a mainstay of vitiligo treatment.

- Psoralen and ultraviolet A (PUVA) with topical or oral 5-methoxypsoralen or 8-methoxypsoralen
- Narrow-band UVB

ORAL THERAPY

Oral therapies include

- Oral 5- or 8-methoxypsoralen in combination with gradual, limited sun exposure
- Pulse therapy with corticosteroids

SURGICAL TREATMENTS

Autologous skin grafting can be a helpful treatment for vitiligo recalcitrant to other therapies. It is not a first- or second-line treatment. Split-thickness grafts, epidermal blister grafts, cultured melanocyte grafts, single hair grafts, and noncultured epidermal suspension grafts have all been examined. Pain after graft procedures is common, particularly at the harvest site (Fig. 28.3).

- A majority of patients employing the epidermal suction graft technique showed improvement.
- Split-thickness grafting and dermabrasion have also achieved repigmentation within an average of 6 months in one study of 22 patients.
- Single hair grafts are most effective in localized or segmental vitiligo. Success in generalized vitiligo is poor.
- Both cultured pure melanocyte suspension as well as cultured epidermal grafting after treatment with CO_2 laser have been shown to be successful in treating vitiligo.
  - Results were best in localized cases of vitiligo.

LASER THERAPY

■ Excimer Laser

An excimer laser emits UVB range light at 308 nm, close to the wavelength of narrow-band UVB therapy that has been used to successfully treat vitiligo. Beginning with a starting dose of 100 mJ/cm^2, with increasing doses in standard phototherapy increments, there was good improvement in recalcitrant vitiligo after 30 weeks of treatments.

- Acral lesions were most refractory to treatment.
- Few adverse effects.
- Best results are produced on the face > neck, extremities, trunk, and genitalia > hands, feet.
- More expensive than many traditional therapies. Combination treatment with tacrolimus 0.1% is more effective than treatment with excimer laser alone.

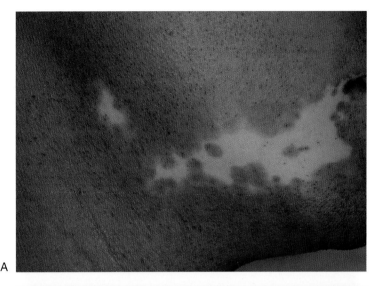

A

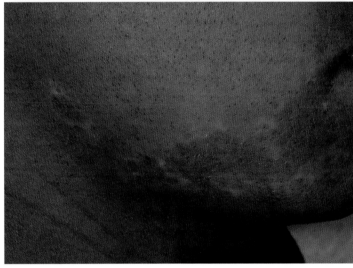

B

Figure 28.3 (A) *Depigmented patch of skin on right mandible.* **(B)** *Significant improvement after multiple 1-mm punch grafts (Courtesy of Pearl E. Grimes, MD)*

PITFALLS TO AVOID/COMPLICATIONS/ MANAGEMENT/OUTCOME EXPECTATIONS

- Vitiligo is a difficult disease to treat.

- There are multiple first- and second-line therapies that should be employed before seeking surgical or laser treatments.

- It is especially difficult to produce long-term significant cosmetic improvement in extensive cases.

- Frequently, repigmentation may be confined to perifollicular areas creating a "spotty" appearance.

- Patients need to be educated that any therapy may not succeed.

- The excimer laser is not widely available, making its use particularly difficult.

BIBLIOGRAPHY

Chen YF, Yang PY, Hu DN, Kuo FS, Hung CS, Hung CM. Treatment of vitiligo by transplantation of cultured pure melanocyte suspension: Analysis of 120 cases. *J Am Acad Dermatol.* 2004;51(1):68-74.

Hadi SM, Spencer JM, Lebwohl M. The use of the 308-nm excimer laser for the treatment of vitiligo. *Dermatol Surg.* 2004;30(7):983-986.

Koga M. Epidermal grafting using the tops of suction blisters in the treatment of vitiligo. *Arch Dermatol.* 1988;124(11):1656-1658.

Na GY, Seo SK, Choi SK. Single hair grafting for the treatment of vitiligo. *J Am Acad Dermatol.* 1998;38(4):580-584.

Ozdemir M, Cetinkale O, Wolf R, et al. Comparison of two surgical approaches for treating vitiligo: A preliminary study. *Int J Dermatol.* 2002;41(3):135-138.

Passeron T, Ostovari N, Zakaria W, et al. Topical tacrolimus and the 308 nm excimer laser: A synergistic combination for the treatment of vitiligo. *Arch Dermatol.* 2004;140(9):1065-1069.

Taneja A, Trehan M, Taylor CR. 308-nm excimer laser for the treatment of localized vitiligo. *Int J Dermatol.* 2003;42(8):658-662.

Toriyama K, Kamei Y, Kazeto T, et al. Combination of short-pulsed CO_2 laser resurfacing and cultured epidermal sheet autografting in the treatment of vitiligo: A preliminary report. *Ann Plast Surg.* 2004;53(2):178-180.

van Geel N, Ongenae K, De Mil M, Haeghen YV, Vervaet C, Naeyaert JM. Double-blind placebo-controlled study of autologous transplanted epidermal cell suspensions for repigmenting vitiligo. *Arch Dermatol.* 2004;140(10): 1203-1208.

SECTION SIX

Vascular Alterations

CHAPTER 29 | Angiokeratoma

Angiokeratomas are telangiectasias with keratotic elements. They present in different clinical scenarios including (a) solitary or multiple angiokeratomas occurring predominantly on lower extremities; (b) angiokeratoma of Fordyce affecting the scrotum and the vulva; (c) angiokeratoma of Mibelli, an autosomal dominant disorder affecting dorsum of hands and feet, elbows, and knees; (d) angiokeratoma corporis diffusum associated with Fabry's disease, an X-linked recessive disorder characterized by α-galactosidase-A deficiency and affecting the lower abdomen, buttocks, and genitalia; and (e) angiokeratoma circumscriptum usually grouped on one extremity.

EPIDEMIOLOGY

Age: solitary or multiple angiokeratomas usually affect young adults, angiokeratomas of Fordyce affect middle-aged and elderly individuals. Angiokeratoma of Mibelli and angiokeratoma circumscriptum are usually diagnosed in childhood.

Sex: angiokeratoma of Mibelli and angiokeratoma circumscriptum exhibit female predominance. Otherwise, there is no sex predisposition.

PHYSICAL EXAMINATION

Red to violaceous, well-circumscribed hyperkeratotic papules and plaques.

DIFFERENTIAL DIAGNOSES

Solitary lesions can be mistaken for melanoma, acquired hemangioma, lymphangioma, seborrheic keratosis, and warts.

LABORATORY DATA

■ Dermatopathology

Marked dilated, thin-walled blood vessels in the papillary dermis, associated with an overlying acanthotic hyperkeratotic epidermis.

COURSE MANAGEMENT

Management of angiokeratomas remains a challenge. Many modalities have been reported in the literature with variable success. Treatment modalities include

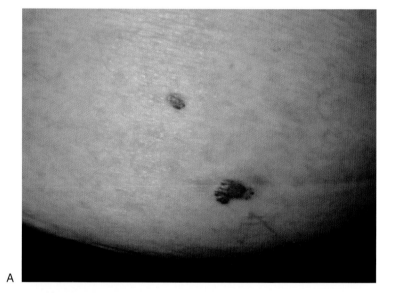

A

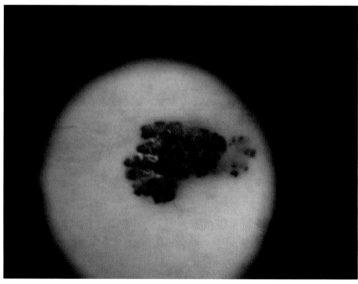

B

Figure 29.1 (A) *Angiokeratomas on the abdomen of a young patient.* **(B)** *Angiokeratoma imaged through an epiluminescence microscope (DermLite)*

- Lasers: angiokeratomas have occasionally been treated successfully with lasers.

  - The pulsed dye laser (PDL) is an effective device for the improvement of the vascular component of angiokeratomas, but frequently some keratosis remains. The target chromophore is hemoglobin. PDL has proven successful at 595 nm, 5-to-7-mm spot, 9 to 11 J/cm^2, DCD 30/20. Covering the angiokeratoma with a glass slide, that is, diascopy, is helpful. The endpoint is lesional purpura. Healing occurs in more than 10 to 14 days. Multiple treatments may be required (Fig. 29.3).

  - Resurfacing lasers such as CO_2 and Er:YAG lasers can be utilized for lesional vaporization. Patients generally require local infiltration with 1% lidocaine with or without epinephrine prior to treatment. The UltraPulse CO_2 (Lumenis, Santa Clara, CA) is employed using a 3-mm collimated handpiece, with an energy of 300 to 500 mJ with nonoverlapping pulses. The various scanned CO_2 lasers such as the Sharplan FeatherTouch are employed using the 125-mm handpiece, 3-mm scan size at 14 to 40 W. The treatment endpoint is ablation to achieve lesional flattening and opalescence. Treatment sites should be cleansed with saline soaked gauze between laser passes. Postoperative care requires twice daily washing with soap and water and application of an antibiotic ointment. Healing occurs in more than 2 to 6 weeks. As with all ablative procedures, scarring may be observed.

  - Other lasers that have been used in the past with variable success include potassium-titanyl-phosphate laser, argon laser, and copper vapor laser. Long-pulsed Nd:YAG (1,064 nm) laser has been shown to be effective in improving angiokeratomas due to its selectivity and its deeper penetration into the skin. Successful treatment with a dual-wavelength laser system (595 and 1,064 nm) has been recently reported (Cynergy with Multiplex™, Cynosure, Westford, MA, USA).

- Other surgical treatments include excision, electrocautery, electrofulguration, or cryosurgery.

PITFALLS TO AVOID

- Patients should be advised that the PDL treatment will cause obvious bruising for up to 14 days.

- Keratotic features may persist after treatment. Improvement is often elusive.

BIBLIOGRAPHY

Gorse SJ, James W, Murison MS. Successful treatment of angiokeratoma with potassium titanyl phosphate laser. *Br J Dermatol*. 2004;150(3):620-622.

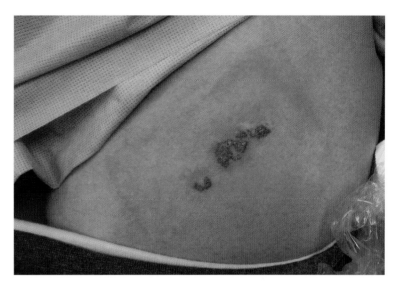

Figure 29.2 *Angiokeratoma on the left thigh resistant to multiple treatments with pulsed dye laser*

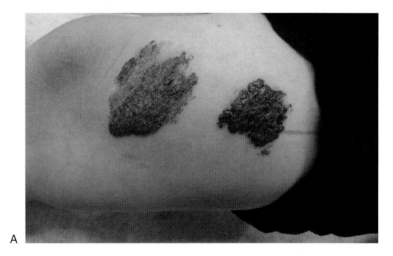

A

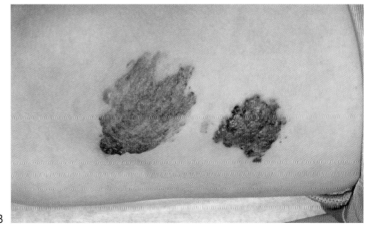

B

Figure 29.3 (A) *Biopsy-proven angiokeratoma on the thigh of a young child.* **(B)** *Some resolution after one treatment with pulsed dye laser at a wavelength of 595 nm with a 10-mm spot, pulse duration of 1.5 ms, a fluence of 7.5 J/cm^2, and DCD 30/20*

Lapins J, Emtestam L, Marcusson JA. Angiokeratomas in Fabry's disease and Fordyce's disease: Successful treatment with copper vapour laser. *Acta Derm Venereol.* 1993;73(2):133-135.

Occella C, Bleidl D, Rampini P, Schiazza L, Rampini E. Argon laser treatment of cutaneous multiple angiokeratomas. *Dermatol Surg.* 1995;21(2):170-172.

Ozdemir M, Baysal I, Engin B, Ozdemir S. Treatment of angiokeratoma of Fordyce with long-pulse neodymium-doped yttrium aluminium garnet laser. *Dermatol Surg.* 2009;35(1):92-97.

Pfirrmann G, Raulin C, Karsai S. Angiokeratoma of the lower extremities: Successful treatment with a dual-wavelength laser system (595 and 1064 nm). *Eur Acad Dermatol Venereol.* 2009;23(2):186-187.

Sommer S, Merchant WJ, Sheehan-Dare R. Severe predominantly acral variant of angiokeratoma of Mibelli: Response to long-pulse Nd:YAG (1064 nm) laser treatment. *J Am Acad Dermatol.* 2001;45(5):764-766.

CHAPTER 30 | Cherry and Spider Angiomas

Cherry angiomas, also known as ruby spots, senile hemangiomas, acquired capillary hemangioma, and Campbell de Morgan spots are very common benign vascular lesions that predominantly affect the trunk. Spider angiomas, also known as nevus araneus, spider telangiectasia, arterial spider, and vascular spider, represent localized telangiectasias radiating from central feeding arterioles. They are common vascular lesions that predominantly affect the face, upper trunk, arms, and hands.

EPIDEMIOLOGY

Incidence: very common

Age: cherry angiomas—middle-aged and elderly people; spider angiomas—all ages

Sex: more common in females

Precipitating factors: cherry angiomas can erupt during pregnancy or with hepatic disease. Spider angiomas are strongly associated with pregnancy, intake of oral contraceptive pills, and hepatocellular disease

PATHOGENESIS

Unknown for both. Association with pregnancy, oral contraceptive use, and liver disease suggest a hormonally mediated angiogenic mechanism.

PHYSICAL EXAMINATION

Cherry angioma presents as a 1-to-3-mm bright red to violaceous, smooth, dome-shaped papule. Spider angioma displays a network of dilated capillaries radiating from a central vessel. Both may bleed when traumatized.

PATHOLOGY

Cherry angiomas show loss of rete ridges as well as congested and ectatic capillaries and postcapillary venules in the papillary dermis. Spider angiomas reveal a central ascending arteriole that branches and communicates with multiple dilated capillaries.

DIFFERENTIAL DIAGNOSES

Cherry angiomas can be mistaken for angiokeratoma, glomeruloid hemangioma, pyogenic granuloma, and nodular melanoma. Spider angiomas can be mistaken for generalized essential telangiectasias and hereditary hemorrhagic telangiectasia.

COURSE

Cherry and spider angiomas arising during pregnancy may regress postpartum. Spider angiomas arising in childhood may also resolve spontaneously. Otherwise, both lesions tend to persist.

MANAGEMENT

Although medically insignificant, cherry and spider angiomas are frequently treated for cosmetic purposes. Multiple effective surgical treatment options exist. Depending on the procedure selected, the cost to the patient may vary significantly. Cherry and spider angiomas that present during pregnancy should not be treated until several months after delivery as they may resolve on their own.

- Electrosurgery
  - Electrodessication with coagulation (monopolar setting, 1–2 W followed by gentle curettage with endpoint of lesional flattening and homostasis) has been the traditional treatment modality for these lesions. It is effective and easily accessible.
  - The potential for scar formation must be considered.
- Laser surgery: different lasers have been used successfully in treatment of cherry and spider angiomas.
  - Pulsed dye laser (PDL) is the treatment of choice. A spot size should be selected that matches diameter of the angioma. With spider angiomas, the central

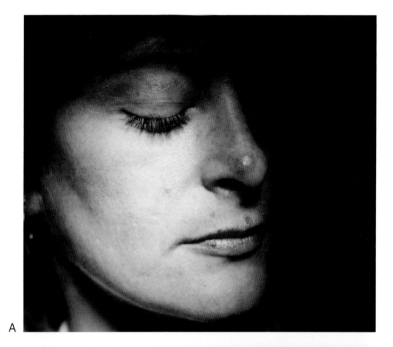

A

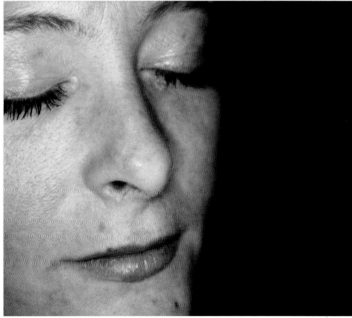

B

Figure 30.1 (A) *Spider angioma, right nose.* **(B)** *Full resolution of spider angioma after a single pulsed dye laser treatment to central vessel and surrounding skin*

feeding vessel as well as the surrounding vessels should be treated. It is best to compress the lesion with a microscope slide to blanch all but the central feeding vessel. A purpuric laser pulse should be delivered. The microscope slide should be removed to allow for cooling of the area. Subsequently, a purpuric laser pulse can be employed to target the telangiectasias radiating from the feeding vessel. The purpuric treatment endpoint represents coagulation of the targeted vessels (Figs. 30.1 and 30.2).

- The potassium-titanyl-phosphate (KTP) 532-nm laser produces a favorable response. Spot size should match the lesion diameter. The vessels should be traced out completely for most effective treatment. Treatment endpoint is lesional clearance or superficial whitening. Erythema can be expected posttreatment, lasting 24 to 48 hours.

- Carbon dioxide laser (UltraPulse 3-mm collimated handpiece, 300–400 mJ/pulse, nonoverlapping pulses; Sharplan FeatherTouch 125-mm handpiece, 14–40 W, 3-mm scan size, nonoverlapping pulses) has been employed as second-line therapy with success. Treatment endpoint is lesional flattening. Potential scar formation must be considered.

- Light therapy

  - Intense pulsed light (IPL) has also been employed with some success. As coagulation is needed for lesional resolution, higher fluences may be required for treatment efficacy.

- Surgical excision

  - Excision should be reserved for lesions that are resistant to other treatments. A postoperative scar is expected which may be less cosmetically pleasing than the angioma.

PITFALLS TO AVOID

- Patients need to be counseled as to the likelihood of obvious purpura following treatment with PDL that may persist for 10 to 14 days, especially off the face. Lesions are less likely to be completely treated at subpurpuric fluences.

- Simple electrocautery may be just as effective as PDL at a reduced cost to the patient.

- Compressing the lesion with a glass slide during PDL or KTP treatment is helpful to minimize its size and allowing for greater laser penetration. This reduces the total energy needed for coagulation and increases the treatment success rate.

- Multiple treatments may be required, in particular for large spider angiomas.

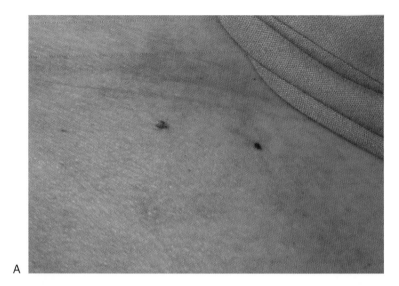

A

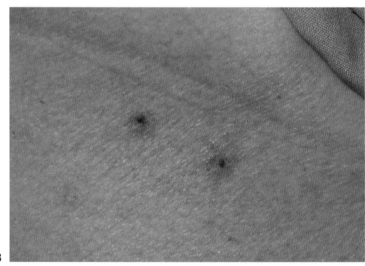

B

Figure 30.2 (A) *Cherry angiomas on the trunk in a middle-aged female.* **(B)** *The appropriate endpoint is purpura obtained after pulsed dye laser treatment (wavelength of 595 nm, 7-mm spot. 1.5-ms pulse duration, fluence of 12 J/cm^2, DCD 30/20)*

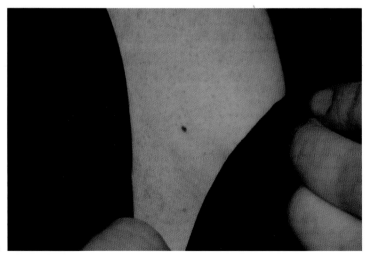

A

Figure 30.3 (A) *Cherry angioma, chest.*

BIBLIOGRAPHY

Dawn G, Gupta G. Comparison of potassium titanyl phosphate vascular laser and hyfrecator in the treatment of vascular spiders and cherry angiomas. *Clin Exp Dermatol.* 2003;28(6):581-583.

Fodor L, Ramon Y, Fodor A, Carmi N, Peled IJ, Ullmann Y. A side-by-side prospective study of intense pulsed light and Nd:YAG laser treatment for vascular lesions. *Ann Plast Surg.* 2006;56(2):164-170.

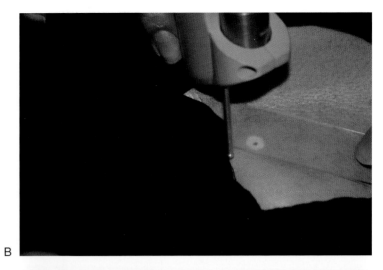

B

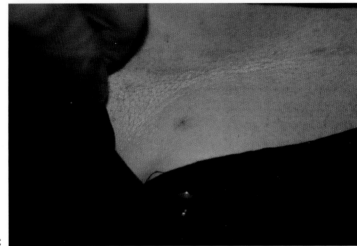

C

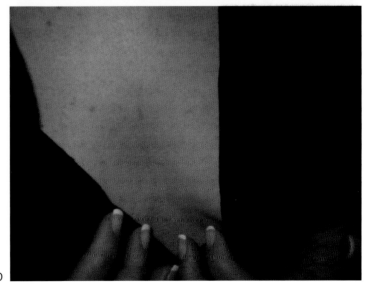

D

Figure 30.3 (*Continued*) (B) *Pulsed dye laser treatment to cherry angioma utilizing diascopy.* **(C)** *Purpura immediately post pulsed dye laser treatment.* **(D)** *Complete resolution of cherry angioma after one pulsed dye laser treatment*

CHAPTER 31 | Granuloma Faciale

Granuloma faciale (GF) was first described by Wigley in 1945 who labeled the disease "eosinophilic granuloma." Pinkus renamed this disorder granuloma faciale in 1952. GF is an idiopathic chronic cutaneous disorder that usually involves the face, particularly the nose. It can present with a single lesion or multiple lesions.

EPIDEMIOLOGY

Incidence: uncommon

Age: 30 to 50 years

Race: primarily seen in Caucasians

Sex: males > females

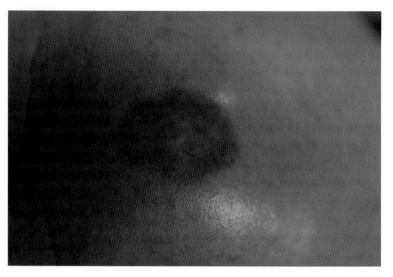

Figure 31.1 *Granuloma faciale on the scalp*

PATHOGENESIS

Unknown, but may be mediated by immune complex deposition.

PHYSICAL EXAMINATION

Single indurated facial brownish-red papule or plaque. Some lesions may have telangiectasia. Multiple lesions may be present. Extrafacial sites rarely observed. Lesions may vary in size from millimeters to centimeters (Fig. 31.1).

DIFFERENTIAL DIAGNOSES

Cutaneous lupus erythematosus, sarcoidosis, lymphoma, pseudolymphoma, cutaneous T-cell lymphoma, fixed drug eruption, rosacea.

DERMATOPATHOLOGY

Dense, polymorphous inflammatory cell infiltrate in the upper two-thirds of the dermis. The infiltrate is composed of numerous eosinophils, neutrophils, lymphocytes, and histiocytes. A prominent grenz zone is characteristically present. Leukocytoclastic vasculitis is frequently observed.

COURSE

The lesions of GF are usually chronic and only occasionally resolve spontaneously.

MANAGEMENT

Difficult to treat with any modality. Any successful treatment often leaves scarring.

■ Topical Treatment

- Corticosteroids: topical, intralesional
- Tacrolimus ointment (0.1%)

■ Systemic Treatment

- Dapsone
- Antimalarials
- Colchicine
- Clofazimine
- Gold injections

SURGICAL TREATMENT

- Cryosurgery: multiple reports indicating successful clearance. Results are unpredictable (Fig. 31.2).
- Surgical excision.
- Dermabrasion.
- Electrosurgery.

■ Light Treatment

- Topical psoralen and ultraviolet A (PUVA) radiation therapy
- Laser therapy: different lasers have been used in the treatment of GF with promising results, either as an ablative therapy with carbon dioxide laser or as a selective therapy targeting the prominent vasculature in GF lesions using the Q-switched argon laser, pulsed dye, diode laser, and potassium titanyl phosphate (KTP) 532-nm laser (Fig. 31.3).

PITFALLS TO AVOID

- GF is often recalcitrant to therapy. Patients should be counseled that successful treatment is often elusive.

BIBLIOGRAPHY

Ammirati CT, Hruza GJ. Treatment of granuloma faciale with the 585-nm pulsed dye laser. *Arch Dermatol.* 1999;135(8):903-905.

Apfelberg DB, Druker D, Maser MR, Lash H, Spence B Jr, Deneau D. Granuloma faciale. Treatment with the argon laser. *Arch Dermatol.* 1983;119(7):573-576.

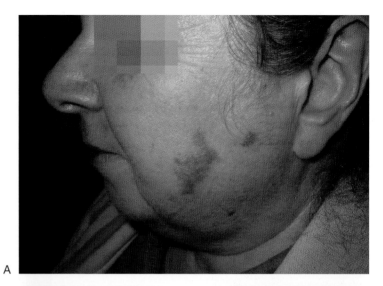

A

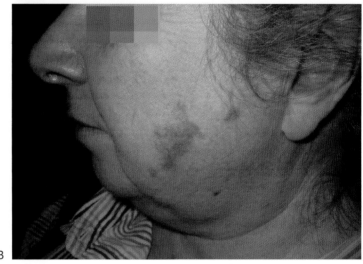

B

Figure 31.2 (A) *Multiple lesions of granuloma faciale on the face.* **(B)** *No significant improvement detected after one treatment with cryotherapy on a 4-month follow-up visit*

Chatrath V, Rohrer TE. Granuloma faciale successfully treated with long-pulsed tunable dye laser. *Dermatol Surg.* 2002;28(6):527-529.

Elston DM. Treatment of granuloma faciale with the pulsed dye laser. *Cutis.* 2000;65(2):97-98.

Khaled A, Jones M, Zermani R, et al. Granuloma faciale. *Pathologica.* 2007;99(5):306-308.

Maillard H, Grognard C, Toledano C, Jan V, Machet L, Vaillant L. Granuloma faciale: Efficacy of cryosurgery in 2 cases. *Ann Dermatol Venereol.* 2000;127(1):77-79.

Tomson N, Sterling JC, Salvary I. Granuloma faciale treated successfully with topical tacrolimus. *Clin Exp Dermatol.* 2009;34(3):424-425.

Wheeland RG, Ashley JR, Smith DA, Ellis DL, Wheeland DN. Carbon dioxide laser treatment of granuloma faciale. *J Dermatol Surg Oncol.* 1984;10(9):730-733.

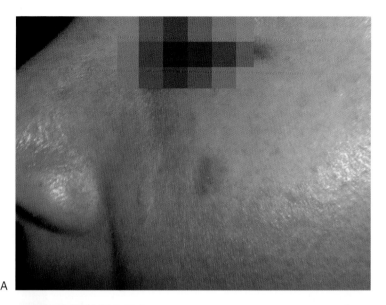

A

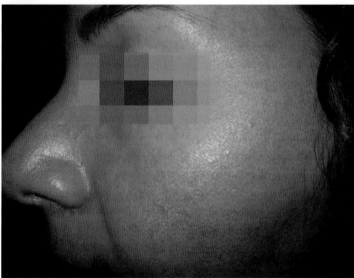

B

Figure 31.3 (A) *Indurated brownish-red plaque on the left cheek of a middle-aged female with granuloma faciale.* **(B)** *Two-year follow-up showing resolution of granuloma faciale after multiple pulsed dye laser treatments*

CHAPTER 32 | Infantile Hemangioma

Infantile hemangioma (IH), also known as strawberry, capillary, or cavernous hemangioma, is a benign endothelial proliferation that represents the most common tumor in infancy. It can be classified into superficial hemangioma (SH, 55% of cases), deep hemangioma (DH, 30% of cases), and mixed superficial and deep hemangioma (MH, 15% of cases). They occur most commonly on head and neck areas.

EPIDEMIOLOGY

Incidence: 1% to 3% are present at birth, 10% to 12% are present by 1 year of age

Age: majority (80%) become apparent between 2 and 5 weeks of age; 20% are noted at birth.

Sex: females are affected two to four times more than males

Precipitating factors: premature infants are more commonly affected

PHYSICAL EXAMINATION

The appearance depends on the depth of the hemangioma and the phase of evolution. SH presents as bright red-colored plaque. DH presents as a soft dermal or subcutaneous nodule with a bluish-purple color. MH shows features of both SH and DH. Multiple truncal hemangiomas may be observed. Involuting hemangiomas demonstrate a flatter surface with a grayish-purple hue that begins centrally and expands outward. The hemangiomas might become ulcerated and hemorrhagic. Residual fatty tissue, atrophy, telangiectasia, scar formation, and hypertrophy may be observed.

DIFFERENTIAL DIAGNOSES

Congenital hemangiomas can be confused with a vascular malformation such as port-wine stain at birth. Hemangiomas are generally present after birth versus vascular malformations, which are generally present at birth.

LABORATORY TESTS

■ Dermatopathology

Proliferations of plump endothelial cells that may extend from the superficial dermis to the deep subcutaneous tissue, depending on the hemangioma subtype.

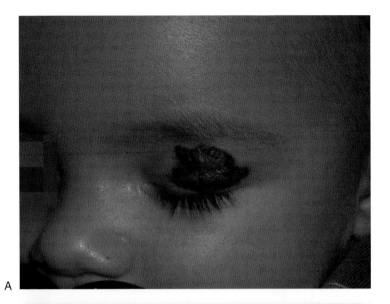
A

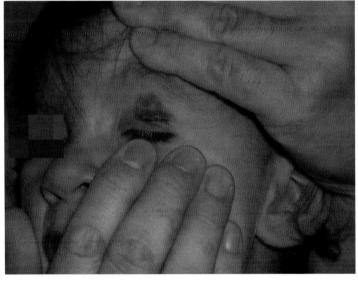
B

Figure 32.1 (A) *Left upper eyelid hemangioma in its early growth phase, a lesion that may threaten the child's vision.* **(B)** *Marked lightening and flattening of the hemangioma after multiple pulsed dye laser treatments*

■ Ancillary Tests

- An abdominal ultrasound should be obtained if more than four truncal hemangiomas are noted prior to 4 months of age.
- An electrocardiogram (ECG) and a cardiac ECHO should be considered for any concern of high cardiac output.

COURSE

Hemangiomas characteristically exhibit three phases of evolution: (a) proliferative phase, (b) involuting phase, and (c) involuted phase. The proliferating phase is characterized by a rapid growth phase that starts at 1 to 2 months of age and lasts until 6 to 9 months of age. This growth phase is followed by the involuting phase that usually starts in the second year of life and persists for several years. More than 90% of untreated hemangiomas involute, that is, attain maximal regression by 9 years of age. Up to 30% of hemangiomas leave postinvolution changes including hypopigmentation, scarring, telangiectasia, and fibrofatty tissue.

COMPLICATIONS

Bleeding and ulceration with secondary infection and scarring, especially in hemangiomas involving the diaper area, are commonly seen. Other serious complications include orbital obstruction and amblyopia with periorbital hemangiomas, upper airway obstruction with hemangiomas in the beard distribution, spinal abnormalities with lumbosacral hemangiomas, posterior fossa malformation in large facial hemangioma (PHACE syndrome), and high output cardiac failure with multiple cutaneous hemangiomas associated with visceral involvement.

KEY CONSULTATIVE QUESTIONS

- Onset of lesion
- Number of lesions noted
- Ulceration noted
- Bleeding noted
- Prior treatments and response

MANAGEMENT

The treatment of IHs is controversial. Given the natural course of IH with spontaneous resolution, many physicians choose to carefully observe the area with no intervention, especially in nonfacial, small, and uncomplicated hemangiomas. Early intervention is recommended for (a) all IHs that interfere with the function of vital organs (eg, periorbital hemangiomas, airway obstruction with hemangiomas in the beard distribution,

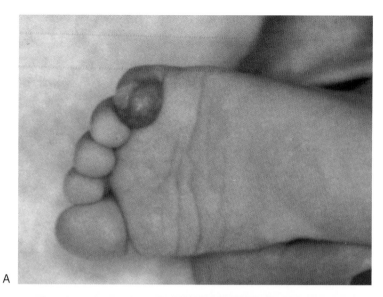

A

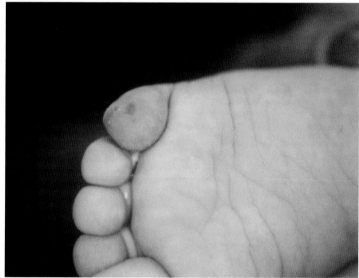

B

Figure 32.2 **(A)** *Hemangioma on the left fifth toe pad, a location that interfered with the child's ability to ambulate.* **(B)** *Significant clearing and near resolution of the hemangioma after multiple pulsed dye laser treatments*

high-output cardiac failure); (b) large facial hemangiomas that usually involute with permanent disfiguring; (c) ulcerated hemangiomas; and (d) hemangiomas in the diaper area that are very likely to ulcerate causing severe pain.

- Medical treatment

  – Steroids including topical steroid application (class 1 corticosteroid applied twice daily with monitoring every 2 weeks), intralesional steroids (triamcinolone acetonide 10 mg/mL administered monthly), and oral steroids (1.5–2 mg/kg/d of prednisone) are the mainstay of treatment. Patients must be monitored closely, especially with oral steroid use given the risk of systemic complications including growth retardation and glucose alterations. Localized side effects include atrophy and yeast infection.

  – Other treatment options include topical imiquimod (applied daily), interferon-α (3 million units/m^2/d, SC), and vincristine (0.05 mg/kg/d if less than 10 kg, IV), especially in steroid-resistant IH. As interferon-α is associated with spastic diplegia, patients must be monitored closely.

- Propranolol at a dose of 2 mg/kg/d has been recently reported to be very effective in treating severe IHs, even in steroid-resistant IHs. This treatment is proposed to replace oral or intravenous steroids that are associated with significant side effects. However, patients on propranolol should be closely monitored for bradycardia, hypotension, and hypoglycemia especially at the onset of the treatment.

- Laser treatment

  – Pulsed dye laser (PDL) treatment induces significantly faster regression of the IH. Fluences lower than those of PWS are effective and are associated with lower risk of laser-induced scarring (Figs. 32.1, 32.2 and 32.3). PDL has been used extensively in the treatment of IH in three clinical scenarios:

    1. Ulcerated hemangiomas respond effectively to PDL. PDL markedly decreases the associated pain and induces rapid healing of the ulceration (75% within 2 weeks) (Fig. 32.4). Residual scar formation from the ulceration is expected.

    2. SHs can respond well to PDL if started either before or early in the proliferative phase. Multiple treatments, every 4 to 6 weeks, are required in the proliferative phase. The only exception is a rapidly proliferating facial hemangioma. PDL treatment may induce ulceration of these variants so treatment should be avoided. IH with deeper components (MH, DH) respond less effectively to PDL because of the limitation of penetration of PDL to 1.2 mm in the skin.

    3. PDL can help treat the residual erythema and telangiectasias on the surface of involuted hemangiomas.

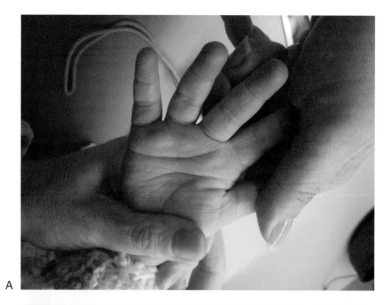

A

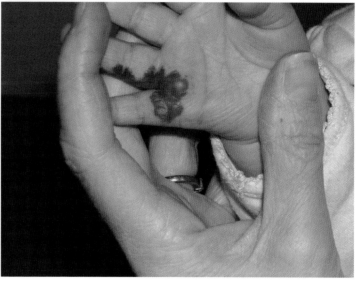

B

Figure 32.3 (A) *Segmental hemangioma involving the hand of a 1-year-old girl.* **(B)** *Complete resolution of the hemangioma after four treatments with 595-nm pulsed dye laser at low fluences*

– Long-pulsed Nd:YAG lasers are useful for photocoagulation of DHs but have a higher incidence of scarring.

• Other interventions include surgical debulking and embolization. The risks and benefits of each surgical approach should be considered carefully before intervention since the scar from spontaneous regression is usually better than the surgical scar. Embolization is utilized in hemangiomas associated with high-output cardiac failure.

PITFALLS TO AVOID

• Use of excessive PDL fluences without skin cooling can cause scar.

• Parents are understandably anxious about their child's hemangioma. A full discussion of the natural course of hemangiomas is mandatory prior to starting therapy. The option of foregoing treatment and clinically monitoring a patient should be reviewed carefully prior to starting treatment.

• Parents should also have a realistic idea of the limitations of therapy. Large hemangiomas respond less successfully to oral, surgical, and laser therapy. Complicated hemangiomas that may interfere with the child's health should be referred to an appropriate pediatric specialist. Parents must be aware that treatment will provide an improvement but may not result in full resolution of the hemangioma.

• Parents need to be educated on proper wound care, especially for ulcerated hemangiomas, in order to improve the child's quality of life.

• Fibrofatty changes are often a sequela of resolved hemangiomas. Such changes can be improved significantly with nonablative and ablative fractional resurfacing.

BIBLIOGRAPHY

Batta K, Goodyear HM, Moss C, Williams HC, Hiller L, Waters R. Randomised controlled study of early pulsed dye laser treatment of uncomplicated childhood haemangiomas: Results of a 1-year analysis. *Lancet.* 2002; 360(9332):521-527.

Léauté-Labrèze C, Dumas de la Roque E, Hubiche T, Boralevi F, Thambo J-B, Taïeb A. Propranolol for severe hemangiomas of infancy. *N Engl J Med.* 2008;358:2649-2651.

Li YC, McCahon E, Rowe NA, Martin PA, Wilcsek GA, Martin FJ. Successful treatment of infantile haemangiomas of the orbit with propranolol. *Clin Experiment Ophthalmol.* 2010;38(6):554-559.

Morelli JG, Tan OT, Yohn JJ, Weston WL. Treatment of ulcerated hemangiomas infancy. *Arch Pediatr Adolesc Med.* 1994;148(10):1104-1105.

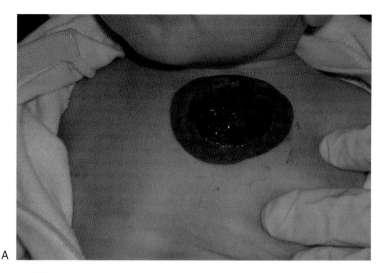

A

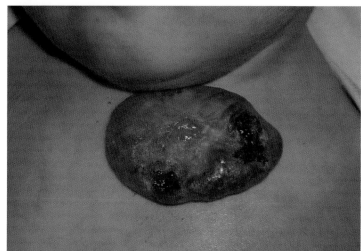

B

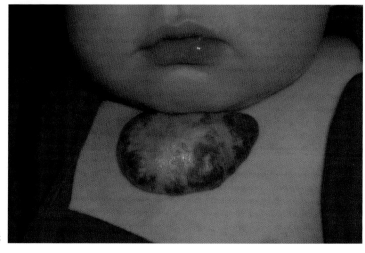

C

Figure 32.4 (A) *Ulcerated hemangioma, isolated nodular type, extremely painful and hemorrhaging, treated twice with pulsed dye laser 6 J/cm², 7-mm spot size, 590 nm.* **(B)** *At 2 months' follow-up, significant healing of the ulceration after a single treatment with pulsed dye laser.* **(C)** *Four months after initial pulsed dye laser treatment and 2 months after second pulsed dye laser treatment, there is complete healing of the ulceration*

CHAPTER 33 | Keratosis Pilaris Atrophicans

Keratosis pilaris atrophicans (KPA) is a group of inherited disorders with three subtypes including (a) keratosis pilaris atrophicans faciei (KPAF), (b) atrophoderma vermiculatum (AV), and (c) keratosis follicularis spinulosa decalvans (KFSD). KPAF and AV present mainly on the face with KFSD often appearing on the eyebrow and AV most commonly seen on the cheeks, sparing the eyebrows and scalp. KFSD can affect the face, scalp, and trunk. Inheritance pattern can be autosomal dominant (KPAF, AV), recessive (AV), or X-linked (KFSD).

EPIDEMIOLOGY

Incidence: very rare; KPAF is the most common subtype

Age: KPAF and KFSD in infancy; AV in childhood

Sex: males are more severely affected in KFSD

PATHOGENESIS

Abnormal follicular keratinization of the upper section of the hair follicle that may later result in atrophic follicular scarring.

PHYSICAL EXAMINATION

Follicular plugging with erythema in early stages (Figure 33.1). Atrophic follicular scar formation with associated alopecia in later stages.

DIFFERENTIAL DIAGNOSIS

Keratosis pilaris, keratosis pilaris rubra, seborrheic dermatitis (KPAF), atopic dermatitis (KFSD), other etiologies of scarring alopecia (KFSD), acne scarring (AV), Rombo syndrome (AV), and KID syndrome (KFSD).

DERMATOPATHOLOGY

Dilated follicles with follicular hyperkeratosis and inflammation in early stages. Follicular fibrosis and atrophy in later stages.

COURSE

The course is chronic with no spontaneous resolution. With time, the erythematous follicular hyperkeratotic papules involute into depressed atrophic follicular scars with alopecia.

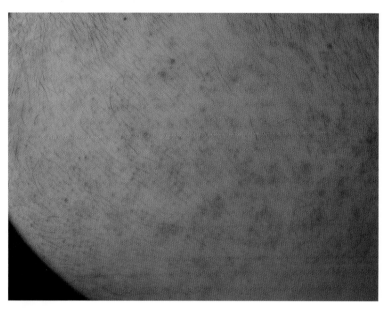

Figure 33.1 *Keratosis pilaris: fine, sandpaper-like follicular papules on the arm of a young man*

MANAGEMENT

There is no completely effective treatment for KPA. Multiple treatment options have been tried with only variable success. Patients should be counseled that therapy may not be effective.

- Topical therapy may, at best, produce modest benefit.
  - Lactic acid and α-hydroxy acid lotions (10%–12%) applied twice daily may improve the textural roughness. However, they may produce irritation.
  - Retinoids (tazarotene, retin-A) applied nightly may improve textural roughness. They may produce irritation.
  - Corticosteroids applied sparingly may show improvement. Risk of facial atrophy limits their use.
- Systemic therapy
  - Other options that have provided variable success include oral retinoids and dapsone.
  - They are most helpful for the inflammatory stage of KPA, but provide minimal improvement in the follicular hyperkeratosis.
  - They require careful monitoring for potential side effects.
- Laser therapy
  - Pulsed dye laser (595 nm, 7-mm spot, 7–10 J/cm^2, DCD 40/20, pulse duration of 1.5–3 ms) can be effective in the treatment of the associated erythema of KPAF but will not significantly improve the textural roughness of KPA (Fig. 33.2A, B).
  - Laser-assisted hair removal with long-pulsed non-Q-switched ruby laser may be an effective treatment in patients with KFSD.

PITFALLS TO AVOID

Patient expectations are generally very high. They must be counseled as to the chronic nature of the condition and minimal response to available therapies.

BIBLIOGRAPHY

Baden HP, Byers HR. Clinical findings, cutaneous pathology, and response to therapy in 21 patients with keratosis pilaris atrophicans. *Arch Dermatol.* 1994;130(4):469-475.

Chui CT, Berger TG, Price VH, Zachary CB. Recalcitrant scarring follicular disorders treated by laser-assisted hair removal: A preliminary report. *Dermatol Surg.* 1999; 25(1):34-37.

Clark SM, Mills CM, Lanigan SW. Treatment of keratosis pilaris atrophicans with the pulsed tunable dye laser. *J Cutan Laser Ther.* 2000;2(3):151-156.

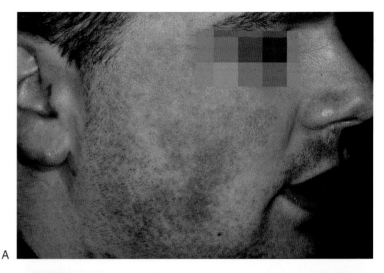

A

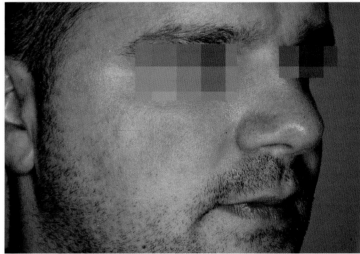

B

Figure 33.2 (A) *Keratosis pilaris atrophicans. Patient is emotionally bothered by persistent erythema.* **(B)** *Marked lightening of erythema 2 years following three pulsed dye laser treatments*

Kaune KM, Haas E, Emmert S, Schön MP, Zutt M. Successful treatment of severe keratosis pilaris rubra with a 595-nm pulsed dye laser. *Dermatol Surg.* 2009;35: 1592-1595.

Marqueling AL, Gilliam AE, Prendiville J, et al. Keratosis pilaris rubra: A common but underrecognized condition. *Arch Dermatol.* 2006;142(12):1611-1616.

Richard G, Harth W. Keratosis follicularis spinulosa decalvans. Therapy with isotretinoin and etretinate in the inflammatory stage. *Hautarzt.* 1993;44(8):529-534.

CHAPTER 34 | Port-wine Stains

Port-wine stains (PWS) are low-flow capillary malformations. They represent the most common type of vascular malformations. Any area of the body can be affected. However, the head and neck areas are most commonly affected.

EPIDEMIOLOGY

Incidence: 3 per 1,000 newborns

Age: present at birth in the majority of patients; rarely appear in adolescence or adulthood

Sex: no sex predilection

Race: less common in Asians and African Americans

Associated syndromes: PWS can be a manifestation of several syndromes including Sturge–Weber syndrome, Klippel–Trenaunay syndrome, Proteus syndrome, and phakomatosis pigmentovascularis

PHYSICAL EXAMINATION

PWS presents at birth as light pink, well-demarcated macular lesions and patches usually in a segmental distribution. They can transform with age into hypertrophic dark red and/or purpuric plaques with nodularity. PWS involves the face most commonly along the trigeminal nerve distribution: ophthalmic branch V1 (upper eyelid and forehead), maxillary branch V2 (upper lip, cheek, lower eyelid), and mandibular branch V3.

DIFFERENTIAL DIAGNOSIS

PWS exhibits characteristic clinical features and is seldom misdiagnosed. It can be confused with the macular stage of hemangioma at birth.

DERMATOPATHOLOGY

Multiple dilated thin-walled vessels in the papillary and reticular dermis.

ANCILLARY TESTS

- The parents should be counseled regarding the possibility of Sturge–Weber syndrome (SWS) in lesions located in a facial V1 or V2 dermatomal distribution. SWS is characterized by the presence of facial PWS with ipsilateral ocular and leptomeningeal anomalies. Ten to fifteen percent of patients with PWS in the V1 distribution will have SWS. Patients with bilateral PWS have even a higher risk of SWS. An ophthalmologic examination to rule out glaucoma and cataract formation with continued followup is necessary for these patients. A head computed tomography (CT) or magnetic resonance imaging (MRI) should be obtained to rule out brain involvement that could affect mental development and result in seizures.

- PWS overlying the spine can be associated with spinal anomaly such as spinal dysraphism or tethered spinal cord. Neurologic evaluation and appropriate imaging studies are recommended.

- Large extremity PWS should raise the consideration of Klippel—Trenaunay syndrome, characterized by capillary-venous malformations or capillary-lymphatic-venous malformations with hypertrophy of the affected extremity. Leg girth and length should be measured and followed over time.

COURSE

PWS grows proportionally with the patient and gradually thickens and darkens in color from pink to dark red to deep purple. Eleven percent may develop nodularity and 24% may develop pyogenic granulomas. PWS may be associated with hypertrophy of underlying soft tissue and bone, particularly in Sturge–Weber syndrome and Klippel–Trenaunay syndrome.

KEY CONSULTATIVE QUESTIONS

- Onset of lesion
- Associated clinical findings
- Is the child meeting developmental milestones?
- Has the child had an eye examination?
- Has the child had a head MRI or CT?
- Past treatments and response
- Bleeding
- Blebs
- Growth of PWS

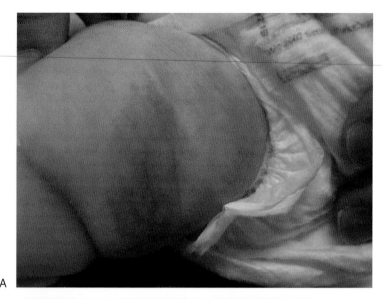

A

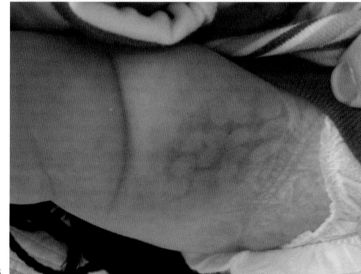

B

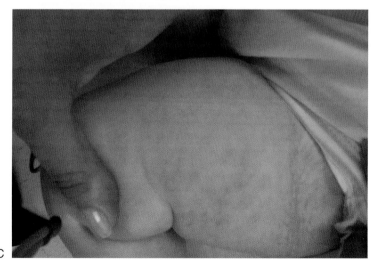

C

Figure 34.1 (A) *PWS on the right inner thigh of an infant girl.*
(B) *Significant lightening of the PWS after a single PDL treatment.*
(C) *Complete resolution of the PWS after PDL treatments*

MANAGEMENT

PWS demonstrates progressive vascular dilatation and hypertrophy with age, thus making treatment during early infancy essential for a better response. Treatment can be started as early as 2 weeks of age. Treatment provides a reduction in the number of vessels and does not completely remove the entire lesion. Therefore, the PWS may exhibit some darkening and thickening over time despite intervention. General anesthesia might be needed for treating large PWS in children.

• Laser treatment (Figs. 34.1–34.5).

Pulsed dye laser (PDL) remains the gold standard for the treatment of PWS. Effective PDL parameters include wavelengths of 585 to 600 nm, fluences of 6 to 15 J/cm^2, pulse durations of 0.45 or 1.5 ms with cryogen spray cooling (CSC). Four to twelve laser sessions with 4-to-8-week intervals are usually required in order to achieve significant blanching of the PWS. Lower fluences are initially utilized for PWS off the face and in darker skin types. The use of CSC concomitantly during PDL treatment significantly decreases the pain associated with the procedure and the incidence of blistering. CSC protects the epidermis and allows for delivery of higher fluences, resulting in more effective blanching of the PWS. PDL treatment is followed by temporary purpura that usually resolves in 7 to 14 days. Complete lightening of PWS with PDL treatment is achieved in less than 20% of PWS.

Resistance to PDL treatment is more frequently encountered in deeper and hypertrophic PWS. Helpful maneuvers to potentiate the efficacy of PDL include increasing the fluences with adequate cryogen cooling to protect the epidermis and increasing the wavelength up to 600 nm to target deeper vessels. A pilot study demonstrated that PWS that are treated with topical *imiquimod* once daily for 1 month after PDL exposure manifest superior blanching response over time as compared to PDL alone. Another report investigated the combined use of PDL and a topical angiogenesis inhibitor, *rapamycin*, using the in vivo rodent window chamber model. There was no reformation and reperfusion of blood vessels after treatment with PDL followed by topical rapamycin for 14 days, in contrast to PDL alone. With extreme caution to avoid scarring and dyspigmentation, it is possible to treat PDL-resistant PWS and deeper or hypertrophic adult PWS successfully with longer wavelength lasers that allow deeper penetration into the skin such as long-pulsed alexandrite (755 nm) laser, long-pulsed Nd:YAG (1,064 nm) laser, and dual 595-nm PDL and 1,064-nm Nd:YAG laser coupled with adequate cooling. Use of the Nd:YAG laser can be treacherous as there is a narrow therapeutic range. Risk of scar can be significant.

• Light treatment: intense pulsed light (IPL) may be effective in treatment of PWS, including PDL-resistant PWS. A green-yellow waveband and lowest available pulse

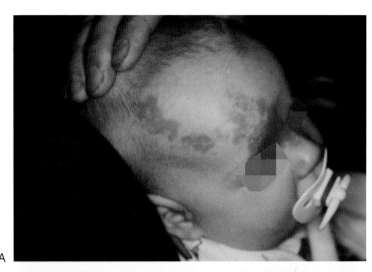

A

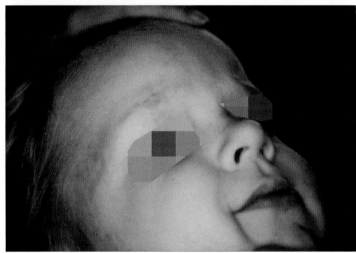

B

Figure 34.2 (A) *Extensive port-wine stain on the right face and forehead of an infant male.* **(B)** *Significant resolution after multiple treatments with pulsed dye laser*

duration should be used, with skin cooling. A recent randomized clinical trial comparing PDL and IPL side by side revealed a better efficacy and higher patient preference after PDL treatment. Photodynamic therapy may also prove to be an alternative efficacious treatment for PWS.

- Other treatment modalities for PWS that can be effective include tattooing and cosmetic makeup.

PITFALLS TO AVOID

- Patients should be counseled that PWS display a variable response to treatment. More extensive and thicker lesions respond less well when compared to superficial lesions. Facial PWS responds best. PWS treatment efficacy decreases as one descends from face to feet, with the lower extremities displaying the least treatment benefit.

- Multiple treatment sessions may be required. Bruising is a necessary side effect to obtain efficacious therapy.

- Laser treatment may produce "footprinting" or only partial improvement.

- Treatments should be ceased when the patient is satisfied with lightening, or when no further benefit has been noted, that is, after two subsequent treatments.

BIBLIOGRAPHY

Alster TS, Tanzi EL. Combined 595-nm and 1,064-nm laser irradiation of recalcitrant and hypertrophic port-wine stains in children and adults. *Dermatol Surg.* 2009;35(5):813-815.

Chang CJ, Hsiao YC, Mihm MC Jr, Nelson JS. Pilot study examining the combined use of pulsed dye laser and topical Imiquimod versus laser alone for treatment of port wine stain birthmarks. *Lasers Surg Med.* 2008;40(9): 605-610.

Chapas AM, Eickhorst K, Geronemus RG. Efficacy of early treatment of facial port wine stains in newborns: A review of 49 cases. *Lasers Surg Med.* 2007;39(7):563-568.

Chiu CH, Chan HH, Ho WS, Yeung CK, Nelson JS. Prospective study of pulsed dye laser in conjunction with cryogen spray cooling for treatment of port wine stains in Chinese patients. *Dermatol Surg.* 2003;29(9):909-915. Discussion 915.

Faurschou A, Togsverd-Bo K, Zachariae C, Haedersdal M. Pulsed dye laser vs. intense pulsed light for port-wine stains: A randomized side-by-side trial with blinded response evaluation. *Br J Dermatol.* 2009;160(2):359-364.

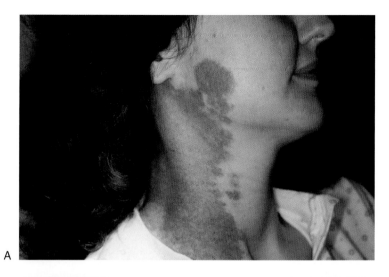

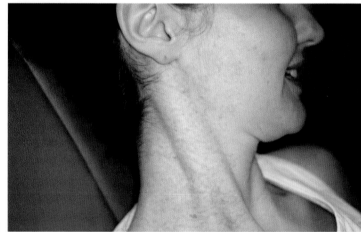

Figure 34.3 (A) *Extensive port-wine stain on the right neck of a young female.* **(B)** *Marked resolution of the port-wine stain after multiple treatments with pulsed dye laser*

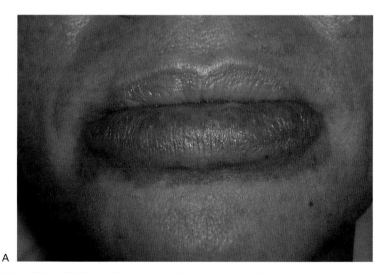

Figure 34.4 (A) *Port-wine stain on the lower mucosal and cutaneous lip.*

Ho WS, Ying SY, Chan PC, Chan HH. Treatment of port wine stains with intense pulsed light: A prospective study. *Dermatol Surg.* 2004;30(6):887-890.

Huikeshoven M, Koster PH, de Borgie CA, Beek JF, van Gemert MJ, van der Horst CM. Redarkening of port-wine stains 10 years after pulsed-dye-laser treatment. *N Engl J Med* 2007;356(12):1235-1240.

Li L, Kono T, Groff WF, Chan HH, Kitazawa Y, Nozaki M. Comparison study of a long-pulse pulsed dye laser and a long-pulse pulsed alexandrite laser in the treatment of port wine stains. *J Cosmet Laser Ther.* 2008;10(1): 12-15.

Phung TL, Oble DA, Jia W, Benjamin LE, Mihm MC Jr, Nelson JS. Can the wound healing response of human skin be modulated after laser treatment and the effects of exposure extended? Implications on the combined use of the pulsed dye laser and a topical angiogenesis inhibitor for treatment of port wine stain birthmarks. *Lasers Surg Med.* 2008;40(1):1-5.

Selim MM, Kelly KM, Nelson JS, Wendelschafer-Crabb G, Kennedy WR, Zelickson BD. Confocal microscopy study of nerves and blood vessels in untreated and treated portwine stains: Preliminary observations. *Dermatol Surg.* 2004;30:892-897.

Yang M, Yaroslavsky A, Farinelli, et al. Long-pulsed neodymium: Yttrium-aluminum-garnet laser treatment for port-wine stains. *J Am Acad Dermatol.* 2005;52(3): 480-490.

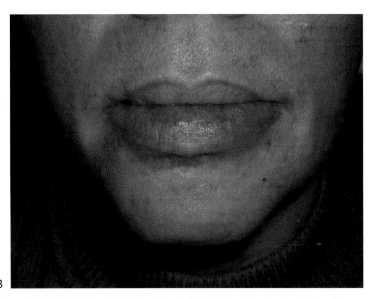

Figure 34.4 (*Continued*) (B) *Significant lightening of port-wine stain after three treatments with a combination of pulsed dye laser to the cutaneous lip and vermilion and long-pulsed 1,064-nm Nd:YAG laser to the inner mucosal lip and vermillion*

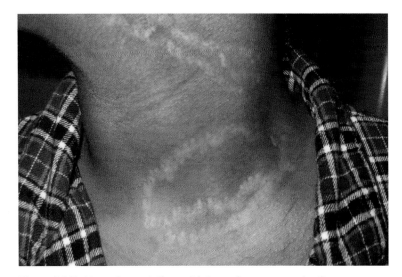

Figure 34.5 *Hypopigmentation, which can be permanent, after aggressive treatment of a PWS in an African-American patient*

CHAPTER 35 | Pyogenic Granuloma

Pyogenic granuloma (PG) can be regarded as a benign vascular tumor or as a reactive vascular process arising at sites of previous trauma or irritation. PG is also known as lobular capillary hemangioma, granuloma telangiectaticum, and granuloma gravidarum when presenting on the gingiva of pregnant women. It commonly occurs in areas of trauma including the face and fingers.

EPIDEMIOLOGY

Incidence: common

Age: most common in children and young adults

Precipitating factors: minor trauma, pregnancy, laser treatment of port-wine stains, isotretinoin

PATHOGENESIS

Reactive neovascularization suggested by common association with preexisting trauma or irritation and limited growth capacity.

PHYSICAL EXAMINATION

Red to violaceous, dome-shaped, friable papule or nodule, 0.5 to 1.5 cm in size, with smooth surface that frequently ulcerates (Figs. 35.1, 35.2 and 35.3).

DIFFERENTIAL DIAGNOSES

Nodular amelanotic melanoma, glomus tumor, hemangioma, squamous cell carcinoma (SCC) (Fig. 35.4), nodular basal cell carcinoma, wart, bacillary angiomatosis, Kaposi's sarcoma, and metastatic cancer.

DERMATOPATHOLOGY

Well-circumscribed exophytic lobular proliferation of capillaries with flattened and sometimes eroded overlying epidermis with peripheral epidermal "collarettes."

COURSE

PG usually grows rapidly over the course of weeks or months and then stabilizes. It bleeds frequently with minor trauma and can persist indefinitely if not treated.

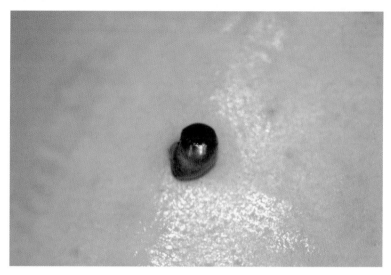

Figure 35.1 *Classic hemorrhagic pyogenic granuloma*

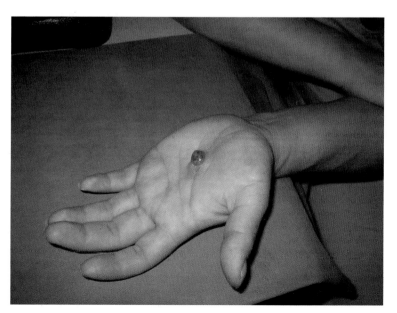

Figure 35.2 *Pyogenic granuloma on the palm of a pregnant woman, bleeding frequently*

MANAGEMENT

- Laser treatment

  - Pulsed dye laser (585–600 nm, 0.45–1.5 ms, 7–10 mm, 6–15 J/cm^2, DCD 20–40/20 with or without diascopy) is a safe and effective device for the treatment of small lesions and for pediatric patients. Serial treatments are usually required. Treatment is well tolerated without anesthesia. A recent report suggested shave excision followed by immediate pulse dye laser (PDL) for larger lesions. PDL has been also reported to be effective in gingival PG. Nd:YAG laser can also be effective.

  - Carbon dioxide is effective. Lesional flattening is the clinical endpoint. Intralesional lidocaine 1% is necessary prior to treatment. Postoperative care requires twice daily cleansing with soap and water and application of antibiotic ointment over a 2 to 6 weeks healing time. Scar formation is likely. A low recurrence rate is noted.

- Surgical treatment: all treatments may result in scar formation.

  - Shave excision followed by electrodessication of the base is the procedure most commonly employed. Recurrence is common (Figs. 35.5 and 35.6)

  - Elliptical excision can be performed with low recurrence but will leave a scar

  - Ligation of the base

  - Cryosurgery

- Alternative treatment options include

  - Imiquimod 5% cream has been recently reported to be effective in pediatric patients and in patients with recurrent PG

  - Intralesional injection of absolute ethanol

  - Sclerotherapy with monoethanolamine oleate

  - Topical alitretinoin (9-*cis*-retinoic cid) gel, a drug that is used for the treatment of Kaposi's sarcoma

PITFALLS TO AVOID

- Patients should be aware that recurrence is common after treatment.

- Patients should be informed that all treatments may result in scarring.

- Amelanotic melanoma as well as SCC and other skin cancers can mimic PG. A biopsy should be performed for any suspicious lesions in the appropriate clinical setting.

BIBLIOGRAPHY

Bourguignon R, Paquet P, Piérard-Franchimont C, Piérard GE. Treatment of pyogenic granulomas with the Nd-YAG laser. *J Dermatolog Treat.* 2006;17(4):247-249.

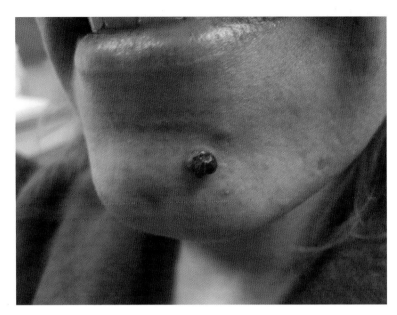

Figure 35.3 *Pyogenic granuloma overlying a dermal nevus*

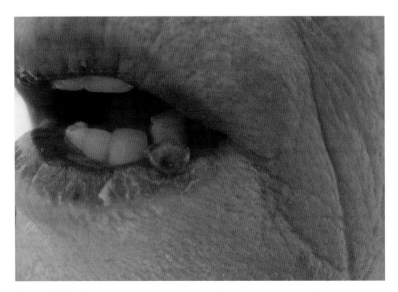

Figure 35.4 *Pyogenic granuloma mimicking a squamous cell carcinoma on the left lower mucosal lip of a patient with multiple nonmelanoma skin cancers*

Fallah H, Fischer G, Zagarella S. Pyogenic granuloma in children: Treatment with topical imiquimod. *Australas J Dermatol.* 2007;48(4):217-220

Khandpur S, Sharma VK. Successful treatment of multiple gingival pyogenic granulomas with pulsed-dye laser. *Indian J Dermatol Venereol Leprol.* 2008;74(3):275-277.

Maloney DM, Schmidt JD, Duvic M. Alitretinoin gel to treat pyogenic granuloma. *J Am Acad Dermatol.* 2002; 47(6):969-970.

Matsumoto K, Nakanishi H, Seike T, Koizumi Y, Mihara K, Kubo Y. Treatment of pyogenic granuloma with a sclerosing agent. *Dermatol Surg.* 2001;27(6):521-523.

Raulin C, Greve B, Hammes S. The combined continuouswave(pulsed carbon dioxide laser for treatment of pyogenic granuloma. *Arch Dermatol.* 2002;138(1):33-37.

Sud AR, Tan ST. Pyogenic granuloma complicating pulsed-dye laser therapy for cherry angioma. *J Plast Reconstr Aesthet Surg.* 2010;63(8):1364-1368.

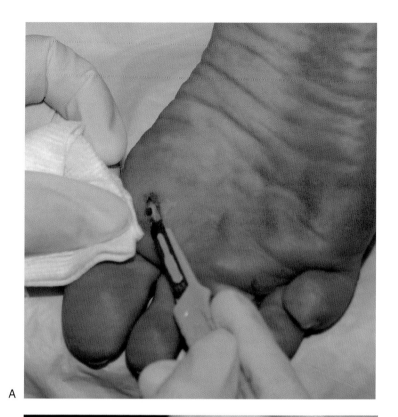

A

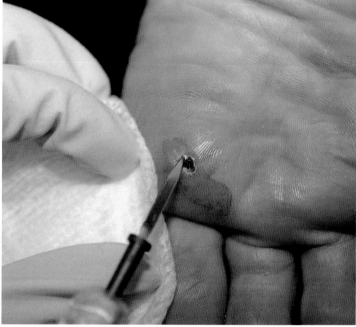

B

Figure 35.5 (A) *Shaving a hemorrhagic and painful pyogenic granuloma on the plantar foot with #15 blade. The specimen was sent for histological confirmation.* **(B)** *Electrodessication of the residual pyogenic granuloma*

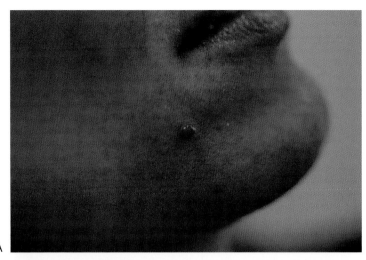

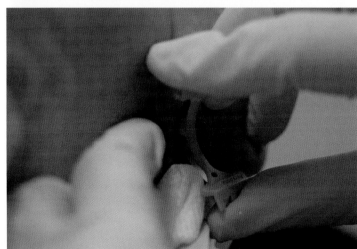

Figure 35.6 (A) *Biopsy-proven pyogenic granuloma on the right chin of a young female.* **(B)** *Shave excision of pyogenic granuloma with Derma Blade (Personna Medical, Verona, VA)*

CHAPTER 36 | Facial Telangiectasias

Facial telangiectasias are dilated vessels appearing superficially in the dermis mostly on the alae nasi. Telangiectasias are also common in scars and various skin lesions.

EPIDEMIOLOGY

Incidence: very common

Age: most common in adults and elderly people

Sex, race: no sex or race predisposition

Precipitating factors: chronic actinic damage, rosacea, and topical steroid use are the most common precipitating factors. Other less common etiologies include hereditary hemorrhagic telengiectasia, Cockayne syndrome, ataxia telengiectasia, Bloom's syndrome, Rothmund–Thomson syndrome, scleroderma, CREST syndrome, lupus, and radiation dermatitis

PHYSICAL EXAMINATION

Telangiectasias consist of fine, tiny, erythematous linear vessels, typically 0.2 to 2 mm in diameter, coursing along the surface of the skin, which blanch easily upon pressure.

DERMATOPATHOLOGY

Dilated, thin-walled vessels in the upper dermis.

COURSE

Facial telangiectasias are usually chronic in nature with no spontaneous resolution.

MANAGEMENT

Facial telangiectasias are frequently treated for cosmetic purposes. Multiple effective treatment options exist.

- Laser treatment: multiple effective options are available. Patients must be aware that over time they are likely to develop more telangiectasias.
  - Pulsed dye lasers (PDL) are the treatment of choice for facial telangiectasias (Figs. 36.1–36.5).
    - The traditional PDL with a short pulse duration of 0.45 or 1.5 ms provides the most effective treatment for facial telangiectasias. However, posttreatment purpura occurs which generally lasts 7 to 14 days

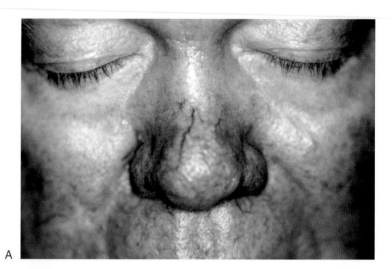

A

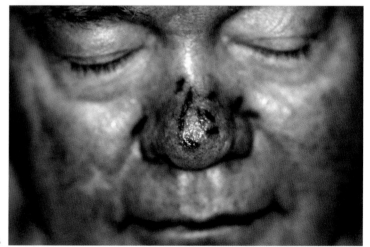

B

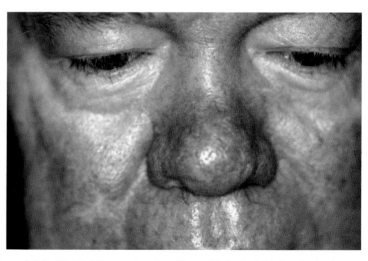

C

Figure 36.1 (A) *Middle-aged male with multiple facial telangiectasias.* **(B)** *Purpura observed immediately after pulsed dye laser treatment.* **(C)** *Significant reduction in telangiectasias after a single-pulsed dye laser treatment*

○ Newer generation 595-nm PDL (ie, V-beam or V-beam Perfecta lasers, Candela Corp., Wayland, MA) with variable pulse durations (0.45, 1.5, 3, 6, 10, 20, 30, 40 ms) can provide a reduced purpura treatment of facial telangiectasias when longer pulse durations are utilized, but is somewhat less effective and usually requires multiple treatments

❏ Commonly, subpurpuric fluences of less than 10 J/cm^2 at pulse duration of 10 ms, with a 7-mm spot size are utilized.

❏ Better efficacy of the variable-pulse PDL in treating facial telangiectasias can be achieved by utilizing purpuric fluences or by pulse stacking with subpurpuric pulses (stacked 2–4 subpupuric pulses at a 1.5-Hz repetition rate, 7.5 J/cm^2, 10-ms pulse duration, 10-mm spot size, DCD of 30/20) or by performing multiple passes during the same session.

❏ Larger thicker linear vessels can be treated with the newest generation 595-nm long-PDL (V-beam Perfecta, Candela Corp., Wayland, MA) using a 3 × 10 mm elliptical spot size, 40-ms pulse duration, 15 to 17 J/cm^2, and DCD 30 to 40/20. The endpoint is transient bluish darkening of the vessel followed by vessel blanching (Figs. 36.4 and 36.5). This treatment may result in mild purpura in around 23% of patients.

○ Facial edema, erythema, and discomfort can occur after extensive treatment with the purpura-free variable-pulse PDL. However, these undesired effects are generally better tolerated when compared to a purpura-inducing laser treatment

– The variable pulse width 1,064-nm Nd:YAG laser has proven to be effective in the treatment of facial telangiectasias. Shorter pulse widths with higher fluences might be necessary for effective treatment of smaller vessels but have an increased risk of blister and scar formation. The sequential delivery of 595- and 1,064-nm wavelength has been reported to be more effective than a single wavelength treatment.

– Frequency-doubled 532-nm Nd:YAG laser also called potassium-titanyl-phosphate (KTP) laser provides effective absorption of hemoglobin with a pulse duration of 1 to 50 ms making it ideally suited to treat superficial vessels without purpura formation. Tracing of individual vessels is a useful technique for patients with a countable number of discrete, visible vessels.

• Flashlamp (intense pulsed light [IPL]) treatment

– IPL provides another effective, purpura-free method for reducing facial telangiectasias and erythema (Fig. 36.6). For example, fluences of 30 to 40 J/cm^2 with 20-ms pulse duration are effective with the Starlux Lux G handpiece (Palomar Medical Technologies,

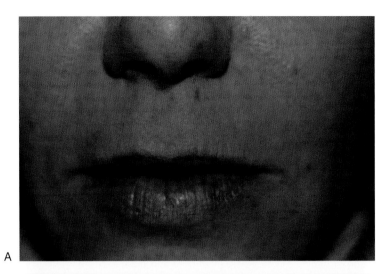

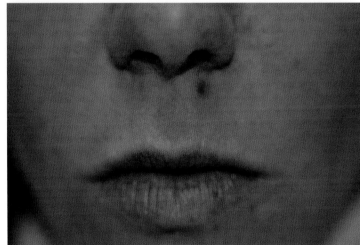

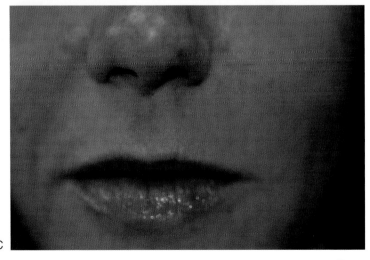

Figure 36.2 (A) *Telangiectasias prior to pulsed dye laser treatment. The setting was 10-mm spot, 595 nm, 8 J/cm^2, 6-ms pulse duration.* **(B)** *Immediately posttreatment.* **(C)** *Ten days after pulsed dye laser treatment*

Burlington, MA). The treatment endpoint is immediate vessel clearance or selective vessel darkening. Multiple treatments may be required for the greatest treatment benefit.

- Other treatment options include electrosurgery, cryotherapy, and infiltration of sclerosing agents. These are less selective, often less effective, and more likely to result in scarring than laser or IPL treatment

PITFALLS TO AVOID

- Treatment typically is well tolerated
- Obvious posttreatment purpura for 7 to 14 days with purpuric settings is expected
- Purpura can be avoided by utilizing nonpurpuric settings at the expense of decreased efficacy
- Facial edema, erythema, and discomfort can occur after extensive treatment with the purpura-free variable-pulse PDL
- Telangiectasias will recur over years
- Caution in darker skin types

BIBLIOGRAPHY

Bernstein EF, Kligman A. Rosacea treatment using the new-generation, high-energy, 595 nm, long pulse-duration pulsed-dye laser. *Lasers Surg Med.* 2008;40(4):233-239.

Jørgensen GF, Hedelund L, Haedersdal M. Long-pulsed dye laser versus intense pulsed light for photodamaged skin: A randomized split-face trial with blinded response evaluation. *Lasers Surg Med.* 2008;40(5):293-299.

Karsai S, Roos S, Raulin C. Treatment of facial telangiectasia using a dual-wavelength laser system (595 and 1,064 nm): A randomized controlled trial with blinded response evaluation. *Dermatol Surg.* 2008;34(5):702-708.

Rohrer TE, Chatrath V, Iyengar V. Does pulse stacking improve the results of treatment with variable-pulse pulsed-dye lasers? *Dermatol Surg.* 2004;30(2, pt 1):163-167. Discussion 167.6.

Ross EV, Uebelhoer NS, Domankevitz Y. Use of a novel pulse dye laser for rapid single-pass purpura-free treatment of telangiectases. *Dermatol Surg.* 2007;33(12):1466-1469.

Sarradet DM, Hussain M, Goldberg DJ. Millisecond 1064-nm neodymium:YAG laser treatment of facial telangiectases. *Dermatol Surg.* 2003;29(1):56-58.

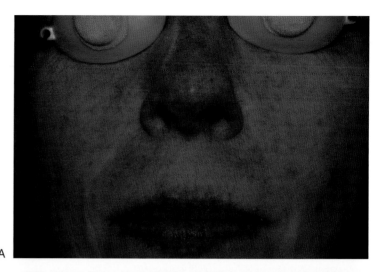

A

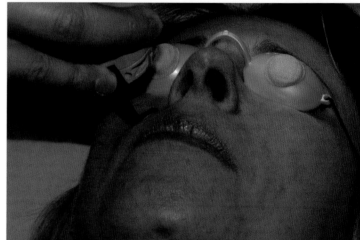

B

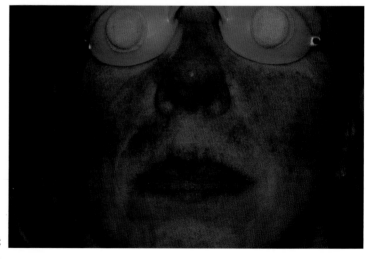

C

Figure 36.3 (A) *Female with centrofacial telangiectasias and erythema prior to pulsed dye laser therapy.* **(B)** *Pulsed dye laser treatment at a wavelength of 595 nm, 10-ms pulse duration, 7 J/cm², 7-mm spot size.* **(C)** *Appropriate clinical endpoint of erythema and slight edema at sites of treatment. No purpura was produced*

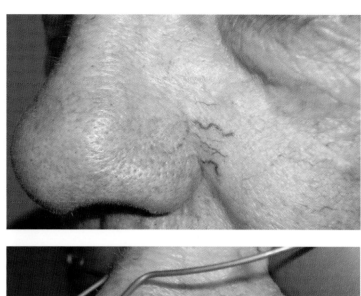

A

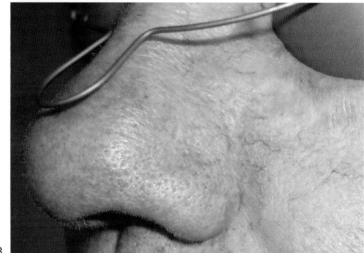

B

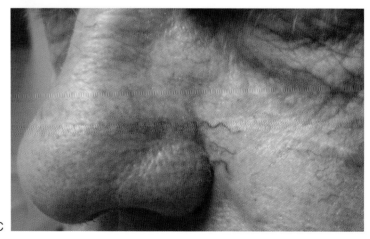

C

Figure 36.4 *Telangiectasias prior to long pulse-duration pulsed dye laser treatment. The settings were 40-ms pulse duration, 7-mm spot, 595 nm, 12J/cm². **(B)** Note the transient vasoconstriction with almost complete disappearance of the telangiectasias immediately posttreatment. **(C)** Slight decrease in diameter of the telangiectasias 1 month after one treatment*

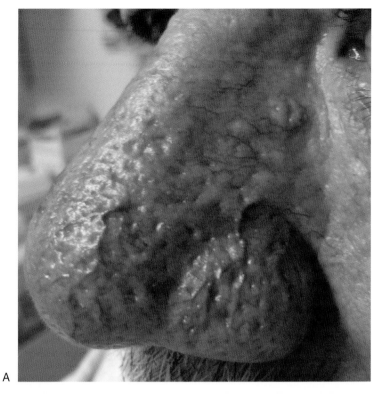

A

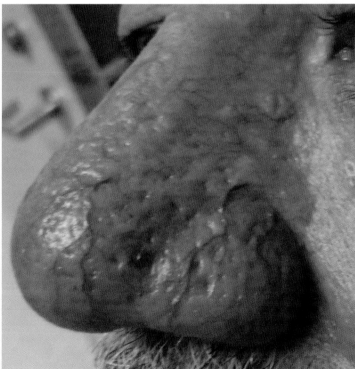

B

Figure 36.5 (A) *Large caliber nasal telangiectasias on the nose prior to long-pulse duration pulsed dye laser treatment. **(B)** Decrease in the diameter of the telangiectasias after six treatments with PDL using long pulse duration of 40 ms, 7-mm spot size, and fluences up to 11.5 J/cm².*

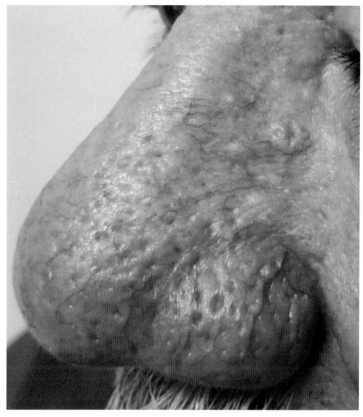

C

Figure 36.5 (*Continued*) **(C)** *Marked resolution of the telangiectasias after an additional four PDL treatments utilizing short pulse duration of 1.5 ms, 7-mm spot size, and 12J/cm²*

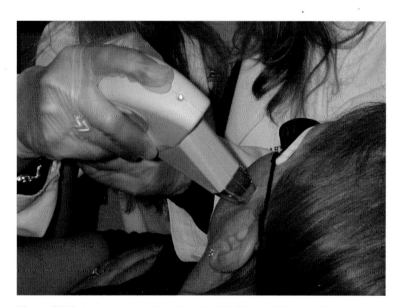

Figure 36.6 *Intense pulsed treatment with Starlux (Palomar Inc., Burlington, MA) of facial telangiectasias. The handpiece is in full contact with the skin*

CHAPTER 37 Lower Extremity Telangiectasias, Reticular and Varicose Veins

Lower extremity telangiectasias, reticular and varicose veins develop as a result of venous system impairment.

EPIDEMIOLOGY

Incidence: very common and the incidence increases with age. Reticular veins can occur in up to 10% of children 10 to 12 years old. The incidence of varicose veins in the seventh decade is 72% in women and 43% in men

Age: more common in adults and elderly

Sex: more common in women

Precipitating factors: familial predisposition, pregnancy, static gravitational pressures, dynamic muscular forces, hormonal influences

PATHOPHYSIOLOGY

Venous pathology develops when venous return is impaired for any reason.

It can develop from venous obstruction (thrombotic or nonthrombotic) or from venous valvular incompetence.

PHYSICAL EXAMINATION

Lower extremity telangiectasias are red to violaceous in color and up to 2 mm in diameter. Reticular veins are blue to blue-green in color and up to 4 mm in diameter. Varicose veins are blue to blue-green in color with a diameter greater than 3 to 4 mm.

LABORATORY DATA

■ Dermatopathology

Dilated vascular channels in the dermis.

■ Vascular Studies

Doppler ultrasound and/or duplex scanning are indicated in the following clinical scenarios:

- Asymptomatic varicosity greater than 4 mm in diameter
- Symptomatic veins
- Reticular, perforating, and/or varicose veins
- Signs of venous insufficiency or stasis changes
- Prior history of deep vein thrombosis or thrombophlebitis
- Prior history of sclerotherapy with recurrences or bad outcome

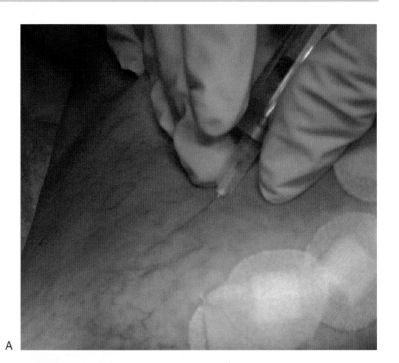

A

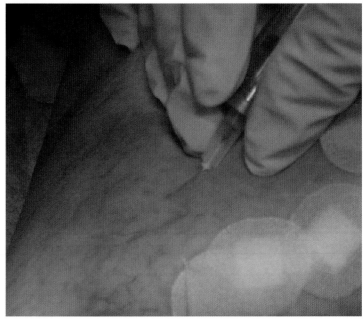

B

Figure 37.1 (A) *Sclerotherapy of spider veins. The needle is bent at a 45-degree angle and the vessel is canalized.* **(B)** *Immediate vessel blanching seen after injecting the sclerosant agent*

MANAGEMENT

■ Sclerotherapy (Figs. 37.1–37.3)

Sclerotherapy is the treatment of choice for lower leg telangiectasias and reticular veins. It should be repeated at 6 to 8 week intervals. Patients may require two to six sclerotherapy sessions to achieve the greatest treatment benefit.

Sclerosing agents

An ideal sclerosing agent causes complete local endothelial destruction of the vessel wall with secondary fibrosis and lumen obliteration, with no systemic toxicity. Sclerosing agents are classified into three groups depending on their mechanism of action of inducing endothelial injury. These include hyperosmotic agents, detergents, and chemical irritants (Tables 37.1 and 37.2). The most commonly used sclerosant agents in the United States are hypertonic saline (HS) and sodium tetradecyl sulfate (STS). Both HS and STS are FDA approved and have lowest incidence of allergenicity. Sodium morrhuate and polidocanol are also FDA approved.

Sclerotherapy technique for telangiectasias and reticular veins

- Fill the sclerosant agent into 3 cm^3 disposable syringes with disposable 30-gauge half inch needles.
- Swab the site to be treated with alcohol to better visualize the vessels.
- Treat larger vessels first.
- Bend the needle at a 30-degree angle to 45-degree angle.
- Stretch the skin overlying the vessels being treated.
- Insert the needle slowly in the vessel wall. You may use the air bolus technique by injecting less than 0.5 cm^3 of air in the vessel or the puncture-fill technique relying on the feel associated with vessel wall perforation while injecting. The empty vein technique, performed by elevating the leg and gently kneading the vein prior to injection, allows for thrombus reduction and need for smaller sclerosant volumes. When treating reticular and varicose veins, aspirate a small amount of blood to confirm intravascular location.
- Inject the sclerosant very slowly to ensure sufficient contact of the sclerosant with the vessel endothelial wall and to prevent distention and rupture. Inject less than 0.5 cm^3 per injection at 3-cm intervals.
- Apply small circular band aids, taped cotton balls or rolls at the injection sites for compression.

Foam sclerotherapy

A treatment modification can be made for larger vessels by vigorously foaming an air-sclerosant solution just prior to injection to induce a solution that displaces blood and remains for an extended time in the target vessel without

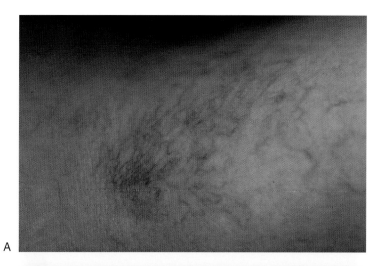

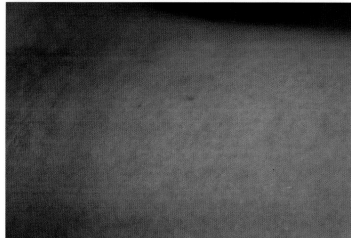

Figure 37.2 (A) *Spider veins, prior to treatment with sclerotherapy.* **(B)** *Marked resolution of the spider veins after sclerotherapy treatment*

being flushed. Theoretically, lower sclerosant concentrations can be used with a lower incidence of pigmentation and matting (Tables 37.2 and 37.3). The foaming detergent of either sotradechol or polidocanol is prepared by mixing the detergent with air (usually 1:4 mL ratio of detergent to air) in a back and forth motion using a three-way stop lock until a foamed emulsion is created. The foam sclerosant is injected in a manner similar to that with other sclerotherapy techniques.

Postoperative care

- Compression increases the efficacy of sclerotherapy and decreases the incidence of hyperpigmentation. Elastic compression stockings (15–60 mmHg) are highly recommended immediately following sclerotherapy and up to 2 to 3 weeks after the procedure, especially posttreatment of larger caliber vessels. Fashion hose (15–18 mmHg) and Class I hose (20–30 mmHg) are the most commonly used graduated compression hose used postsclerotherapy of telangiectasias and reticular veins.

- Encourage walking to avoid thromboembolic diseases.

- Avoid sun exposure to minimize posttreatment hyperpigmentation.

Complications (Table 37.3)

- Postsclerotherapy hyperpigmentation (PSH): The incidence of PSH can be up to 30% depending on the technique used, the size of the treated vessels, the type of sclerosing agent, and the solution concentration. Postsclerotherapy compression decreases the incidence of PSH. PSH is caused by perivascular deposition of hemosiderin rather than melanin and follows the

A

B

Figure 37.3 (A) *Lower leg telangiectasias at baseline.* **(B)** *Marked resolution of the telangiectasias 1 month after one sclerotherapy treatment. Note the development of slight telangiectatic matting superior to the treated area*

TABLE 37.1 ■ Sclerosing Agents

Sclerosant class	Sclerosant types	Mechanism
Hyperosmotic agents	Hypertonic saline (10–30%)	Dehydration
	Hypertonic saline (10%) dextrose (25%) (Sclerodex)	
Detergents	Sodium tetradecyl sulfate (Sotradechol, Thromboinject)	Surface tension change
	Polidocanol (Aethoxysclerol, Aetoxisclerol, Sclerovein)	
	Sodium morrhuate (Scleromate)	
	Ethanolamine oleate	
Chemical irritants	Polyiodide iodide (Varigloban, Variglobin, Sclerodine)	Corrosives
	Glycerin (72%) with 8% chromium potassium alum (Chromex)	

TABLE 37.2 ■ Recommended Sclerosant Concentration

Sclerosant/recommended concentration	Telangiectasias	Reticular veins	Varicose veins	Dose limitation
Hypertonic saline	11.7–23.4%	23.4%	Not commonly used	6–10 mL of 18–30% solution
Sodium tetradecyl sulfate	0.1–0.5%	0.3–0.5%, 0.1–0.25% foam	0.5–3%, 0.5–1% foam	10 mL of 3% solution

TABLE 37.3 ■ Complications of Sclerotherapy

Sclerosant	Allergenicity	Cramping	Pain	Hyperpigmentation	Telangiectatic matting	Skin necrosis
Hypertonic saline	–	+	+	+	+	+
Sodium tetradecyl sulfate	+ Anaphylaxis (rare, < 0.01%)	–	+	+	+	+

course of the treated site. The pigmentation usually resolves in 6 to 12 months. It can improve with the use of intense pulsed light (IPL).

- Telangiectatic matting (TM): The incidence of TM can be up to 16%. It consists of a network of blush-like, fine (<0.2 mm) telangiectatic vessels surrounding a previously treated area, occurring within days to months after sclerotherapy. They usually resolve within 3 to 12 months. Predisposing factors include pregnancy, obesity, hormonal therapy, and family history of telangiectasias. TM can improve with pulsed dye laser or IPL. Ways to avoid this complication include

  - Lower injection pressure

  - Lower sclerosant volume (up to 1.0 mL per injection site)

  - Lower sclerosant concentration

  - Limiting blanching (up to 1–2 cm)

- Skin necrosis and ulceration: Necrosis can occur secondary to extravasation of the sclerosing agent into the tissue, regardless of the technique used or the sclerosant type. To minimize extravasation, the surgeon should stop the injection when encountering

  - Even slight resistance to injection

  - Bleb formation

  - Increased pain reported by the patient

If extravasation is recognized immediately, the surgeon can inject normal saline at the site or apply 2% nitroglycerin paste.

- Other complications include pain and cramping (common), allergic reactions (rare), superficial thrombophlebitis (up to 1%), and thromboembolic reactions (very rare).

■ Laser and Intense Pulsed Light Therapies (Figs. 37.4 and 37.5)

Lasers and IPL sources can occasionally be successful in the treatment of lower extremity telangiectasias and reticular veins, especially when coupled with longer pulse duration and cooling devices. They are considered second-line treatment after sclerotherapy. Wavelengths in the range of 500 to 1,100 nm are most effective, with shorter wavelengths [eg, pulsed dye laser (PDI), potassium titanyl phosphate (KTP)] being used for red superficial blood

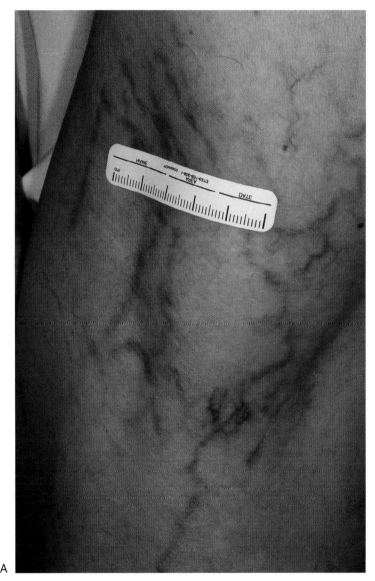

A

Figure 37.4 (A) *Marked erythema immediately after pulsed dye laser treatment to lower extremity spider veins.*

vessels and longer wavelengths (eg, 755-nm Alexandrite laser with around 60 ms pulse duration, 1064 Nd:YAG laser) for bluish deeper blood vessels. Indications for laser/IPL treatments include the following:

- Needle phobic patients
- Vessels resistant to sclerotherapy
- Vessels located below the ankle
- TM
- Propensity for PSH or TM

▪ Ambulatory Phlebectomy, Endovascular Techniques, Surgical Ligation/Stripping

Multiple treatment options exist for varicose veins including ambulatory phlebectomy, endovascular laser ablation, endovascular radiofrequency obliteration, as well as surgical ligation and stripping procedures. Ambulatory phlebectomy can be used for large varicosities. Endovenous occlusion can be achieved with radiofrequency (RF) or laser sources. Either a laser fiber or an RF catheter is inserted into the saphenous vein at or just below the knee. Laser systems include 810-nm diode, 940-nm diode, 980-nm diode, and 1,320-nm Nd:YAG lasers. These devices spare the need for general anesthesia and extended recovery time associated with vein stripping and ligation. There is little downtime, with patients resuming normal activities on the same day of the procedure.

BIBLIOGRAPHY

Barrett JM, Allen B, Ockelford A, Goldman MP. Microfoam ultrasound-guided sclerotherapy of varicose veins in 100 legs. *Dermatol Surg.* 2004;30(1):6-12.

Coleridge Smith P. Sclerotherapy and foam sclerotherapy for varicose veins. *Phlebology.* 2009;24(6):260-269.

Kahle B, Leng K. Efficacy of sclerotherapy in varicose veins—prospective, blinded, placebo-controlled study. *Dermatol Surg.* 2004;30(5):723-728.

Kern P, Ramelet AA, Wütschert R, Hayoz D. Compression after sclerotherapy for telangiectasias and reticular leg veins: A randomized controlled study. J Vasc Surg. 2007;45(6):1212-1216.

Morrison N, Neuhardt DL. Foam sclerotherapy: Cardiac and cerebral monitoring. *Phlebology.* 2009;24(6):252-259.

Ross EV, Meehan KJ, Gilbert S, Domankevitz Y. Optimal pulse durations for the treatment of leg telangiectasias with an alexandrite laser. *Lasers Surg Med.* 2009;41(2): 104-109.

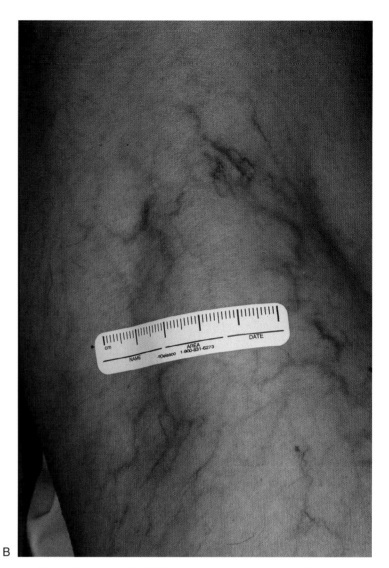

B

Figure 37.4 (*Continued*) (B) *Mild reduction in spider veins after a single pulsed dye laser treatment*

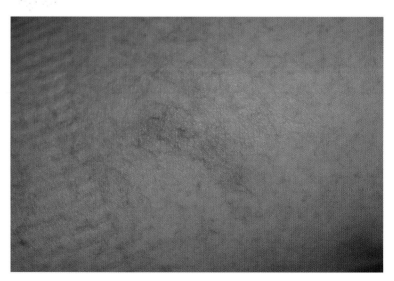

Figure 37.5 *Postinflammatory changes after laser leg vein treatment*

CHAPTER 38 | Venous Lakes

Venous lakes are benign vascular lesions that result from dilated venules. They commonly affect the lips, face, and ears.

EPIDEMIOLOGY

Incidence: common

Age: most commonly observed in the elderly

Precipitating factors: may be related to sun exposure

PHYSICAL EXAMINATION

Venous lake presents as dark blue to violaceous, elevated, soft, and easily compressible *papule or nodule.*

DIFFERENTIAL DIAGNOSES

Pyogenic granuloma, melanoma, *labial melanotic macule, atypical nevus,* hemangioma.

DERMATOPATHOLOGY

Dilated thin-walled venules in the superficial dermis. Thrombosis may be observed.

EPILUMINESCENCE MICROSCOPY

Epiluminescence microscopy (ELM) reveals erythematous globules with no pigmentary network. It is helpful in differentiating this vascular lesion from a melanocytic lesion.

COURSE

They usually persist for years and can bleed after trauma.

MANAGEMENT

Venous lakes are frequently treated for cosmetic purposes. Multiple treatment options exist.

- Light treatment
  - Lasers (Figs. 38.1 38.3)
    - Pulsed dye laser (585–595 nm, 0.45–1.5 ms, 5–10 mm spot, 7–10 J/cm², DCD 30–40/20, with and without diascopy). *Pulsed dye laser provides inconsistent benefit for venous lakes.*

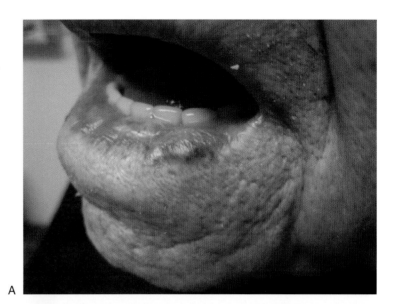

A

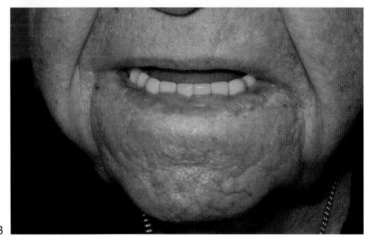

B

Figure 38.1 (A) *Venous like on the lower lip of an elderly man.* **(B)** *Marked resolution of the venous lake after multiple treatment sessions with the pulsed dye laser*

○ Diode laser (800–810 nm, 30 ms, 30–50 J/cm²) can also be a very effective treatment. It is helpful to allow 3 seconds of compression of the lesion with the chill tip prior to the laser pulse. A physical "kickback" is often felt by the laser surgeon at the time of the pulsation. The clinical endpoint is immediate purpura.

○ Long-pulsed Nd:YAG laser and intense pulsed light (IPL) have also been reported to be effective.

• Sclerotherapy: In one study, intralesional injections with 1% polidocanol have been shown to be effective in clearing two venous lakes after two sessions of sclerotherapy. *A scar* was noted to occur in one patient.

• Electrosurgery, surgical excision, cryotherapy are other alternate treatment options. However, these modalities can result in a scar.

PITFALLS

• Often requires several treatments with laser.

• All therapeutic modalities may produce a scar.

BIBLIOGRAPHY

Bekhor PS. Long-pulsed Nd:YAG laser treatment of venous lakes: Report of a series of 34 cases. *Dermatol Surg.* 2006;32(9):1151-1154.

Jay H, Borek C. Treatment of a venous-lake angioma with intense pulsed light. *Lancet.* 1998;351(9096):112.

Kuo HW, Yang CH. Venous lake of the lip treated with a sclerosing agent: Report of two cases. *Dermatol Surg.* 2003;29(4):425-428.

Wall TL, Grassi AM, Avram MM. Clearance of multiple venous lakes with an 800-nm diode laser: A novel approach. *Dermatol Surg.* 2007;33(1):100-103.

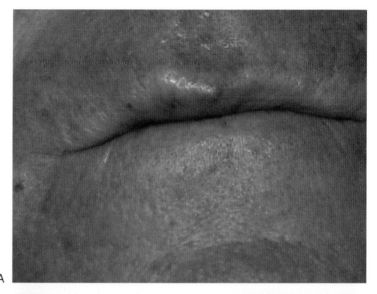

A

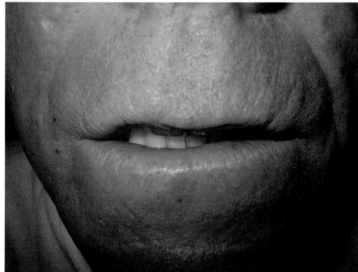

B

Figure 38.2 (A) *Venous lake on the upper lip.* **(B)** *Five-month follow-up demonstrating complete resolution of the venous lake after a single treatment with an 800-nm diode lase, 30-ms pulse duration, at energy settings of 45 J/cm² (one pulse), and 50 J/cm² (one pulse)*

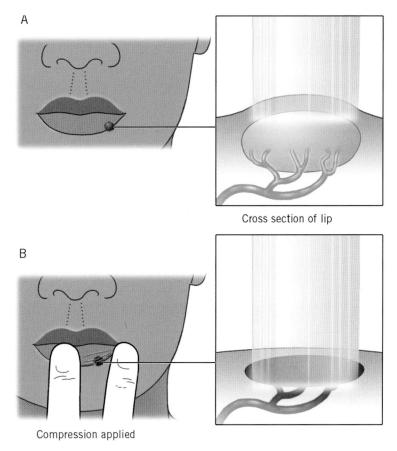

A

Cross section of lip

B

Compression applied

Figure 38.3 *Clinical efficacy of pulsed dye laser for a venous lake with compression of the vessels during treatment versus no compression*

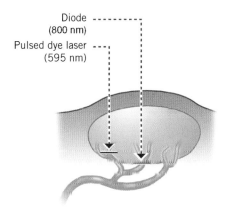

Diode - - - - - - - - -
(800 nm)
Pulsed dye laser - - - -
(595 nm)

Laser penetration: pulsed dye vs diode

Figure 38.4 *Pulsed dye laser does not penetrate deep enough. Compression is needed. Diode laser penetrates deeper and therefore is more effective than PDL*

CHAPTER 39 | Warts

Viral warts are caused by human papillomaviruses (HPV). Various types of HPV-induced warts exist including common warts (70% of all warts), palmoplantar warts, plane warts, and genital warts.

EPIDEMIOLOGY

Incidence: common

Age: children and adults

Precipitating factors: skin trauma, immunosuppression (HIV and transplant patients), genetic predisposition (epidermodysplasia verruciformis)

PATHOGENESIS

HPVs are nonenveloped double-stranded DNA viruses that produce infection and induction of hyperproliferation when the virus enters proliferating basal epithelial cells. Avoidance of host immune surveillance occurs. Exact mechanisms of infection, latency, and reactivation of HPV are unknown.

PHYSICAL EXAMINATION

Warts present as single or multiple hyperkeratotic, exophytic, skin-colored papules, nodules or plaques. They can have finger-like projections (filiform warts) or can be flat-topped (plane warts). Black punctate dots representing thrombosed capillaries are observed frequently. They most commonly present on fingers, dorsal hands, plantar surfaces, and pressure areas.

DIFFERENTIAL DIAGNOSES

Hypertrophic actinic keratosis, seborrheic keratosis, squamous cell carcinoma, verrucous carcinoma, and acral amelanotic melanoma. Plantar warts can also be mistaken for corns or calluses.

DERMATOPATHOLOGY

The epidermis features hyperkeratosis, acanthosis, papillomatosis, with tiers of parakeratosis, valleys of hypergranulosis and koilocytosis. The dermis features dilated capillary loops and hemorrhage.

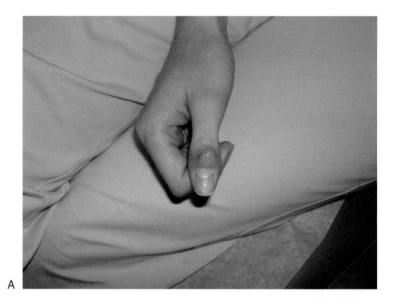

A

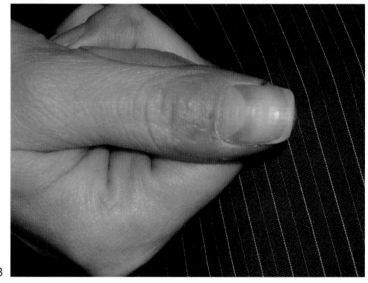

B

Figure 39.1 (A) *Verruca vulgaris on the left thumb immediately posttreatment with pulsed dye laser, 590-nm wavelength, 7-mm spot size, 10 J/cm², with pulse stacking.* **(B)** *Five-month follow-up with complete resolution of the wart after single pulsed dye laser treatment*

COURSE

They generally resolve spontaneously in immunocompetent patients, but this may take years. They tend to persist and resist treatment in immunosuppressed patients. Autoinoculation by scratching may occur.

MANAGEMENT

There is no current specific antiviral therapy for HPV. There are multiple treatment options that either induce local physical destruction of the warts or stimulate the immune response against HPV infection or both. Squamous cell carcinoma can arise from some lesions, that is, condylomata and epidermodysplasia verruciformis and require continuous monitoring. Histological evaluation should be considered for warts that are unresponsive to multiple treatment modalities to rule out malignancy.

■ Topical Treatment

Patients should be educated as to the viral, infectious, and recurrent nature of HPV despite therapeutic intervention. Patients must also be informed of the need for repetitive treatments for all treatment modalities employed. Multiple effective topical treatments exist. There is no current treatment of choice.

- Localized tissue destruction: salicylic acid, 5% cantharone, trichloracetic acid, and 0.5% podophyllotoxin are employed daily. Localized wart occlusion with duct tape has demonstrated efficacy in a study. Surrounding normal tissue may demonstrate temporary maceration during treatment.

- Viral cell division alteration: intralesional bleomycin (0.4 mg/mL) in normal preserved saline; 5-fluorouracil cream.

- Immune modulation: topical imiquimod has demonstrated efficacy.

■ Surgical Treatment

Lasers (Table 39.1)

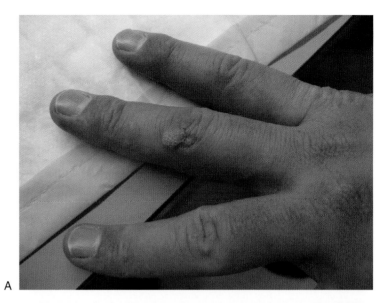

A

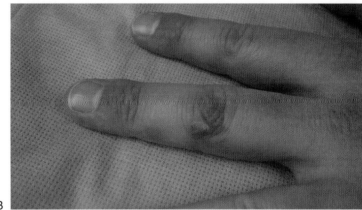

B

Figure 39.2 (A) *Verruca vulgaris on the left middle finger resistant to multiple treatments with cryotherapy.* **(B)** *Marked resolution of the wart after three PDL treatments.*

TABLE 39.1 ■ Laser Treatment of Warts

	PDL	CO_2
Efficacy	Variable	Effective
Average number of sessions	2–12	1–3
Anesthesia needed	Occasionally	Yes
Scarring risk	Low	High
Dyschromia risk	Low	Moderate
Infection risk	Low	Low
Pain	Moderate to high	Minimal to high

- Pulsed dye laser (PDL) (Figs. 39.1–39.4)
  - PDL is the most commonly employed laser for warts. It may induce a therapeutic response by vascular absorption of laser light producing thermal necrosis of wart tissue as well as by induction of a host immune response. Clinical improvement is variable. PDL is generally utilized after failure of first-line therapies.
  - PDL protocol
    ○ Protective laser masks, gloves, and gowns as well as use of a smoke evacuator are recommended to avoid transmission of the wart virus.
    ○ The hyperkeratotic portion of the wart should be pared prior to treatment. Bleeding is to be avoided, as this will minimize laser light absorption by the wart.
    ○ High fluences (585–595 nm, 0.45–1.5 ms pulse duration, 8–15 J/cm^2) are typically required for effective treatment. Multiple pulses are most effective, but should be performed with caution. Diascopy with pulses should be considered. Treat 1 to 2 mm of surrounding healthy skin.
    ○ Treat until lesional purpura is apparent.
    ○ Repetitive treatments spaced 3 weeks apart are generally optimal. Longer intervals between treatment sessions may facilitate wart regrowth and shorter intervals may prevent complete healing.
- Carbon dioxide laser (CO$_2$)
  - CO$_2$ laser treatment is generally reserved for recalcitrant, widespread, painful, or hyperkeratotic warts
  - Advantages: high success rate usually after one or two sessions, no bleeding
  - Disadvantages: unknown hazard of HPV in laser plume, risks of dyschromia, recurrence and infection; prolonged healing time of weeks to months; residual scarring that can be painful; risk of permanent nail dystrophy with periungual treatment
  - CO$_2$ protocol
- Protective laser masks, gloves, and gowns as well as use of a smoke evacuator are recommended to avoid transmission of the wart virus.
- Administer intralesional infiltrative anesthesia or a digital block (1% lidocaine with or without 1:100,000 epinephrine).
- Vaporize the wart and a 2- to 5-mm margin until the surface is charred (Ultrapulse CW defocused, 15–20 W; Sharplan superpulsed mode, 1–2 mm spot, 5–15 W).
- Remove the char by rubbing a saline-soaked gauze pad. Allow the area to dry.
- Revaporize the wart as above with char removal between passes until tissue separation occurs and normal tissue is observed.

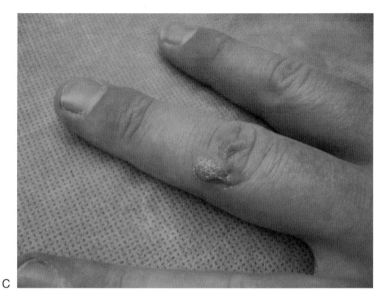

Figure 39.2 *(Continued)* **(C)** *Recurrence of the wart after six PDL treatments*

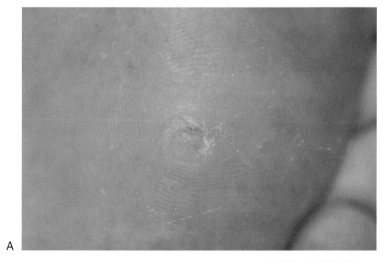

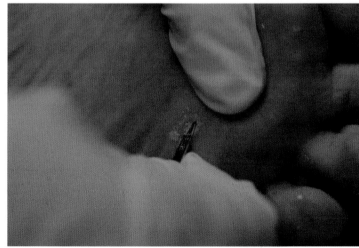

Figure 39.3 (A) *Plantar verruca with characteristic thrombosed capillaries.* **(B)** *Paring of wart with #15 blade prior to pulsed dye therapy*

Nonlaser surgical modalities

- Cryotherapy with liquid nitrogen is the most commonly employed surgical treatment modality employed. Treatment benefit is dependent on ice crystal-induced cell death as well as the induction of a host immune response.

  - Treatment may be delivered via a cryosurgical unit (Brymill Cryogenic Systems, Ellington, CT) or via a cotton-tipped applicator, dipstick, or forceps.

  - A single or double 5 to 15 seconds freeze–thaw cycle may be delivered depending on the treatment site and lesion thickness. Thicker lesions and plantar lesions require more aggressive treatment. Multiple treatment sessions are generally required.

  - Treatment may induce temporary or permanent hyperpigmentation and hypopigmentation, blistering and scar formation.

- Electrodessication and curettage and surgical excision have also been employed with variable response.

PITFALLS TO AVOID

- Be very aware of the depth of destruction with CO_2 laser. As you go below the papillary dermis, the risk of scarring and dyschromia increases.

- Patients must be aware that scar formation is likely and may be painful. Painful scarring is most common on pressure-bearing areas.

- Recurrences most frequently occur at the wound edge. Treating a margin of normal skin minimizes this risk.

  - Cryotherapy can produce pigment changes and scar

  - Improvement is variable with any treatment modality

  - Warts can recur after any treatment

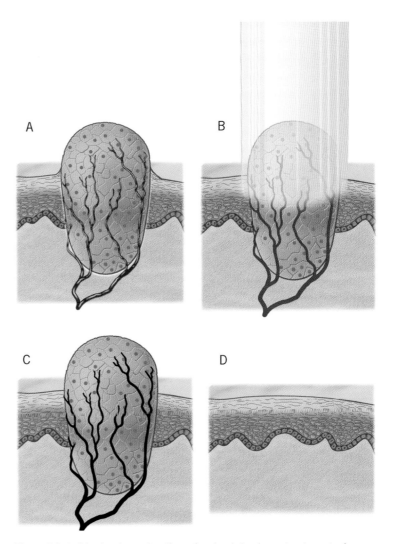

Figure 39.4 *Mechanism of action of pulsed dye laser treatment of verruca. (A) The verruca is characterized by a rich vascular supply. (B) The pulsed dye laser selectively targets the vascular component of the verruca. (C) The laser light is selectively absorbed by the blood leading to coagulation of the vessels (D) and resolution of the wart*

BIBLIOGRAPHY

Park HS, Choi WS. Pulsed dye laser treatment for viral warts: A study of 120 patients. *J Dermatol.* 2008;35(8): 491-498.

Schellhaas U, Gerber W, Hammes S, Ockenfels HM. Pulsed dye laser treatment is effective in the treatment of recalcitrant viral warts. *Dermatol Surg.* 2008;34(1):67-72.

Serour F, Somekh E. Successful treatment of recalcitrant warts in pediatric patients with carbon dioxide laser. *Eur J Pediatr Surg.* 2003;13(4):219-223.

Sethuraman G, Richards KA, Hiremagalore RN, Wagner A. Effectiveness of pulsed dye laser in the treatment of recalcitrant warts in children. *Dermatol Surg.* 2010; 36(1):58-65.

Shumer SM, O'Keefe EJ. Bleomycin in the treatment of recalcitrant warts. *J Am Acad Dermatol.* 1983;9:91.

SECTION SEVEN

Benign Growths

CHAPTER 40 | Angiofibroma

Angiofibroma is a descriptive term for a group of lesions with different clinical presentations but with the same histopathology. These lesions include fibrous papule, facial angiofibroma, pearly penile papule, adenoma sebaceum, periungual fibroma, and Koenen's tumor. This chapter will focus on facial angiofibroma. Generally, an angiofibroma presents as a 1 to 5 mm skin-colored to erythematous dome-shaped papule on the face. When it presents as multiple facial lesions, it can be associated with tuberous sclerosis or multiple endocrine neoplasia type 1 (MEN 1).

EPIDEMIOLOGY

Incidence: common

Age: majority in early to mid childhood

Race: none

Sex: equal

Precipitating factors: tuberous sclerosis, MEN 1

PATHOGENESIS

Unknown.

PHYSICAL EXAMINATION (Fig. 40.1)

Firm skin-colored to erythematous papules (1–5 mm) on the nose, chin, and cheeks, which may be arranged bilaterally. Individuals with tuberous sclerosis can also have periungual fibromas, fibrous plaques, and ash-leaf macules.

DIFFERENTIAL DIAGNOSIS

Intradermal melanocytic nevi, appendageal tumors, basal cell carcinoma, acne vulgaris

DERMATOPATHOLOGY

A symmetric, well-circumscribed papule with a normal to slightly atrophic epidermis. The papillary and reticular dermis features a proliferation of varying degrees of normal blood vessels within a fibrotic stroma. The collagen fibers are arranged perpendicularly to the epidermis and concentrically around the vessels and hair follicles. Stellate-shaped multinucleated fibroblasts may be seen.

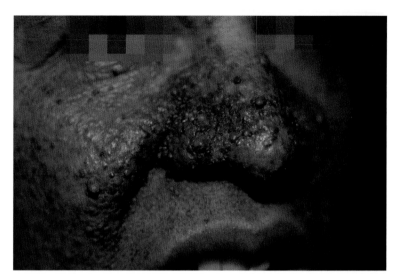

Figure 40.1 *Patient with numerous facial angiofibromas. He is noted to have associated tuberous sclerosis*

LABORATORY EXAMINATION

In the setting of multiple facial and/or periungual angiofibromas, tuberous sclerosis and MEN 1 must be investigated. This is best performed by referral to pediatric specialists.

COURSE

Multiple facial angiofibromas typically present in childhood and may be associated with tuberous sclerosis (Fig. 40.2). Isolated lesions remain unchanged. Further angiofibromas may develop in adulthood.

KEY CONSULTATIVE QUESTIONS

- Onset and location of lesions
- Family history of similar lesions
- Family history of cancer
- Associated central nervous system disorders

MANAGEMENT

There is no medical indication to treat angiofibromas. Their cosmetic appearance, however, may be striking and understandably concerning to some individuals.

■ Treatment

Multiple treatment modalities are available. Recurrence rate is high with the majority of the treatment options. Treatment options may be combined for the best treatment outcome.

- Surgical
  - Shave excision—outline lesion prior to applying local anesthesia as the lesion may blanch after the anesthesia is injected
  - Punch or elliptical excision—limited to isolated few lesions. Residual scar expected
  - Electrodessication and curettage—may leave residual scar
- Laser surgery–best for multiple lesions
  - Pulsed dye laser—reduces the erythematous component of the lesion only. Possible lesional flattening with use of 5-aminolevulinic acid blue light photodynamic therapy followed by pulsed dye laser treatment
  - Carbon dioxide laser (Fig. 40.3)—continuous wave mode most effective. Long-term improvement has been seen. Adverse reactions including temporary and/or permanent dyspigmentation especially in Fitzpatrick skin phototypes III and IV, as well as scar formation. Lesional recurrence is expected over time

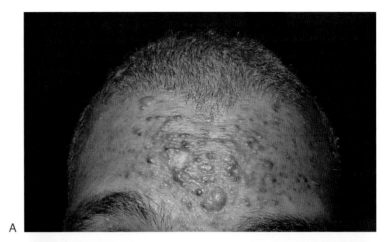

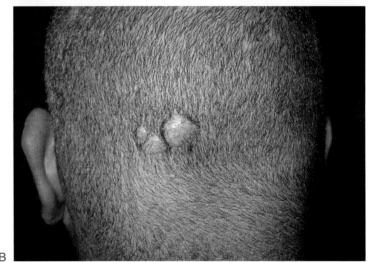

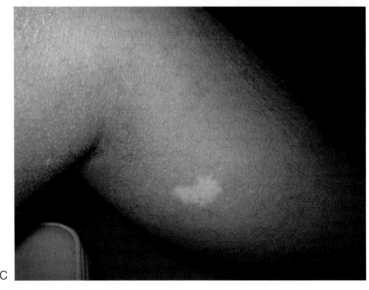

Figure 40.2 (A) *Fibrous plaques on the forehead in an adult patient with tuberous sclerosis.* **(B)** *Fibrous plaques on the scalp.* **(C)** *Ash leaf macule on the leg of the same patient*

– KTP laser—stacked pulses without cooling has been utilized with some success. Requires two to five sessions for lesional flattening. Dyspigmentation and scar formation are possible. Lesional recurrence is expected

- Dermabrasion—similar outcome to continuous wave carbon dioxide laser treatment

PITFALLS TO AVOID

- Though there are many treatment modalities for the improvement of angiofibromas, the endpoint is generally lesional flattening and not clearance. Setting realistic expectations prior to treatment is key

- Patients must be aware of the likelihood of lesional recurrence over time. With underlying tuberous sclerosis, new lesions are likely to occur

- Ablative therapies carry a risk of scarring and dyspigmentation. Use of conservative parameters are paramount to avoid potential side effects

BIBLIOGRAPHY

Bittencourt RC, Huilgol SC, Seed PT, Calonje E, Markey AC, Barlow RJ. Treatment of angiofibromas with a scanning carbon dioxide laser: a clinicopathologic study with long-term follow-up. *J Am Acad Dermatol.* 2001;45(5):731-735.

Boixeda P, Sanchez-Miralles E, Azana JM, Arrazola JM, Moreno R, Ledo A. CO_2, argon, and pulsed dye laser treatment of angiofibromas. *J Dermatol Surg Oncol.* 1994;20(12):808-812.

Papadavid E, Markey A, Bellaney G, Walker NP. Carbon dioxide and pulsed dye laser treatment of angiofibromas in 29 patients with tuberous sclerosis. *Br J Dermatol.* 2002;147(2):337-342.

Tope WD, Kageyama N. "Hot" KTP-laser treatment of facial angiomata. *Lases Surg Med.* 2001;29(1):78-81.

Weinberger, CH, Endrizzi B. Hook KP, Lee PK. Treatment of angiofibromas of tuberous sclerosis with 5-aminolevulinic acid blue light photodynamic therapy followed by immediate pulsed dye laser. *Dermatol Surg.* 2009;35(11):1849-1851.

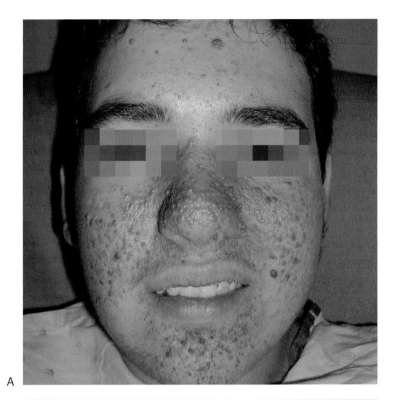

A

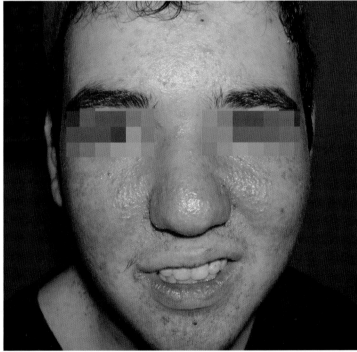

B

Figure 40.3 (A) *Multiple angiofibromas on a 16-year-old male with tuberous sclerosis.* **(B)** *Improvement 2 months after single treatment with CO_2 laser.*

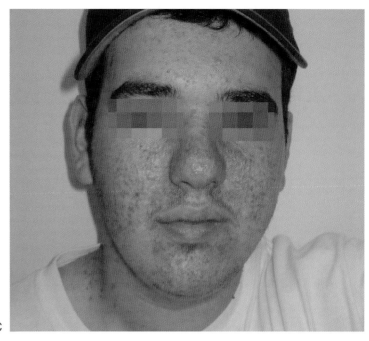

C

Figure 40.3 *(Continued)* **(C)** *Partial recurrence of angiofibromas noted 13 months after CO$_2$ laser treatment*

CHAPTER 41 | Becker's Nevus

Becker's nevus is a sharply demarcated tan to brown patch or slightly raised verrucous plaque that most commonly appears on the shoulder, chest, or upper back. It typically presents unilaterally and is frequently associated with overlying hypertrichosis. It is a benign hamartoma.

EPIDEMIOLOGY

Incidence: 0.5% of males

Age: teens to thirties, rarely congenital, familial cases reported

Race: all races

Sex: males > females (6:1)

Precipitating factors: none

PATHOGENESIS

Unclear etiology. Postulated to have a localized increase in androgen receptors and heightened sensitivity to androgens.

PATHOLOGY

There is papillomatosis, hyperkeratosis, acanthosis, and basal layer hyperpigmentation. There is an increase in the melanin content of keratinocytes with little or no change in the number of melanocytes. A smooth muscle hamartoma is frequently present in the dermis.

PHYSICAL LESIONS

They occur most often on the upper trunk as a well-demarcated unilateral tan to dark brown patch with a block-like configuration ranging from a few to >15 cm. Hypertrichosis usually develops after the hyperpigmentation (Figs. 41.1 and 41.2). Acneiform lesions strictly limited to areas of hyperpigmentation have been reported.

DIFFERENTIAL DIAGNOSIS

Congenital nevus, café au lait macule, epidermal nevus, plexiform neurofibroma

LABORATORY EXAMINATION

Physical examination should be performed to rule out associated hypoplasia of the ipsilateral arm, breast, areola, or ipsilateral arm shortening as well as pectus carinatum or thoracic scoliosis.

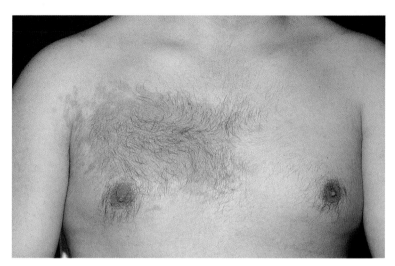

Figure 41.1 *Becker's nevus. A slightly raised light-tan plaque with sharply defined and highly irregular border and hypertrichosis on the chest of a 35-year-old male (Wolff K, Johnson RA, Suurmond D. Fitzpatrick's Color Atlas & Synopsis of Clinical Dermatology, 5th ed. New York: McGraw-Hill; 2005)*

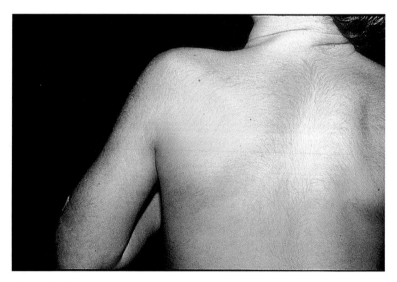

Figure 41.2 *Becker's nevus. Large brown plaque that becomes noticeable at puberty with increased pigment followed by hair growth (Wolff K, Johnson RA, Suurmond D. Fitzpatrick's Color Atlas & Synopsis of Clinical Dermatology, 5th ed. New York: McGraw-Hill; 2005)*

COURSE

It most commonly presents at puberty as a unilateral tan patch. Over time, it may develop into a plaque and display a darker brown hue. Hair growth, which becomes darker and coarser over time, follows pigmentary changes. They tend to enlarge slowly for a few years, then remain stable over time. The color may fade with time; however, the hair growth usually persists.

KEY CONSULTATIVE QUESTIONS

Onset of lesion?

Is the lesion stable?

Is the pigment, the hair growth, or both cosmetically troubling?

MANAGEMENT

There is no medical indication to treat Becker's nevus. The cosmetic appearance, however, may displease some individuals—most often females who note its hypertrichosis. Treatment options are multiple, but not always effective including camouflage makeup, electrolysis, waxing, laser therapy, and surgical excision. Surgical excision is impractical for larger lesions. Laser therapies can be tailored for hair removal or pigment resolution (Fig. 41.3).

■ Laser Treatment

- A test site is recommended before initiating any laser therapy to assess for efficacy and side effects.
- Pigment: Q-switched ruby (694 nm), Q-switched Nd:YAG (532 nm or 1,064 nm), and Q-switched alexandrite (755 nm) lasers have been reported effective in treating the pigmentary component of a Becker's nevus (Fig. 41.4).

  - In general, response is poor. Multiple treatments are usually required for lightening.

  - There is a high rate of repigmentation. This is likely due to deep hair follicle melanocytes.

- Fractionated laser treatment: the 1,550-nm wavelength fractionated laser has been shown to safely and effectively reduce the pigmentary component. Multiple treatments spaced 4 weeks apart were employed.

- Hair removal: long-pulsed alexandrite and diode (800 nm) lasers can produce hair reduction but are less effective with long-term pigment lightening.

- Ablative therapy: Erbium: YAG laser (2,940 nm) has been demonstrated to be more effective than long-pulsed Nd:YAG laser (1,064 nm) in side by side comparison treatment of Becker's nevus. Both lasers

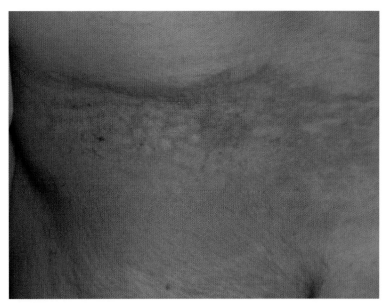

Figure 41.3 *Incomplete improvement of Becker's nevus on upper buttock after three treatments with Q-switched ruby laser. Associated pigmentary changes noted*

produce erythema which clears within 15 days. The long-term clinical and histological clearance has been noted.

– It is important to note that there is a high risk of texture change and/or scar formation associated with ablative therapy.

• Intense pulsed light has demonstrated mixed success in improving pigmentation and hair loss.

PITFALLS TO AVOID/COMPLICATIONS/ MANAGEMENT/OUTCOME EXPECTATIONS

• Treatment of the pigmentary component of the nevus is often ineffective and recurrences are common

• Laser hair removal can improve overlying hypertrichosis and is generally permanent in nature

• Postinflammatory hypo- and hyperpigmentation occur frequently, therefore a conservative laser approach is vital to minimize any associated pigmentary change

• Patients with dark skin phototypes (types IV and V) should be treated cautiously and at lower fluences, as their threshold response occurs at lower energies. A conservative laser approach is best to avoid postinflammatory hyperpigmentation and/or hypopigmentation

• Laser treatment should be limited to nontanned individuals to avoid temporary or permanent dyspigmentation

• Surgical excision is dependent on the size and location of a lesion and is generally limited to very small lesions

BIBLIOGRAPHY

Choi JE, Kim JW, Seo SH, Son SW, Ahn HH, Kye YC. Treatment of Becker's Nevi with a Long-pulse Alexandrite laser. *Dermatol Surg.* 2009;35(7):1105-1108.

Glaich AS, Goldberg LH, Dai T, Kunishige JH, Friedman PM. Fractional Resurfacing: A new therapeutic modality for Becker's nevus. *Arch Dermatol.* 2007;143(12):1488-1490.

Kopera D, Hohenleutner U, Landthaler M. Quality-switched ruby laser treatment of solar lentigines and Becker's nevus: A histopathological and immunohistochemical study. *Dermatology.* 1997;194(4):338-343.

Nanni CA, Alster TS. Treatment of a Becker's nevus using a 694-nm long-pulsed ruby laser. *Dermatol Surg.* 1998;24(9):1032-1034.

Trelles MA, Allones I, Moreno-Arias GA, Velez M. Becker's nevus: A comparative study between erbium:YAG and Q-switched neodymium:YAG; clinical and histopathological findings. *Br J Dermatol.* 2005;152 (2):308-313.

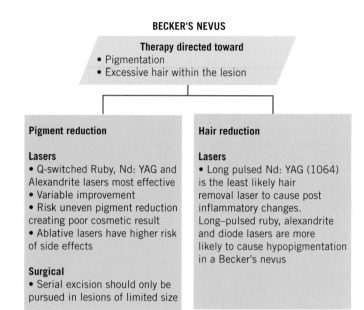

Figure 41.4 *Becker's nevus treatment diagram*

CHAPTER 42 Epidermal Inclusion Cyst

The epidermal inclusion cyst (EIC), also known as sebaceous cyst and epidermoid cyst, is the most common cyst of the skin. It ranges in size from a few millimeters to a few centimeters and originates from the follicular infundibulum. Its contents are a cheesy, malodorous mixture of degraded lipid and keratin. It often ruptures, with associated pain and inflammation.

EPIDEMIOLOGY

Incidence: very common

Age: adults

Race: none

Sex: equal

Precipitating factors: develop spontaneously or as a result of trauma

PATHOGENESIS

Arise from epidermal cells in the dermis. These cells may be implanted as a result of trauma or arise from follicular infundibular cells. These cells may proliferate as a result of pilosebaceous occlusion. Multiple lesions have associated with Gardner syndrome and basal cell nevus syndrome.

PATHOLOGY

Within the dermis or subcutaneous fat, there is a well-demarcated cyst containing laminated keratin debris. The cyst wall is lined by stratified squamous epithelium featuring a granular cell layer. In ruptured cysts, there is a foreign body granulomatous reaction with multinucleated giant cells.

PHYSICAL LESIONS

An EIC is a dome-shaped, smooth, firm, well-circumscribed mobile nodule frequently protruding above the skin surface with a central pore (Fig. 42.1). They range in size from a few millimeters to a few centimeters. They typically present on hair-bearing skin, such as the upper trunk, neck, earlobes, and face. After rupture, these cysts develop a strong inflammatory reaction as a result of the spillage of cyst contents into the dermis. In this setting, the cysts become red, inflamed, tender, and enlarged. Perilesional fibrosis may develop with chronic inflammation.

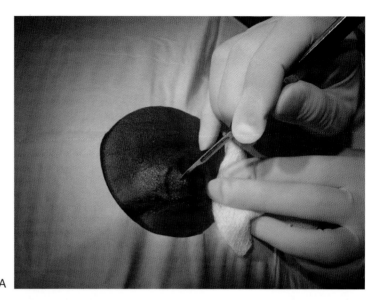

A

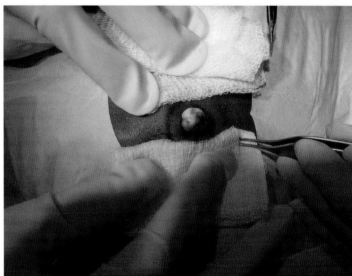

B

Figure 42.1 (A) *Elliptical excision around epidermal inclusion cyst punctum.* **(B)** *Cyst sac being "delivered" from excision site.*

DIFFERENTIAL DIAGNOSIS

Pilars cyst, dermoid cyst, branchial cleft cyst, nodular fibroma, and dermal tumors may cause confusion with EICs. Of these lesions, only EICs feature central pores.

LABORATORY EXAMINATION

In the event of uncertainty of diagnosis, a biopsy can be performed to rule out neoplasm.

COURSE

EICs may increase in size over time, especially with physical manipulation. These lesions frequently become inflamed, resulting in discomfort. Frank purulence may arise, requiring incision and drainage.

KEY CONSULTATIVE QUESTIONS

• Is the lesion recurrently inflamed and painful?
• Is the lesion symptomatic?
• Is the lesion increasing in size?
• Has the lesion been inflamed before?
• Has the lesion been drained or excised in the past?
• Would the patient prefer a surgical scar rather than keeping the cyst?

MANAGEMENT

There is no medical indication to treat EICs if they are not symptomatic. The cosmetic appearance, however, may displease some individuals. In these instances, surgical excision is the treatment of choice. Ruptured EICs can produce recurrent discomfort and repeated infections for some patients. For these lesions, surgical removal is beneficial. Cyst recurrence is highest for cysts that have been inflamed with the development of associated fibrosis.

TREATMENT

• Patient education is paramount to avoid cyst enlargement. Discontinuation of cyst manipulation reduces the risk of cyst enlargement and cyst rupture
• Surgical excision is the treatment of choice for cyst removal
• For noninflamed EICs
   – The cyst margins should be palpated and delineated prior to anesthesia
   – The surgical incision line should transect the epidermal pore as possible

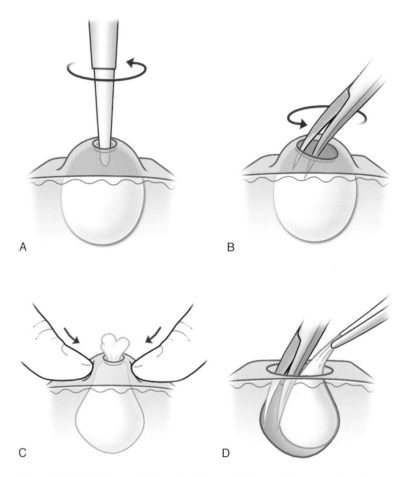

Figure 42.2 (A) *Removal of cyst with punch biopsy,* **(B)** *dissection of cyst from surrounding skin,* **(C,D)** *extrusion of cyst sac*

- Typically, a small elliptical-shaped excision or a small punch biopsy is performed over the cyst around the central pore (Figs. 42.1 and 42.2)
- The cyst sac is then identified and carefully dissected to keep the sac intact
- Sac removal may require lateral compression to extrude the cyst. A portion of the cyst contents may be removed to assist in sac removal
- It is important to note that short of full removal of the entire sac wall, there is a likelihood of recurrence. Consider irrigation of the wound with saline if cystic contents are noted in the wound
- The patient must be aware of the potential dead space that may result from cyst removal. Healing in these instances may result in an indentation of the affected skin

- For inflamed EICs
  - In the event of an inflamed, infected, or newly ruptured cyst, surgical removal should be postponed until the infection and inflammation have resolved
  - Inflamed EICs are more difficult to excise as they become more firmly adherent to the surrounding dermal structures
  - Drainage of contents is important prior to treating larger inflamed cysts
  - Intralesional corticosteroids, warm compresses, and antibiotics (in the event of infection) can aid in decreasing inflammation
  - When the inflammation has subsided, surgical excision can proceed
  - Consider a course of postexcisional oral antibiotics when cysts are inflamed or have drainage

PITFALLS TO AVOID/COMPLICATIONS/ MANAGEMENT/OUTCOME EXPECTATIONS

- It is important to discuss with the patient that while surgical excision of an EIC is a routine surgical procedure, the scar left from the surgery may be more cosmetically disturbing than the EIC itself.
- Patients must be aware that cyst recurrence may occur.
- Chronically inflamed EICs should be excised to avoid further inflammation/infection.

BIBLIOGRAPHY

Mehrabi D, Leonhardt JM, Brodell RT. Removal of keratinous and pilar cysts with the punch incision technique: Analysis of surgical outcomes. *Dermatol Surg.* 2002;28: 673-677.

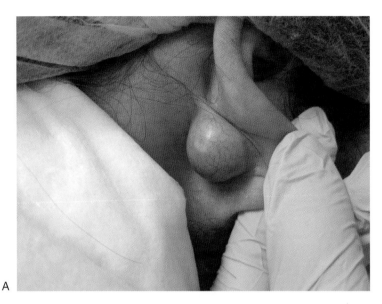

A

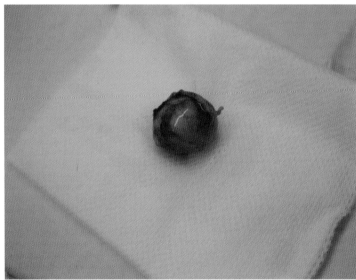

B

Figure 42.3 **(A)** *Epidermal inclusion cyst prior to punch biopsy* **(B)** *Epidermal inclusion cyst immediately following removal. An intact cyst sac decreases the risk of cyst recurrence.*

Rao K, Tehrani H. Excision of epidermoid cysts with a minimal linear incision. *Dermatol Online J.* 2006; 12(1):21.

Smoot EC. Removal of large inclusion cysts with minimal incision scars. *Plast Reconstr Surg.* 2007;119(4):1395.

Wade CL, Haley JC, Hood AF. The utility of submitting epidermoid cysts for histologic examination. *Int J Dermatol.* 2000;39:314-315.

CHAPTER 43 Epidermal Nevus

Epidermal nevus (EN) is a benign hamartomatous growth. It presents as a group of verrucous, closely grouped, skin-colored to brown papules often in a linear arrangement following the Lines of Blaschko (Fig. 43.1). It develops primarily in childhood. There are several variations of EN including localized nevus unius lateris, systematized EN, EN syndrome, and inflammatory verrucous epidermal nevus (ILVEN) (Fig. 43.2).

EPIDEMIOLOGY

Incidence: 0.1% of births

Age: majority in the first year of life; few develop in puberty

Race: none

Sex: female predominance in ILVEN

Precipitating factors: usually sporadic; familial cases reported

PATHOGENESIS

EN is created by overproduction of keratinocytes from pluripotent embryonic epidermal basal keratinocytes. Genetic mosaicism is thought to be responsible for most epidermal nevi.

PATHOLOGY

Papillomatosis, acanthosis, epidermal hyperplasia, and hyperkeratosis along with elongated rete ridges are present. In some lesions, epidermolytic hyperkeratosis and variable parakeratosis may be present. If this finding is made in the setting of multiple epidermal nevi, genetic counseling should be offered in order to educate patients as to the risk of epidermolytic hyperkeratosis in offspring. Neoplasms such as keratoacanthoma, basal cell carcinoma, and squamous cell carcinoma may rarely develop in association with epidermal nevi.

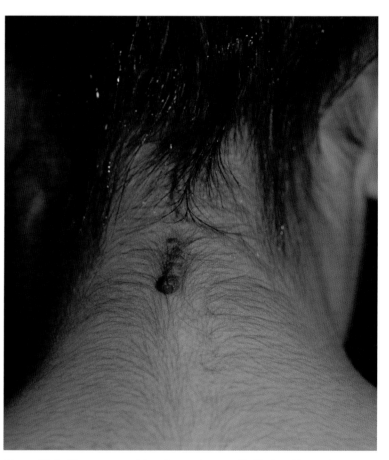

Figure 43.1 *Young man with epidermal nevus limited to his neck nape*

PHYSICAL LESIONS

Commonly present as a single linear lesion, although unilateral or bilateral linear plaques may be present. Most consist of multiple, well-defined, closely grouped linear, yellow, pink, or brown verrucous papules on any body site. EN often follows the Lines of Blaschko on the trunk and travels longitudinally on the extremities. Size can vary from a few millimeters to multiple centimeters. May thicken and become more verrucous over time, especially in flexural regions. Erythema is a common feature of ILVEN.

DIFFERENTIAL DIAGNOSIS

Nevus sebaceous, seborrheic keratosis, verruca vulgaris, lichen striatus, melanocytic nevus, lichen planus, psoriasis.

LABORATORY EXAMINATION

A biopsy may be indicated to distinguish from nevus sebaceous or lichen striatus. Rarely, basal cell and squamous cell carcinoma may arise in EN.

COURSE

An EN generally presents at birth or childhood as macules initially which thicken over time. Eighty percent of ENs appear within the first year of life. At puberty, they tend to enlarge, darken, and become more verrucous. ILVEN may be pruritic in nature.

KEY CONSULTATIVE QUESTIONS

- Age of onset
- CNS abnormalities
- Skeletal defects
- Pruritus
- Family history

MANAGEMENT

In patients with multiple ENs, a thorough examination for systemic abnormalities is indicated. There is no medical indication to treat EN. The cosmetic appearance, however, may be bothersome to the affected individual or parents of children with disfiguring growths. There are multiple treatment modalities for EN including surgery, dermabrasion, topical therapy, and laser therapy (Fig. 43.3). Patients should be counseled that treatment results are variable. The physician needs to consider whether treatment will produce a superior

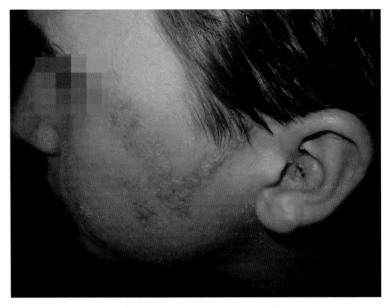

Figure 43.2 *An extensive epidermal nevus on the left face and left ear*

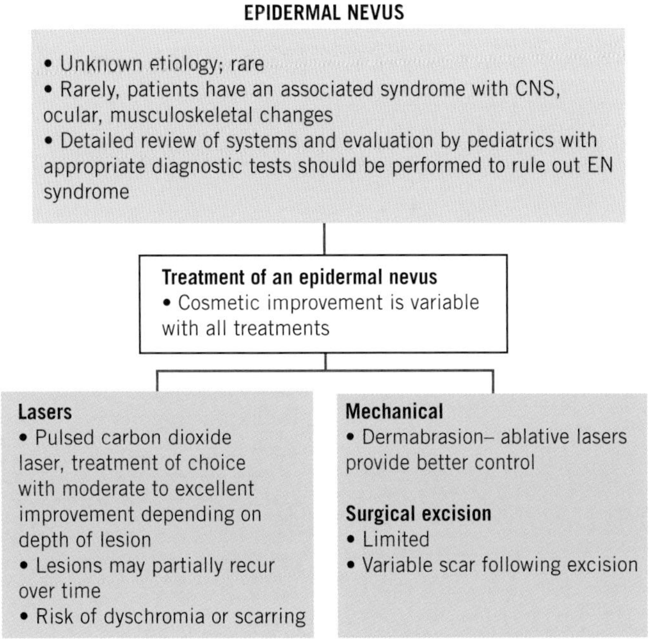

EPIDERMAL NEVUS

- Unknown etiology; rare
- Rarely, patients have an associated syndrome with CNS, ocular, musculoskeletal changes
- Detailed review of systems and evaluation by pediatrics with appropriate diagnostic tests should be performed to rule out EN syndrome

Treatment of an epidermal nevus
- Cosmetic improvement is variable with all treatments

Lasers
- Pulsed carbon dioxide laser, treatment of choice with moderate to excellent improvement depending on depth of lesion
- Lesions may partially recur over time
- Risk of dyschromia or scarring

Mechanical
- Dermabrasion– ablative lasers provide better control

Surgical excision
- Limited
- Variable scar following excision

Figure 43.3 *Epidermal nevus treatment diagram*

outcome to nonintervention. The most aggressive forms of therapy, laser ablation and surgical excision, carry a high risk of scar formation and/or dyspigmentation (Fig. 43.4).

TOPICAL TREATMENTS

The following topical therapies provide limited success for lesional improvement and may best utilized for symptomatic relief of pruritus: high-potency corticosteroids, tretinoin, anthralin, 5-fluorouracil, podophyllin, calcipotriol, and 5% 5-fluorouracil.

SURGERY

- Full-thickness surgical excision of EN is curative
- Postoperative scar is expected
- Cosmesis is variable
- Possibility of hypertrophic or keloidal scarring
- Surgical outcome is best for smaller lesions
- Excision may be difficult for young children to tolerate
- Shave biopsy and curettage may be too superficial, recurrences likely

CRYOTHERAPY/ELECTROCAUTERY/ DERMABRASION

Cryotherapy, electrocautery, and dermabrasion have limited efficacy, a high rate of recurrence, and high risk of a permanent pigmentary alteration and scarring.

LASER TREATMENT

Laser therapy can be effective in treating EN. A test site is recommended prior to treatment

- CO_2 laser (Fig. 43.5)
  - Laser ablation can provide good control of the depth of treatment
  - Treatment depth is limited to the papillary dermis in order to avoid scar formation
- Erbium:YAG laser
- Fractionated ablative laser
  - Most effective for more superficial lesions
  - Treatment depth is limited to the papillary dermis
- With ablative laser treatment, there is a narrow margin between successful treatment and harmful side effects such as scarring and permanent dyspigmentation
- Recurrences are common after laser treatment
- Q-switched lasers

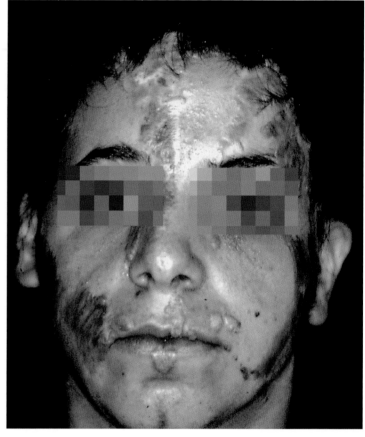

A

Figure 43.4 **(A)** *Young patient with epidermal nevus syndrome. Note the extensive nature of these lesions even after several surgical procedures*

The Q-switched alexandrite (755 nm) and frequency-doubled Q-switched Nd:YAG 532-nm lasers may be effective for improvement of thin ENs.

PITFALLS TO AVOID

- It is important to inform patients that treatment may only be partially successful and may recur
- Laser treatment of the epidermis alone will result in incomplete removal
- Laser treatment beyond the papillary dermis may result in scar formation and/or dyspigmentation
- There is always the risk that treatment will produce an inferior result to nonintervention
- Adverse side effects as described above must be explained in detail to patients for realistic expectations regarding treatment outcome

BIBLIOGRAPHY

Boyce S, Alster TS. CO$_2$ laser treatment of epidermal nevi: Long-term success. *Dermatol Surg.* 2002;28(7): 611-614.

Kim JJ, Chang MW, Schwayder T. Topical tretinoin and 5-fluorouracil in the treatment of linear verrucous epidermal nevus. *J Am Acad Dermatol.* 2000;43(1 pt 1):129-132.

Lee BJ, Mancini AJ, Renucci J, Paller AS, Bauer BS. Full-thickness surgical excision for the treatment of inflammatory linear verrucous epidermal nevus. *Ann Plast Surg.* 2001;47(3):285-292.

Mitsuhashi Y, Katagiri Y, Kondo S. Treatment of inflammatory linear verrucous epidermal naevus with topical vitamin D3. *Br J Dermatol.* 1997;136(1):134-135.

Moreno Arias GA, Ferrando J. Intense pulsed light for melanocytic lesions. *Dermatol Surg.* 2001;27(4):397-400.

Panagiotopoulos A, Chasapi V, Nikolaou V, et al. Assessment of cryosurgery for the treatment of verrucous epidermal naevi. *Acta Derm Venereol.* 2009;89(3): 292-294.

Park JH, Hwang ES, Kim SN, et al. Er:YAG laser treatment of verrucous epidermal nevi. *Dermatol Surg.* 2004; 30(3):378-381.

Toyozawa S, Yamamoto Y, Kaminaka C, Kishioka A, Yonei N., Furukawa F. Successful treatment with trichloroacetic acid peeling for inflammatory linear verrucous epidermal nevus. *J Dermatol.* 2010;37(4):384-386.

Zvulunov A, Grunwald MH, Halvy S. Topical calcipotriol for treatment of inflammatory linear verrucous epidermal nevus. *Arch Dermatol.* 1997;133(5):567-568.

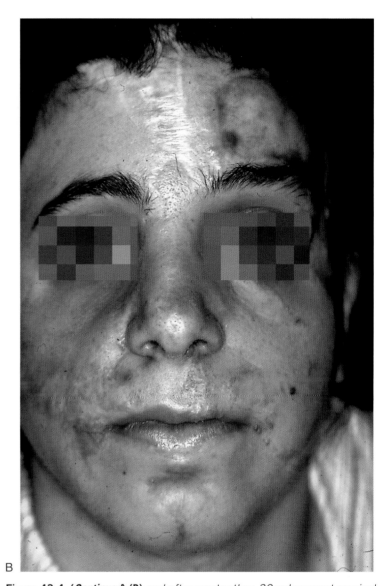

B

Figure 43.4 (*Continued*) (B) *and after greater than 30 subsequent surgical procedures including flaps and skin grafts (Courtesy of Richard Bennett, Muba Taher, and Mathew Avram)*

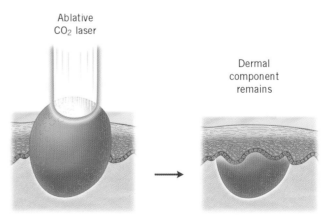

Ablative CO$_2$ laser

Dermal component remains

Figure 43.5 *Effect of ablative CO$_2$ laser on removing an epidermal nevus. With the dermal component remaining, there is a risk of recurrence*

CHAPTER 44 | Lipoma

Lipoma is a benign tumor of mature fat. It presents as a soft subcutaneous flesh-colored tumor that freely moves against overlying skin. Most often, it presents as a solitary lesion on the trunk, neck, and proximal extremities (Fig. 44.1). Infrequently, individuals may present with multiple lipomas, rarely as a part of an inherited syndrome.

EPIDEMIOLOGY

Incidence: very common

Age: can present at any age but most commonly in the fourth decade

Race: none

Sex: equal

Precipitating factors: most frequently, there is no precipitating factor. Multiple lipomas can be associated with syndromes such as Dercum's disease, familial multiple lipomatosis, Madelung's disease, Gardner's syndrome, Bannayan—Zonana and Proteus syndrome

PATHOGENESIS

Unknown.

PATHOLOGY

Well-circumscribed, lobulated tumor of uniform, mature adipocytes in the subcutaneous fat, often with a thin surrounding fibrous capsule and eccentric nuclei.

PHYSICAL LESIONS

A lipoma presents as a soft, freely mobile flesh-colored oval or round subcutaneous nodule with a normal overlying epidermis. Its size can vary greatly from millimeters to many centimeters. It is nontender unless presenting as part of Dercum's disease, as an angiolipoma or if impinging on a nerve.

DIFFERENTIAL DIAGNOSIS

Epidermal inclusion cyst, pilar cyst, hibernoma, angiolipoma, and other fatty tumors including liposarcoma must be considered. If the lesion is greater than 10 cm or fixed, malignancy should be considered.

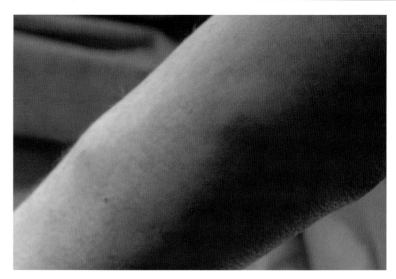

Figure 44.1 *A middle-aged female with two lipomas on her arms*

LABORATORY EXAMINATION

In normal circumstances, no workup is indicated. In the event of rapid or extensive growth, however, biopsy may be indicated if malignancy is suspected. Caution is indicated in the event of excising a lipoma located in the midline sacrococcygeal region. It may represent spinal dysraphism. In this circumstance, consider radiological and neurosurgical evaluation. Do not perform a biopsy.

COURSE

They tend to grow slowly to a certain size and do not involute without intervention.

KEY CONSULTATIVE QUESTIONS

• Number and location of lipomas

• Family history of similar lesions

• History of keloids/hypertrophic scarring

• Associated pain

• Recent lesional growth

MANAGEMENT

There is no medical indication to treat lipomas unless they produce pain or constriction of movement or demonstrate accelerated growth. Many patients, however, request treatment for cosmesis. Surgical removal, via excision or liposuction, is the mainstay of therapy. If the lesion is located in the midline sacrococcygeal region, consider spinal dysraphism.

TREATMENT

• Surgical excision: best for small lipomas (Figs. 44.2 and 44.3)

  – Depending on the size of the lipoma, a small elliptical excision is performed over the tumor. Once the lipoma is encountered, it is dissected from its surrounding tissue.

  – After removal, a layered closure with subcutaneous sutures is generally required to repair the cavity produced by the procedure.

  – Recurrence is common due to the difficulty of distinguishing tumor from normal subcutaneous fat.

  – Surgical excision is preferred for smaller lipomas and is less expensive than liposuction.

• Liposuction: best for large lipomas

  – A small incision is created within the center of the lipoma after regional anesthesia and liposuction of the lipoma is performed.

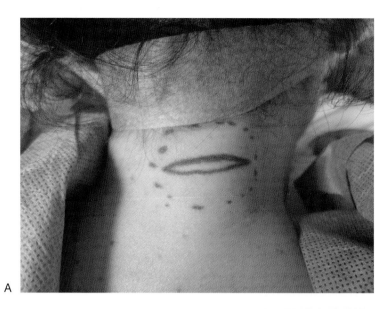

A

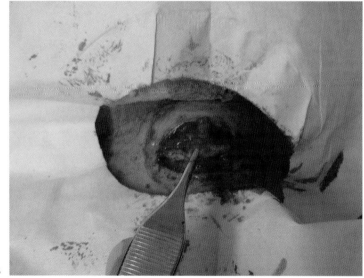

B

Figure 44.2 (A) *Lipoma on posterior neck prior to surgical excision.* **(B)** *Excision of lipoma.*

– The entire tumor is not necessarily removed. Rather, portions of the lipoma are removed until the affected area lies flush with the surrounding skin.

– Postprocedure fibrosis can ensure a persistent flattened contour of the remaining lipoma tissue.

– The advantage of liposuction over excision is that it produces a smaller scar.

– It is more expensive than standard excision.

Low concentration deoxycholate injections have been shown to be effective for the treatment of lipomas in a limited study. These injections obviate the need for surgery, and thus scarring. Nonetheless, further study is recommended before this alternative treatment can be recommended.

PITFALLS TO AVOID/COMPLICATIONS/ MANAGEMENT/OUTCOME EXPECTATIONS

• The physician should inform the patient that all surgical interventions produce some degree of scarring.

• Scarring may bother patients more than the lipoma itself.

• Additionally, removal of large lipomas frequently results in a postoperative skin depression.

• Recurrence is common, especially with liposuction.

BIBLIOGRAPHY

Harrington AC, Admot J, Chesser RS. Infiltrating lipomas of the upper extremities. *J Dermatol Surg Oncol.* 1990; 16:834-836.

Rotunda AR, Ablon G, Kolodney MS. Lipomas treated with subcutaneous deoxycholate injections. *Dermatol Surg.* 53(6):73-78.

Salasche SJ, McCollough ML, Angeloni VL, Grabski WJ. Frontalis-associated lipoma of the forehead. *J Am Acad Dermatol.* 1989;20:462-468.

Sanchez MR, Golomb FA, Moy JA, Potozkin JR. Giant lipoma: case report and review of the literature. *J Am Acad Dermatol.* 1993;28:266-268.

Truhan AP, Garden JM, et al. Facial and scalp lipomas: case reports and study of prevalence. *J Dermatol Surg Oncol.* 1985;11:91.

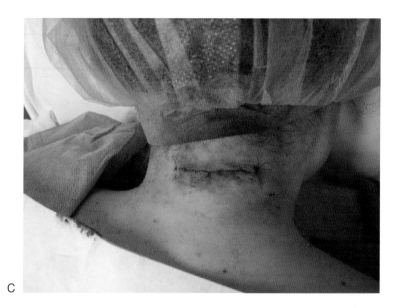

C

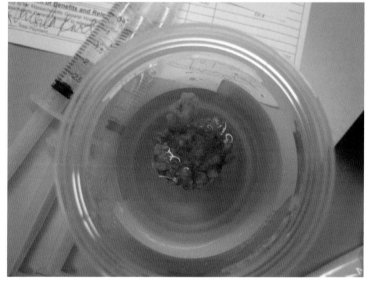

D

Figure 44.2 (*Continued*) (C) *Subcutaneous suture for closure.* **(D)** *Gross path specimen of lipoma*

CHAPTER 45 | Milium

Milia are benign superficial white-yellow keratinaceous cysts that typically present on the eyelids, forehead, and face but may present anywhere (Fig. 45.1). They occur at all ages and are very common.

EPIDEMIOLOGY

Incidence: very common

Age: any age; most common in newborns and adults

Race: none

Sex: equal

Precipitating factors: These are most frequently sporadic lesions but they can be associated with subepidermal blistering diseases such as porphyria cutanea tarda, epidermolysis bullosa acquisita, varicella zoster virus, bullous pemphigoid, and bullous lichen planus. They are also associated with skin trauma such as abrasions, burns, dermatologic surgery, ablative and nonablative fractional resurfacing, CO_2 resurfacing, and radiation therapy. They may also occur following treatment with topical 5-fluorouracil, topical corticosteroids, and microdermabrasion

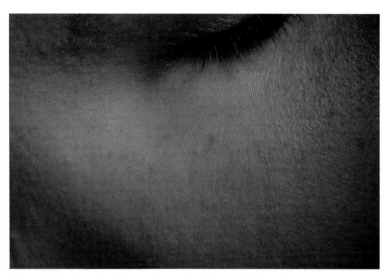

Figure 45.1 *Small milia on face of a 37-year-old female*

PATHOGENESIS

Milia are believed to be retention cysts derived from vellus hair follicles. Milia secondary to trauma or bullous diseases arise from ectopic hair follicles.

PATHOLOGY

They represent small epidermoid cysts and feature characteristic stratified squamous epithelium with laminated keratin debris. A granular layer is present in the cyst wall.

PHYSICAL LESIONS

Milia present as 1 to 4 mm superficial white-yellow cysts that most commonly appear on the eyelids, cheeks, and forehead.

DIFFERENTIAL DIAGNOSIS

Their clinical appearance is characteristic.

LABORATORY EXAMINATION

None.

COURSE

They can present at any age and do not resolve without intervention.

KEY CONSULTATIVE QUESTIONS

Is there any history of blistering or trauma?

MANAGEMENT

There is no medical indication to treat milia. The cosmetic appearance, however, may displease some individuals.

TREATMENT

- Incision and expression: treatment of choice (Fig. 45.2)
  - Local anesthesia may be required.
  - Incision with a #11 blade and removal of keratinaceous debris with pressure from comedone extractor, microvascular forceps, or cotton swab tips.
  - The procedure is fast, simple, and effective.
- Topical medications
  - Topical tretinoin can be effective for multiple milia.
- Other treatments
  - Electrical fulguration.
  - Ablative or fractional ablative lasers can be effective but are far more expensive with a higher rate of side effects and recovery time.

EXPECTATIONS

Treatment of milia is straightforward. Incision and expression is fast, simple, and successful. It remains the treatment of choice. In cases of multiple milia, topical tretinoin is a good choice, particularly if the lesions are small (Fig. 45.1). Laser plays no practical role in the treatment of milia.

BIBLIOGRAPHY

Marra DE, Pourrabbani S, Fincher EF, Moy RL. Fractional photothermolysis for the treatment of adult colloid milium. *Arch Dermatol.* 2007;143(5):572-574.

Dmovsek-Olup B, Vedlin B. Use of Er-YAG laser for benign skin disorders. *Lasers Surg Med.* 1997;21(1): 13-19.

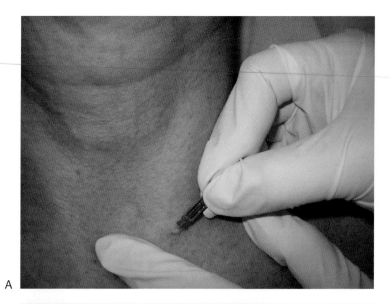

A

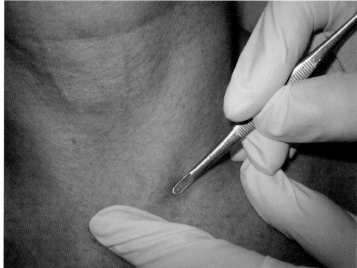

B

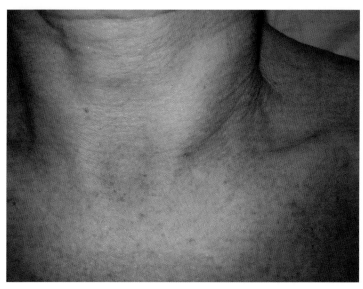

C

Figure 45.2 (A) *Lancet piercing a milium on the left lower anterior neck of a patient.* **(B)** *Comedone extractor extruding keratinaceous debris from milium.* **(C)** *Postprocedure resolution of milium after comedone extraction*

CHAPTER 46 | Neurofibroma

Neurofibromas (NFs) are benign, soft, pink, neuromesenchymal tumors that can be solitary or multiple (Fig. 46.1). Solitary tumors are not associated with systemic findings. Multiple NFs are associated with neurofibromatosis types I and II, both neurocutaneous disorders with important systemic manifestations including malignancies. Plexiform NFs are seen in patients with neurofibromatosis type I.

EPIDEMIOLOGY

Incidence: common

Age: young adults

Race: none

Sex: equal

Precipitating factors: multiple NFs are seen in association with neurofibromatosis I and II. There are no precipitating factors for solitary NFs

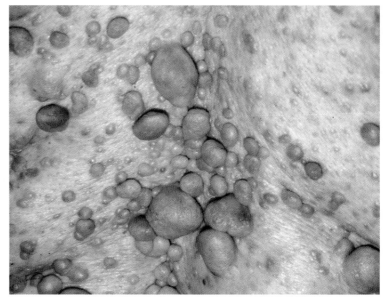

Figure 46.1 *Multiple nonfacial neurofibromas*

PATHOGENESIS

The pathogenesis of solitary lesions is unknown. Multiple germline and somatic mutations have been identified for patients with neurofibromatosis types I and II.

PATHOLOGY

NF is characterized by a well-circumscribed, unencapsulated dermal and subcuticular collection of small nerve fibers and loosely arranged spindle cells possessing wavy nuclei in an eosinophilic matrix. Mast cells are commonly seen. Mitoses are absent.

PHYSICAL LESIONS

NFs present as skin colored to pink to brown soft or rubbery, papules or nodules (Fig. 46.2). The ability to easily invaginate the lesion with pressure, known as "buttonholing," is a characteristic physical finding. They range in size from a few millimeters to a few centimeters. Plexiform NFs are characterized by large, bag-like masses that may have associated hyperpigmentation.

DIFFERENTIAL DIAGNOSIS

Dermal nevi; congenital nevi; dermatofibromas; neuromas; and fibromas

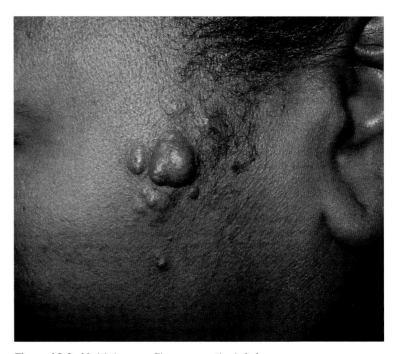

Figure 46.2 *Multiple neurofibromas on the left face*

LABORATORY EXAMINATION

A solitary NF does not merit a workup. Biopsy may be indicated of a clinically atypical NF. Multiple NFs merit referral to neurologic, ophthalmologic, genetics, and orthopedic specialists to assess for neurofibromatosis I or II. Complete skin and eye examination of the patient and immediate relatives is indicated as well. Skin examination should assess for axillary freckling, café au lait macules, plexiform NFs, juvenile xanthogranulomas, and Lisch nodules.

COURSE

They tend to grow indolently and painlessly. Plexiform NF require continuous monitoring for potential malignant change.

KEY CONSULTATIVE QUESTIONS

• Number of lesions

• Family history

• Central nervous system (CNS) abnormalities

• Scoliosis

• Eye abnormalities

• Bone defects

• Loss of hearing

MANAGEMENT

There is no medical indication to treat NFs unless they produce pain or are cosmetically disfiguring or are changing in growth. Many patients, however, request treatment for improvement of cosmetic appearance.

TREATMENT (Fig. 46.3)

• Surgical excision

 – While there are many methods for removing NFs, surgical excision is the most common and efficient means of removal. Recurrence is likely if the NF is not completely excised

 – Elliptical excision is an effective, inexpensive treatment and is particularly appropriate for management of a few number of lesions. As with any surgery, an expected scar will result (Fig. 46.4)

• Laser ablation

 – Not first-line therapy

 – Carbon dioxide (CO_2) laser resurfacing can be utilized for facial lesions. CO_2 laser treatment of nonfacial lesions is generally not recommended given risk of hypertrophic scar/keloid formation

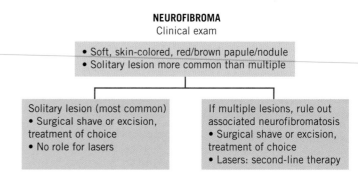

Figure 46.3 *Neurofibroma diagram*

- A cutting technique can be utilized to excise tumors. CO_2 treatment in a focused continuous wave beam, 15 to 30 W is performed along the marked margin. Reincise along the margin until the desired depth is obtained. Tissue undermining and hemorrhage control can be obtained utilizing the same laser parameters with the handpiece held away from the wound to defocus the beam. Wound closure is performed in a standard fashion

- A vaporization technique may be utilized to flatten and remove tumors. CO_2 treatment with a defocused beam and 3 to 6 W is performed to the level of adjacent normal skin. It may be necessary to manually extract large residual dermal tumor once visualized. Char should be debrided between passes with a wet gauze and dried fully prior to continuing treatment

- Several treatment sessions may be required for patients with numerous NFs

- Postinflammatory hyperpigmentation, atrophic scarring, hypertrophic scarring, and incomplete removal have been reported as side effects. A test site should be considered, in particular in patients with Fitzpatrick skin phototypes III–VI

- Erbium: yttrium aluminum garnet laser resurfacing can be utilized for facial lesions

  - Surface vaporization to flatten tumors. This treatment modality is less effective than the CO_2 laser in lesional removal. However, this laser may be more appropriate for patients with darker Fitzpatrick skin phototypes to minimize postinflammatory pigmentary changes

  - Interstitial photocoagulation can be performed for the treatment of bulkier lesions, including nonfacial lesions

PITFALLS TO AVOID/COMPLICATIONS/ MANAGEMENT/OUTCOME EXPECTATIONS

- The physician should inform the patient that any surgical or laser intervention produces some degree of scarring.

- Removal of NFs via laser ablation may produce postinflammatory hyperpigmentation and/or scarring. Recurrence is common.

- CO_2 laser incisional treatment can lead to decreased tensile wound strength during the wound healing phase when compared to standard surgical excision due to laser thermal damage at the wound margin. Sutures should be left in for an additional week to assist in wound healing.

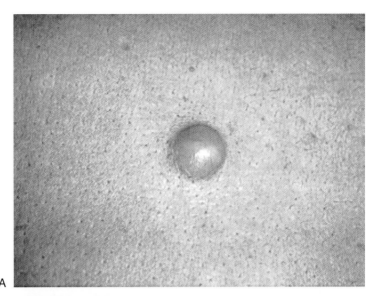

A

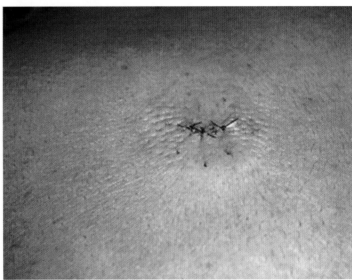

B

Figure 46.4 (A) *Solitary neurofibroma preop.* **(B)** *Solitary neurofibroma following simple excision. This is the treatment of choice for solitary neurofibromas. It is also a good option for removal of limited neurofibromas*

• CO$_2$ laser vaporization treatment should be limited to facial NFs, given an increased risk of scar formation with use on nonfacial sites.

BIBLIOGRAPHY

Cole RP, Widdowson D, Moore JC. Outcome of erbium:yttrium aluminum garnet laser resurfacing treatments. *Lasers Med Sci*. 2008;23(4):427-433.

Elwakil TF, Samy NA, Elbasiouny MS. Non-excision treatment of multiple cutaneous neurofibromas by laser photocoagulation. *Lasers Med Sci*. 2008;23(3):301-316.

Moreno JC, Mathoret C, Lantieri L, Seller J, Revuz, J, Wolkenstein P. Carbon dioxide laser for removal of multiple cutaneous neurofibromas. *Br J Dermatol*. 2001; 144(5):1096-1098.

Neville HL, Seymour-Dempsey K, Slopis J, et al. The role of surgery in children with neurofibromatosis. *J Pediatr Surg*. 2001;36(1):25-29.

CHAPTER 47 | Seborrheic Keratosis

Seborrheic keratosis (SK) are the most common benign cutaneous tumors, and in adults SK are warty, keratotic skin growth that first present after the fourth decade. The measure from a few millimeters to centimeters The color ranges from pink to tan to dark brown. Lesions can be solitary or multiple (Fig. 47.1). Over time, patients develop anywhere from a few to hundreds of SKs. Many patients request removal of SKs, particularly when multiple or large, because of their unsightly appearance.

EPIDEMIOLOGY

Incidence: very common

Age: usually in fourth decade and become more numerous in middle age and beyond

Race: more common in Caucasians

Sex: equal

Precipitating factors: family history with likely autosomal dominant inheritance

PATHOGENESIS

Unknown.

PATHOLOGY

Classically, SKs are well-circumscribed epidermal growths that rise above the surface of the surrounding skin. All feature hyperkeratosis, papillomatosis, and acanthosis. The epidermis contains basaloid cells that show squamous differentiation. Squamous eddies may be present.

PHYSICAL LESIONS

There are many clinical variants of SKs. They range in size from a few millimeters to a few centimeters and most commonly occur on the face, neck, and trunk. They typically first present as well-demarcated tan or light brown macules. With time, they rise to become plaques and develop a warty and stuck-on appearance. Horn cysts become apparent within the lesions. They can occur anywhere on hair-bearing skin and are not seen on the palms and soles.

DIFFERENTIAL DIAGNOSIS

Lentigines, verruca, acrochordons, condyloma acuminatum, acrokeratosis verruciformis, dermatosis papulosa nigra, Bowen's disease, nevus, epidermal nevus, lentigo maligna, melanoma, and squamous cell carcinoma. The clinical appearance and presence of horn cysts in SKs makes the diagnosis straightforward.

LABORATORY EXAMINATION

None; skin biopsy if suspect malignancy.

COURSE

They present in the fourth decade and persist for years. Over time, they become larger, more pigmented and feature a more verrucous appearance. They typically become more numerous with age. Infrequently, they can regress spontaneously.

KEY CONSULTATIVE QUESTIONS

• Family history of skin cancer

• History of bleeding

• Time of onset

• Was there a rapid onset of numerous SKs?

MANAGEMENT

There is no medical indication to treat SKs, unless they are irritated. Still, the cosmetic appearance bothers many patients. There are multiple modalities for treating SKs

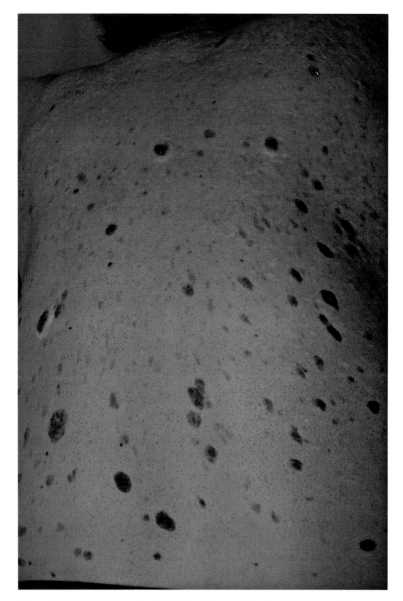

Figure 47.1 *Multiple seborrheic keratoses on back of elderly male*

including cryotherapy, electrodesiccation, curettage, Q-switched and ablative laser therapy. Most often, the traditional methods of treating SKs are most appropriate. If there is a rapid onset of widespread lesions, perform a review of systems and consider a full physical examination to rule out any underlying medical condition or carcinoma (Sign of Leser Trelet).

TRADITIONAL TREATMENTS

Emphasize risk of incomplete removal and recurrence with any treatment modality.

- Cryotherapy
  - Light cryotherapy is a quick, inexpensive, and effective method of treating SKs. Risk hypo- or hyperpigmentation and low risk of scarring
  - If the lesion does not resolve, retreatment is necessary in 3 to 4 weeks
- Currettage and light cautery
  - Electrodesiccation of SKs is another quick and effective method of treatment. Slight discomfort associated with local anesthesia
  - Curetting the lesion after electrodesiccation can ensure removal
  - Light, quick electrodesiccation of the base may also enhance efficacy and prevent recurrence
  - Postprocedure wound care is needed with emollient for 7 to 10 days
- Shave excision
  - Shave excision can effectively remove SKs

LASER TREATMENTS

Laser is not a first-line treatment for SKs. Rather, it should be considered an alternative treatment and only used in the correct clinical setting.

- Melanin targeting lasers for thin SKs
  - Q-switched ruby (694 nm) and Q-switched alexandrite (755 nm), and the long-pulsed 532 nm lasers can effectively treat thin SKs (Fig. 47.2)
  - Sometimes ineffective, especially as thickness increases; repeat treatments may be required
  - Risk of hypopigmentation
  - Expensive compared to traditional therapies, but may be more tolerable to a patient with multiple lesions
- Ablative lasers
  - CO_2 and erbium:YAG lasers can ablate SKs
  - Repigmentation of SKs occurs infrequently after treatment
  - Expensive compared to traditional therapies

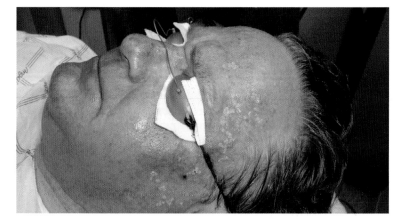

Figure 47.2 *Posttreatment whitening of seborrheic keratoses after treatment with a 755-nm Q-switched alexandrite laser with a fluence of 10 J/cm² and a 3-mm spot size. The procedure was performed after fractional resurfacing, which explains the blue dye remnants apparent on his face*

PITFALLS TO AVOID/COMPLICATIONS/ MANAGEMENT/OUTCOME EXPECTATIONS

- SKs can be treated with a number of different and effective modalities.
- The physician should educate the patient that any therapy has possible adverse effects such as pigmentary changes, scarring, and recurrence.
- Traditional therapies such as light cryotherapy or curettage are simple, quick, and effective (Fig. 47.3).
- Laser therapy is an alternative treatment at a higher expense.

BIBLIOGRAPHY

Brodsky J. Management of benign skin lesions commonly affecting the face: actinic keratosis, seborrheic keratosis, and rosacea. *Curr Opin Otolaryngol Head Neck Surg.* 2009;(4):315-320.

Culbertson GR. 532-nm diode laser treatment of seborrheic keratoses with color enhancement [published online ahead of print January 29, 2008]. *Dermatol Surg.* 2008;34(4):525-528; discussion 528.

Kilmer SL. Laser eradication of pigmented lesions and tattoos. *Dermatol Clin.* 2002;20(1):37-53.

Mehrabi D, Brodell RT. Use of the alexandrite laser for treatment of seborrheic keratoses. *Dermatol Surg.* 2002;28(5):437-439.

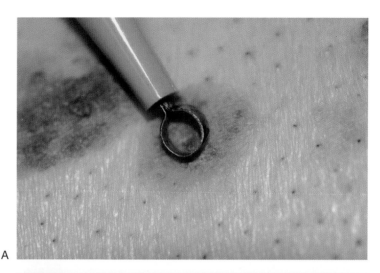

A

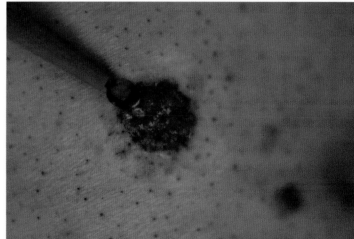

B

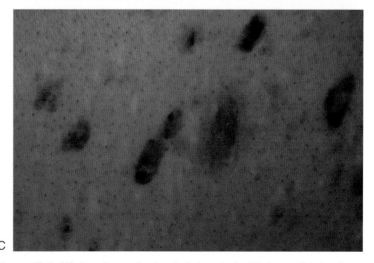

C

Figure 47.3 **(A)** *Curettage of seborrheic keratosis.* **(B)** *Immediately after curettage of seborrheic keratosis.* **(C)** *Postinflammatory erythema 1 month after curettage of seborrheic keratosis*

CHAPTER 48 | Syringoma

Syringomas are common benign adnexal neoplasms of eccrine duct derivation that present most frequently in females on the face, especially around the eyes (Fig. 48.1). They may also be seen on the chest, umbilicus, axillae, and vulva.

EPIDEMIOLOGY

Incidence: common

Age: usually present at puberty

Race: none

Sex: female > male

Precipitating factors: more common in Down's syndrome

PATHOGENESIS

Unknown.

PATHOLOGY

These benign symmetric, well-circumscribed dermal tumors are composed of multiple small ducts with two layers of cuboidal epithelium, often with a "tail" giving a "tadpole," or comma-like appearance in the upper dermis. These ducts are sometimes dilated and are lined by an eosinophilic cuticle. There is a surrounding dense fibrous eosinophilic stroma.

PHYSICAL LESIONS

Skin-colored to yellow, 1- to 3-mm firm papules. They are seen most frequently around the eyes, especially the lower eyelid. Typically, they are multiple and symmetric. They can also be seen on the chest, umbilicus, axillae, and genitalia (Fig. 48.2). Acral lesions are seen in eruptive syringomas.

DIFFERENTIAL DIAGNOSIS

Milia, sebaceous hyperplasia, basal cell carcinoma, trichoepithelioma, fibrous papule,

LABORATORY EXAMINATION

Biopsy may be indicated if basal cell carcinoma is suspected. No other laboratories are indicated.

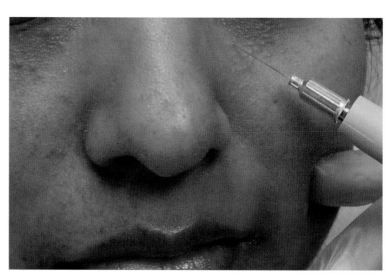

Figure 48.1 *Infraorbital syringomas being treated with low setting electrocautery on a young female. The treatment was not effective.*

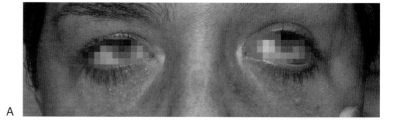

A

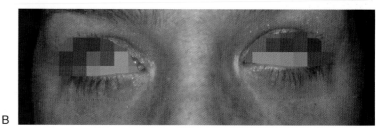

B

Figure 48.2 (A) *Infraorbital syringomas in a young female.* **(B)** *Follow-up picture at 1 week after ablative fractional CO_2 laser resurfacing showing improvement of the syringomas. This improvement is attributed mostly to the postprocedure edema. No significant improvement was noted at a later follow up*

COURSE

They present at puberty and do not resolve without intervention.

KEY CONSULTATIVE QUESTIONS

Time of onset

MANAGEMENT

There is no medical indication to treat syringomas. Many patients, however, request treatment for cosmetic appearance. Syringomas are therapeutically challenging. Although there are multiple treatment modalities available, none is completely successful in complete or permanent removal of syringomas. Often, the side effects of treatment will bother patients more than the syringomas themselves. Ideally, the treatment of syringomas should produce destruction of the tumor with minimal scarring and no recurrence. There are no effective topical medications.

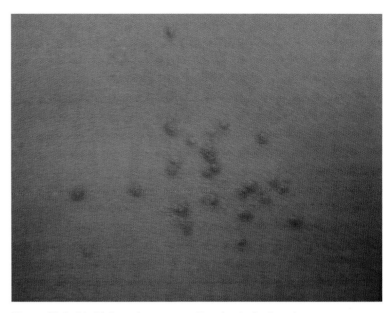

Figure 48.3 *Multiple syringomas on the chest of a female*

TREATMENT

- Surgical excision: best reserved for solitary lesions.
  - Scar will be produced
- Electrocautery: can be successful
  - Localized anesthesia with 1% lidocaine with or without epinephrine may be employed.
  - Low-energy setting electrocautery performed at 1 to 2 W with the electrode placed in the center of the syringoma.
  - Clinical endpoint is lesional flattening.
  - Light settings are advised to avoid pigmentary changes or scarring.
  - Gentle curretage is recommended to ensure that effective removal of the syringoma has been obtained.
- Carbon dioxide (CO_2) laser is an effective means of improving these lesions. The goal is to flatten rather than remove the lesions.
  - Limited to patients with skin phototypes I–III.
  - Individual lesions or multiple syringomas with the same cosmetic unit may be treated.
  - CO_2 treatment in a defocused mode, 3 to 6 W, 3-mm spot, 0.1 to 0.2 seconds may be employed.
  - Multiple passes are performed with removal of residual char between passes with saline-soaked gauze pads. Lesions are treated to the level of adjacent normal skin.

– Lesional recurrence is common. Postinflammatory hyperpigmentation and scarring may occur.

• Other treatments: include cryosurgery and dermabrasion. There is little data with which to judge their efficacy and side-effect profile.

PITFALLS TO AVOID/COMPLICATIONS/ MANAGEMENT/OUTCOME EXPECTATIONS

• Although there are multiple treatment modalities, they are often resistant to therapy. Recurrence is common (Figs. 48.3 and 48.4).

• Caution should be exercised with each of the above-listed modalities.

• Patients must also be informed that the side effects of treatment may be more cosmetically undesirable than the syringomas themselves. These side effects include scarring, hyperpigmentation, recurrence, and erythema.

• When treating syringomas, care should be taken to not overtreat the lesions. It is not necessary to completely eliminate the lesions, as some dermal fibrosis is expected with healing, with residual lesions becoming less apparent over time.

• Great care should be given to the treatment of patients with skin phototypes IV and higher to avoid temporary and permanent pigmentary changes.

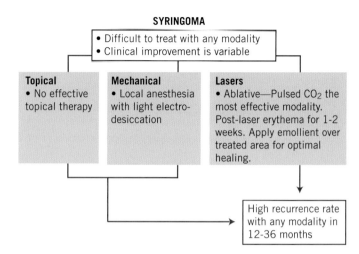

Figure 48.4 *Diagram of syringoma treatment*

BIBLIOGRAPHY

Akita H, Takasu E, Washimi Y, Sugaya N, Nakazawa Y, Matsunaga K. Syringoma of the face treated with fractional photothermolysis. *J Cosmet Laser Ther.* 2009; 11(4):216-219.

Frazier CC, Camacho AP, Cockerell CJ. The treatment of eruptive syringomas in an African American patient with a combination of trichloroacetic acid and CO_2 laser destruction. *Dermatol Surg.* 2001;27(5):489-492.

Kang WH, Km NS, Kim YB, Shim WC. A new treatment for syringoma. Combination of carbon dioxide laser and trichloroacetic acid. *Dermatol Surg.* 1998;24(12):1370-1374.

Karam P, Benedetto AV. Syringomas: new approach to an old technique. *Int J Dermatol.* 1996;35(3):219-220.

Sajben FP, Ross EV. The use of the 1.0 mm handpiece in high energy, pulsed CO_2 laser destruction of facial adnexal tumors. *Dermatol Surg.* 1999;25(1):41-44.

Wang JI, Roenigk HH Jr. Treatment of multiple facial syringomas with the carbon dioxide (CO_2) laser. *Dermatol Surg.* 1999;25(2):136-139.

CHAPTER 49 | Dermatosis Papulosa Nigra

Dermatosis papulosa nigra (DPNs) are very common benign brown warty papules that appear in African Americans and other patients with dark skin phototypes, DPNs usually affect the cheeks, neck, and upper chest (Fig. 49.1). DPNs are a type of seborrheic keratosis. Many patients request removal of DPNs, particularly when multiple or large, due to their unsightly appearance.

EPIDEMIOLOGY

Incidence: very common in African Americans and Asians

Age: second decade to middle age

Race: more common in African Americans and Asians

Sex: females > males (2:1)

Precipitating factors: strongly associated with family history

PATHOGENESIS

Unknown.

PATHOLOGY

DPNs feature hyperkeratosis, papillomatosis, and acanthosis as seen in seborrheic keratoses. No squamous eddies are present.

PHYSICAL LESIONS

They present in a symmetric fashion as small brown smooth sessile papules on the face, neck, and upper trunk of African Americans and Asians. They range from 1 to 5 mm in diameter and are often pedunculated.

DIFFERENTIAL DIAGNOSIS

Seborrheic keratosis, lentigo, verruca, acrochordon, melanocytic nevus, angiofibroma, and adnexal tumors are all in the differential diagnosis.

LABORATORY EXAMINATION

None.

COURSE

They present during teenage years. Over time, they become larger and more numerous, peaking in middle age. They do not regress spontaneously.

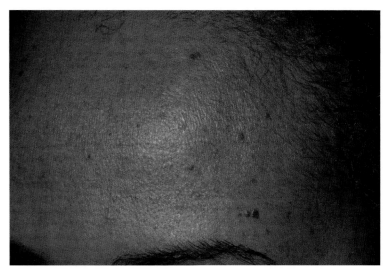

Figure 49.1 *Dermatosis papulos nigra on the forehead of an African American female*

KEY CONSULTATIVE QUESTIONS

Family history of DPNs.

MANAGEMENT

There is no medical indication to treat DPNs, unless they are irritated. Still, the cosmetic appearance bothers many patients particularly when numerous. There are multiple modalities for treating DPNs including cryotherapy, electrodessication, gradle scissor removal, curettage, and ablative laser therapy. Primary consideration before treatment should be the effective removal of the DPNs without producing pigmentary change.

TREATMENTS

- Shave or gradle scissor excision can effectively remove DPNs
  - Local infiltration with local anesthesia followed by gradle scissor removal is safe, fast and has the lowest risk of postinflammatory dyschromia
- Cryotherapy
  - Light cryotherapy is a quick, inexpensive, slightly painful, and effective method of treating DPNs
  - Caution: cryotherapy can produce hypopigmentation by destroying melanocytes. Hyperpigmentation can also occur
- Light electrodesiccation and curettage
  - Light electrodesiccation of DPNs is another quick and effective method of treatment. There is a risk of postinflammatory dyschromia
  - With light electrodesiccation, the lesion will turn white
- Only light electrodesiccation should be employed to decrease the risk of pigmentary changes

LASER TREATMENTS

- Melanin targeting lasers for thin DPNs
  - Q-switched ruby (694 nm) and Q-switched alexandrite (755 nm) can sometimes effectively treat thinner DPNs.
  - Spot size should be less than the size of the lesion.
  - Repeat treatments may be required.
  Risk of hypopigmentation and hyperpigmentation should be explained carefully to patient.
  - Expensive compared to traditional therapies.
- Ablative lasers
  - CO_2, fractional ablative and erbium:YAG lasers can ablate these epidermal lesions.

- Expensive compared to traditional therapies.
- Risk of hypopigmentation and hyperpigmentation should be explained carefully to the patient.

PITFALLS TO AVOID/COMPLICATIONS/ MANAGEMENT/OUTCOME EXPECTATIONS

- Any therapy has possible adverse effects such as pigmentary changes, scarring, and recurrence. Gradle scissor removal has the lowest risk of dyschromia.
- DPNs can be treated with a number of different and effective modalities.
- Traditional therapies such as scissor excision, curettage, or light cryotherapy are simple, quick, and effective.
- Laser therapy is more expensive and carries a higher potential for hyper- or hypopigmentation. Test spot may be appropriate.

BIBLIOGRAPHY

Kilmer SL. Laser eradication of pigmented lesions and tattoos. *Dermatol Clin.* 2002;20(1):37-53.

Schweiger ES, Kwasniak L, Aires DJ. Treatment of dermatosis papulosa nigra with a 1064 nm Nd:YAG laser: Report of two cases. *J Cosmet Laser Ther.* 2008;10(2): 120-122.

CHAPTER 50 | Xanthelasma

Xanthelasmas, also referred to as xanthelasma palpebrarum, are plane xanthomas, occurring on the eyelids.

EPIDEMIOLOGY

Incidence: relatively common

Age: middle-aged adults

Precipitating factors: hyperlipidemia present in 50% of patients with xanthelasmas, family history of hyperlipedima, and xanthelsma. Younger adults who present with xanthelasma are more likely to have lipid abnormalities

PATHOGENESIS

Abnormalities of apolipoprotein E phenotypes or other lipoproteins.

PHYSICAL EXAMINATION

Xanthelasmas commonly present as multiple soft symmetrical oval yellowish papules and plaques on the eyelids.

DIFFERENTIAL DIAGNOSES

Syringomas, sebaceous neoplasms, milia, necrobiotic xanthogranuloma.

DERMATOPATHOLOGY

Collections of foam cells in the superficial dermis.

COURSE

They are generally permanent with tendency to increase in number and coalesce with time.

MANAGEMENT

Xanthelasmas often recur after treatment with any modality.

■ Surgical Excision

Surgical excision is the treatment of choice for xanthelasmas. The lesion is lifted and then excised using a blade or a Gradle scissor. The defect is either left to heal by second intention or sutured using silk or ethilon sutures (Fig. 50.1). This procedure usually results in a very cosmetically acceptable outcome.

■ Localized Tissue Destruction

CO_2 or erbium laser vaporization, trichloroacetic acid, electrosurgery, or cryotherapy.

PITFALLS TO AVOID

• Although 50% of patients with xanthelasmas are normolipemic, it is crucial to screen new patients with xanthelasmas for the presence of hyperlipidemia. This is particularly important in younger patients who present with xanthelasma since they are more likely to have associated lipid abnormalities.

• Patients must be made aware that complete removal of the xanthelasmas does not prevent future development of new lesions.

• Extreme caution should be exerted when operating on the eyelids in order to avoid eye injury.

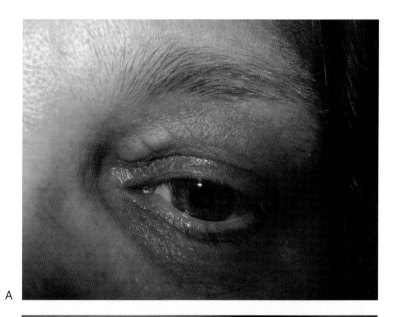
A

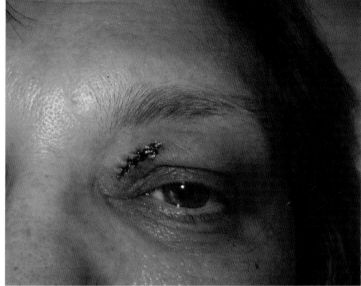
B

Figure 50.1 *Xanthelasma on the left upper medial eyelid in a middle-aged woman. (B) The resulting defect is sutured using ethilon sutures. This procedure produced a very good cosmetic result*

BIBLIOGRAPHY

Eedy DJ. Treatment of xanthelasma by excision with secondary intention healing. *Clin Exp Dermatol.* 1996;21:273-275.

Ghosh YK, Pradhan E, Ahluwalia HS. Excision of xanthelasmata—clamp, shave, and suture. *Int J Dermatol.* 2009;48(2):181-183.

Hawk JL. Cryotherapy may be effective for eyelid xanthelasma. *Clin Exp Dermatol.* 2000;25:351.

Mannino G, Papale A, De Bella F, et al. Use of erbium:YAG laser in the treatment of palpebral xanthelasmas. *Ophthalmic Surg Lasers.* 2001;32:129-133.

Nahas TR, Marques JC, Nicoletti A, Cunha M, Nishiwaki-Dantas MC, Filho JV. Treatment of eyelid xanthelasma with 70% trichloroacetic acid. *Ophthal Plast Reconstr Surg.* 2009;25(4):280-283.

Ullmann Y, Har-Shai Y, Peled IJ. The use of CO_2 laser for the treatment of xanthelasma palpebrarum. *Ann Plast Surg.* 1993;31:504-507

SECTION
EIGHT

Cutaneous Carcinomas

CHAPTER 51 | Actinic Keratosis

Actinic keratosis (AK) present as single or multiple discrete, scaly lesions, found most frequently in habitually sun-exposed skin of adults.

EPIDEMIOLOGY

Age: most commonly noted in middle age, occasionally occurs in patients under 30 years

Sex: more common in males

Incidence: very common; in Australia 1:1,000 persons

Race: skin phototypes I–III, rarely seen in skin phototypes IV–VI

Occupation: outdoor workers (eg, farmer, rancher, sailor) and outdoor sports (golf, tennis, sailing)

PATHOGENESIS

Prolonged and repeated sun exposure in susceptible persons results in cumulative keratinocyte damage. The principle sun damage is secondary to ultravoilet B (UVB) (290–320 nm) light.

PHYSICAL EXAMINATION

AKs present as single or multiple skin-colored, erythematous, or brown scaly patches. There is a predilection for sun-exposed areas including the face, ears, neck, forearms, and dorsal hands. AKs may become thickened, forming a cutaneous horn. More easily palpated than seen. They are generally asymptomatic but may be tender or pruritic. Actinic cheilitis develops on the vermilion border as diffuse scaling or dryness. Associated telangiectasia, solar elastosis, and lentigines are frequently observed.

DERMATOPATHOLOGY

Epidermal proliferation with mild-to-moderate basilar keratinocyte pleomorphism, parakeratosis, and dyskeratotic keratinocytes. Cytologically, atypical keratinocytes are usually confined to the epidermal basal layer.

DIFFERENTIAL DIAGNOSIS

- Eczematous dermatitis
- Extramammary Paget's
- Squamous cell carcinoma
- Basal cell carcinoma

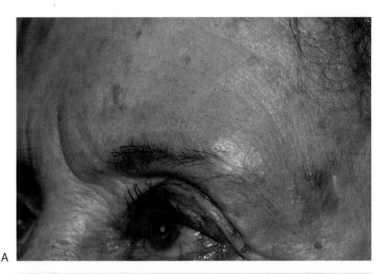

A

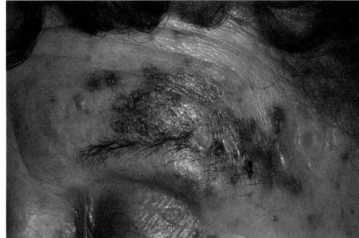

B

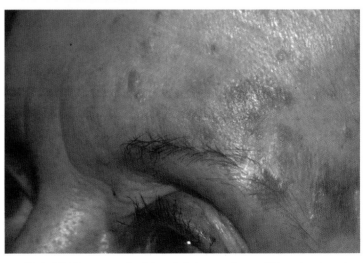

C

Figure 51.1 (A) *Numerous facial actinic keratosis pre-Aldara treatment.* **(B)** *Expected erythema and crusting during Aldara treatment.* **(C)** *Facial actinic keratosis post-Aldara treatment applied twice weekly for 4 weeks (Courtesy of Richard Johnson, MD)*

COURSE

AKs can self-resolve, but generally are persistent in nature. The progression to skin cancer within preexisting AKs is unknown but is estimated at less than 1% of individual lesions. Biopsy warranted for pigmented AKs (superficial pigmented actinic keratosis) or nodular keratosis.

KEY CONSULTATIVE QUESTIONS

- Duration of lesion(s)
- Lesional rate of growth
- Prior treatment for lesions and response
- Personal and family history of prior skin cancers
- History of prior radiation treatment to the area
- Current medical history
- Medication use
- Evidence of immunosuppression
- Predisposing syndromes

MANAGEMENT

Assessment of the number, size, location, frequency of development, and any underlying immunosuppressed state should be obtained. A biopsy should be obtained of any lesion that is suspicious for skin cancers. Consideration may then be given to treatment of individual or multiple lesions, prophylactic therapy, and determination of the need for clinical follow-up.

TREATMENT

- Prevention
  - Application of daily sunscreen with UVA/UVB protection
  - Topical tretinoin applied nightly
- Topical
  - Once daily (Carac) or twice daily (Efudex) application of 5-fluorouracil for 3 to 4 weeks
  - Twice weekly or every third day application of imiquinod (Aldara 3M St. Paul, MN) for 4 weeks (Fig. 52.1)
  - Diclofenac (Solaraze) 3% sodium topical gel twice daily for 2 to 3 months
  - Ingenol mebutate applied on 2 subsequent days or twice 1 week apart
- Gentle cryosurgery with a single freeze–thaw cycle. Blister formation possible. Repeat treatment may be required. Risk of temporary hyperpigmentation and

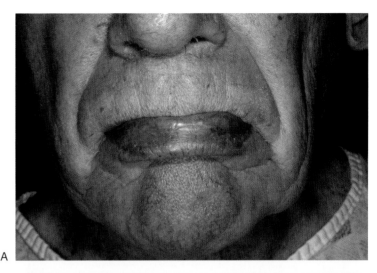

A

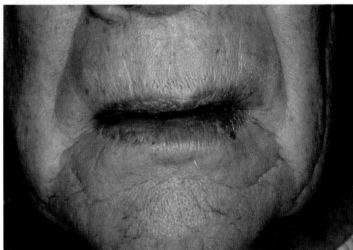

B

Figure 51.2 (A) *Actinic cheilitis, lower lip. Patient complained of frequent peeling that was poorly responsive to cryosurgery and efudex.* **(B)** *Reduction in actinic damage following carbon dioxide resurfacing. Patient reported complete resolution of peeling*

permanent depigmentation must be addressed with the patient. This modality is best for isolated number of lesions

- Systemic
  - Long-term low-dose oral retinoid has been used, this treatment requires close follow-up to avoid potential side effects. Beneficial only while on medication
  - Oral vitamin A has been used, requires close follow-up to avoid potential side effects. Beneficial only while on medication
- Surgical
  - Photodynamic therapy with topical aminolevulinic acid (Levulen, Dusa Pharmaceuticals, Inc., Wilmington, MA) has been successfully utilized. The pulsed dye laser 595 nm, blue light 415 nm, near-infrared 830 nm, intense pulsed light source, and light-emitting diode have been employed for delivery of treatment. Multiple treatments are usually required. Topical levulan applied 1 hour prior to light treatment may be used. Photosensitivity posttreatment prominent
  - Chemical peels—serial medium-depth peels including Jessner/10% to 35% trichloroacetic acid peels are highly beneficial in reducing lesion count. Postoperative peeling may last up to 2 weeks depending on the strength utilized
  - Fractionated ablative carbon dioxide laser—serial treatments may be required to reach treatment endpoint of lesional reduction
  - Pulsed carbon dioxide laser—highly effective in management of actinic cheilitis (Fig. 52.2). The vermilion border is outlined prior to the administration of mental block and/or localized infiltrative anesthesia with 1% lidocaine with 1:100,000 epinephrine. Passes are performed until removal of epidermis is observed. Area wiped with saline soaked sponges between the passes. Postoperative care requires soaking the treatment site with water and a clean washcloth to remove any crusting and application of vaseline three to four times a day. Risk of scar formation and infection must be considered

PITFALLS TO AVOID

- With actinic cheilitis, it is essential to avoid vaporization of the vermilion border to prevent scarring. Delineating the border prior to administration of anesthesia is helpful.

- Patients must be aware that any treatment administered does not eliminate the development of future premalignant and malignant growths. Strict photoprotection and sun avoidance is mandatory.

- Patients utilizing topical treatments must be made aware of the expected erythema, crusting, and discomfort that will persist during the duration of treatment and for 1 to 2 weeks posttreatment. A mild topical corticosteroid may be prescribed posttreatment completion to assist in the resolution of these findings.

BIBLIOGRAPHY

Alberts D, Ranger-Moore J, Einspahr J, et al. Safety and efficacy of dose-intensive oral vitamin A in subjects with sun-damaged skin. *Clin Cancer Res.* 2004;10(6):1875-1880.

Ericson MB, Sandberg C, Stenquist B, et al. Photodynamic therapy of actinic keratosis at varying fluence rates: Assessment of photobleaching, pain and primary clinical outcome. *Br J Dermatol.* 2004;151(6): 1204-1212.

Hadley G, Derry S, Moore RA. Imiquimod for actinc keratosis: Systemic review and meta-analysis. *J Invest Dermatol.* 2006;126(6):1251-1255.

Jarvis B, Figgitt DP. Topical 3% diclofenac in 2.5% hyaluronic acid gel: A review of its use in patients with actinic keratosis. *Am J Clin Dermatol.* 2003;4(3):203-213.

Jorizzo J, Weiss J, Furst K, VandePol C. Effect of a 1-week treatment with 0.5% topical fluorouracil on occurrence of actinic keratosis afater cryosurgery: A randomized, vehicle-controlled clinical trial. *Arch Dermatol.* 2004;140(7):813-816.

Rolf-Markus S, Matheson R, Davis S, et al. Topical methyl aminolevulinate photodynamic therapy using red llight-emitting diode light for multiple actinic keratosis: A randomized study. *J Dermatol Surg.* 2009;35(4):586-592.

Siller G, Gebauer K, Welburn P, Katsamas J, Ogbourne SM. PEP005 (ingenol mebutate) gel, a novel agent for the treatment of actinic keratosis: Results of a randomized, double-blind, vehicle-controlled, multicentre phase IIa study. *Australas J Dermatol.* 2009;50(1):16-22.

Thai KE, Fergin P, Freeman M, et al. A prospective study of the use of cryosurgery for the treatment of actinic keratosis. *Int J Dermatol.* 2004;43(9):687-692.

CHAPTER 52 | Basal Cell Carcinoma

Basal cell carcinoma (BCC) is a slow-growing malignant skin tumor that presents in distinct histological subtypes including nodular, superficial, micronodular, infiltrating, and morpheaform. Nodular BCC is the most common type occurring predominantly on the head and neck regions.

EPIDEMIOLOGY

Incidence: the most common skin cancer in Caucasians with approximately 800,000 cases/year diagnosed in the United States

Age: most common in patients over 40 years

Race: most common in Caucasians

Sex: higher incidence in males

Precipitating factors: chronic ultraviolet radiation and fair skin are the most significant predisposing factors. Other factors include ionizing radiation, arsenic exposure, immunosuppression, PUVA, and genetic predisposition.

PATHOGENESIS

The most common altered gene in BCC is the *PTCH* tumor suppressor gene with a resultant altered Hedgehog signaling pathway leading to unregulated cell proliferation and altered cell differentiation. Mutations in the *p53* tumor suppressor gene are also frequently observed leading to cellular immortality and resistance to apoptosis.

PHYSICAL EXAMINATION

Pink, erythematous, pearly translucent papule, nodule, or plaque with a rolled border and overlying telangiectasias (Fig. 52.1). Superficial BCC presents as a pink or erythematous thin scaly plaque. The center may become ulcerated and covered by a crust, that is, "rodent ulcer." Morpheaform BCC exhibits a scar-like appearance with ill-defined borders. They most commonly present in photodistributed areas.

DIFFERENTIAL DIAGNOSES

Dermal melanocytic nevi, sebaceous hyperplasia, squamous cell carcinoma (SCC).

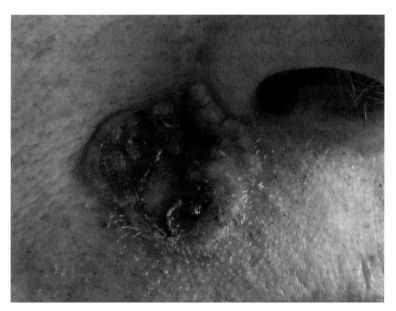

Figure 52.1 *Large BCC on the face. Note the characteristic rolled borders, overlying telangiectasias, and the central ulceration*

LABORATORY DATA

■ Dermatopathology

Lobules, nests, or cords of neoplastic basaloid cells with peripheral palisading, clefting, and mucinous stroma.

COURSE

Locally invasive and slow growing over months and even years. Metastasis is an exceedingly rare occurrence.

KEY CONSULTATIVE QUESTIONS

Excessive sun exposure and other predisposing factors, prior history of BCC or SCC, personal and family history of skin cancer, immunosuppression.

MANAGEMENT

There are multiple methods for treating BCC. Treatment selection should be based upon the age, health, and preferences of the patient after a full discussion of treatment options, risks, and benefits. Given the locally destructive nature of BCC, histological confirmation of complete removal is optimal. Surgical excision and histological evaluation remain the treatment of choice in most cases. Tumors fixed to underlying bone, especially the scalp, merit radiological workup prior to surgical excision or Mohs micrographic surgery. Topical therapies require close follow-up for any evidence of treatment failure or recurrence. Patient education regarding the benefits of sun avoidance, sunscreen use, and regular self-examinations are important preventive measures.

■ First-line Therapies

- Excisional surgery: generally with 4-mm margins is the treatment of choice for nonsuperficial BCC that do not meet the criteria of Mohs micrographic surgery
- Mohs micrographic surgery is the treatment of choice for high-risk anatomical locations (ie, "mask" area of the face), locations where tissue conservation is crucial for functional or cosmetic reasons, recurrent tumors, ill-defined clinical margins, histologically aggressive subtypes, tumors in immunosuppressed patients, tumors larger than 2 cm, irradiated skin, and perineural invasion on biopsy (Figs. 52.2–52.4). Mohs micrographic surgery has the highest cure rate of any treatment of BCC
- Electrodessication and curettage
- Cryotherapy

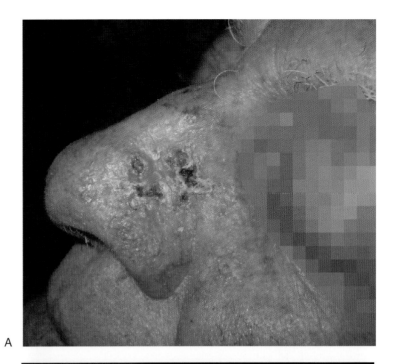

A

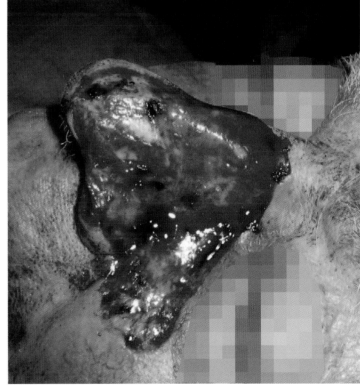

B

Figure 52.2 (A) *BCC on the nose with very ill-defined clinical margins.* **(B)** *Large defect after Mohs micrographic surgery. Mohs micrographic surgery is the ideal treatment for this type of skin cancer providing the highest cure rate among all other treatment modalities*

- Radiation therapy is another treatment option especially when surgery is not feasible or contraindicated. It can also be used as an adjuvant therapy when perineural invasion is identified

■ Alternate Therapies

- Topical imiquimod, applied five times a week for a total duration of 6 weeks. It is FDA approved for treatment of superficial BCC. Recurrence rates are significantly higher than surgical excision.

- Topical 5-fluorouracil is primarily reserved for treatment of superficial BCC. However, recurrence rates are high.

- Photodynamic therapy produces a photochemical reaction that requires the presence of a photosensitizing agent, tissue oxygen, and light with photoactivating wavelength. The most common topical photosensitizer is 5-aminolevulinic acid (5-ALA). 5-ALA is a precursor of the intrinsic intracellular hemebiosynthetic pathway, which results in the production of a photoactive porphyrin, protoporphyrin IX. The methyl derivative of 5-ALA, methyl aminolevulinic acid (MAL) is also very commonly used and demonstrates a better selectivity for malignant cells. The light sources are usually in the visible light range and they include laser (coherent) light sources (eg, pulsed dye lasers) or noncoherent light sources (red, blue light). Red light provides the deepest penetration of these light based treatment modalities. PDT can provide 76% to 97% clearance rates for superficial BCC. It is particularly useful in patients who are poor surgical candidates or those who have multiple BCCs that require multiple surgeries. Close clinical follow-up after treatment is required for any evidence of recurrence or incomplete removal

- Intralesional interferon is rarely performed

- Carbon dioxide laser—may be effective for superficial BCC and patients with multiple shallow tumors such as in basal cell nevus syndrome

PITFALLS TO AVOID

– Infection, bleeding, pain, nerve damage, poor cosmesis following surgical repair, hypertrophic or atrophic scarring, and recurrence are all common pitfalls of BCC surgical therapy and should be fully discussed with the patient prior to treatment.

– Nonsurgical therapies may provide better cosmesis but significantly higher rates of recurrence. Furthermore, nonsurgical interventions do not provide the opportunity for histological confirmation of complete removal. They are best for patients who have numerous BCCs and in those who are poor surgical candidates.

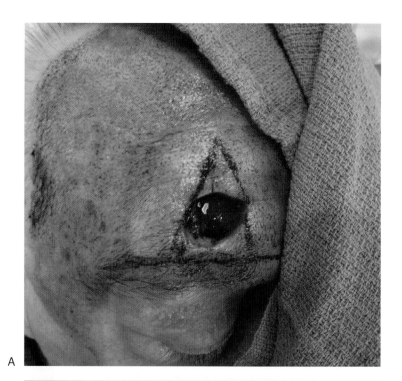

A

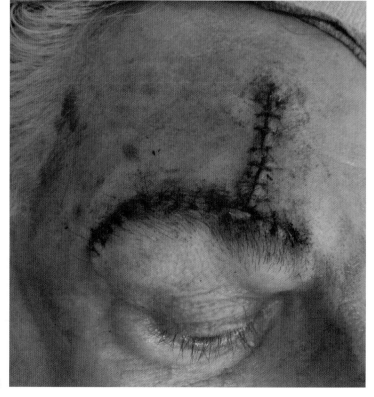

B

Figure 52.3 (A) *Surgical defect after Mohs micrographic surgery of BCC on the right forehead.* **(B)** *Repair of the defect with an A to T advancement flap. Notice that the horizontal incision line is hidden within the eyebrow hairs for a better cosmetic outcome*

BIBLIOGRAPHY

Attili SK, Lesar A, McNeill A, et al. An open pilot study of ambulatory photodynamic therapy using a wearable low-irradiance organic light-emitting diode light source in the treatment of nonmelanoma skin cancer. *Br J Dermatol.* 2009.

Muller FM, Dawe RS, Moseley H, Fleming CJ. Randomized comparison of mohs micrographic surgery and surgical excision for small nodular basal cell carcinoma: Tissue-sparing outcome. *Dermatol Surg.* 2009.

Rowe DE, Carroll RJ, Day CL Jr. Long term recurrence rates in previously untreated (primary) basal cell carcinoma: Implications for patient follow-up. *J Dermatol Surg Oncol.* 1989;15:315-328.

Tierney E, Barker A, Ahdout J, Hanke CW, Moy RL, Kouba DJ. Photodynamic therapy for the treatment of cutaneous neoplasia, inflammatory disorders, and photoaging. *Dermatol Surg.* 2009;35(5):725-746.

Wolf DJ, Zitelli JA. Surgical margins for basal cell carcinoma. *Arch dermatol.* 1987;123:340-344.

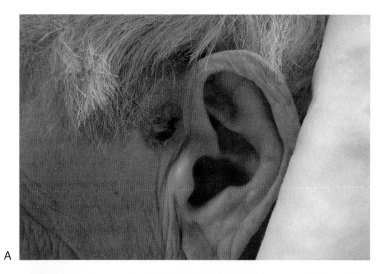

A

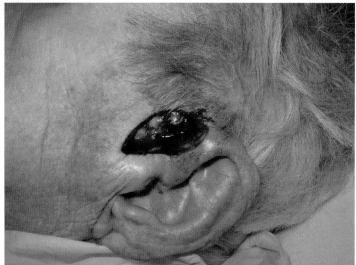

B

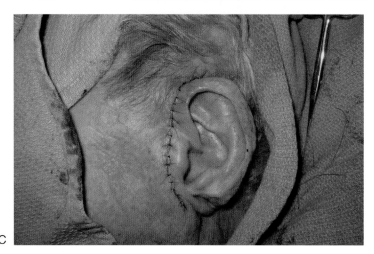

C

Figure 52.4 (A) *Nodular basal cell carcinoma on the left preauricular area.* **(B)** *Clearance of basal cell carcinoma after Mohs surgery.* **(C)** *Primary closure of the Mohs defect with dog-ear repair*

CHAPTER 53 | Squamous Cell Carcinoma

Squamous cell carcinoma (SCC) most commonly originates from keratinocytes in sun-damaged skin either de novo or from a preexisting actinic keratosis or SCC in situ (also known as Bowen's disease), predominantly affecting the head, neck, and arms. It can also arise in non-sun-exposed skin most commonly from chronic leg ulcers and burn scars.

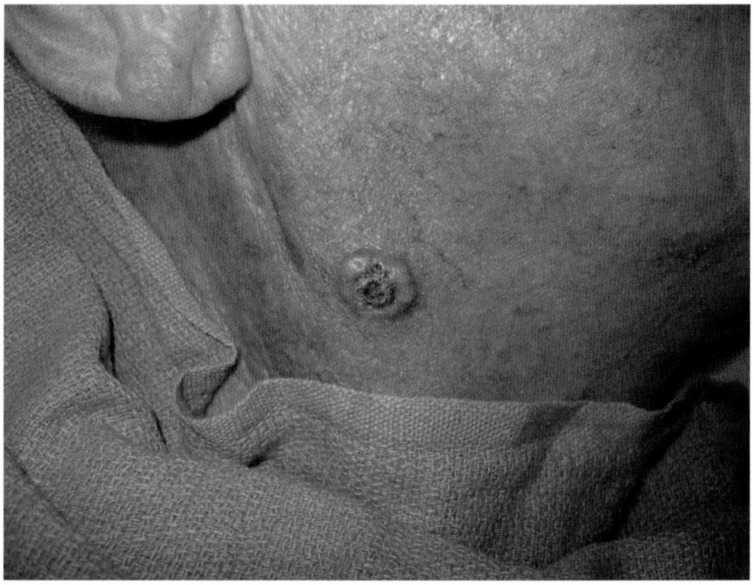

EPIDEMIOLOGY

Incidence: it is the second most common skin cancer in Caucasians and the most common skin cancer in darkly pigmented skin. Approximately 150,000 cases/year are diagnosed in the United States

Age: most common in patients over 55 years

Race: mainly affects Caucasians

Sex: higher incidence in males

Precipitating factors: chronic ultraviolet radiation and fair skin are the most significant predisposing factors. Other factors include immunosuppression, human papilloma virus infection, ionizing radiation, arsenic exposure, genetic disorders (epidermodysplasia verruciformis, albinism, xeroderma pigmentosum, epidermolysis bullosa), PUVA exposure, smoking, and chronic inflammation (ulcers, burn scars, discoid lupus)

PATHOGENESIS

The most common altered gene in SCC is the *p53* tumor suppressor gene, resulting in keratinocyte immortalization and unregulated cell proliferation.

PHYSICAL EXAMINATION

Hyperkeratotic skin-colored to erythematous papule, plaque, or nodule (Figs. 53.1 and 53.2). It can be ulcerated, friable, or exophytic. It most commonly presents within sun-damaged skin.

DIFFERENTIAL DIAGNOSES

Keratoacanthoma (Fig. 53.3), hypertrophic actinic keratosis, basal cell carcinoma (BCC), inflamed seborrheic keratosis.

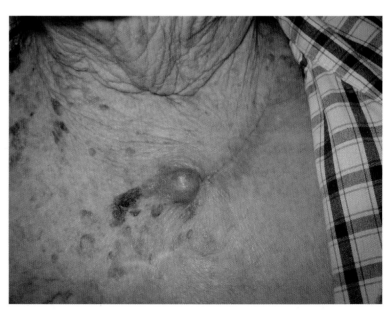

Figure 53.1 *Invasive squamous cell carcinoma on the right neck*

Figure 53.2 *Recurrent squamous cell carcinoma on the chest of an elderly woman*

LABORATORY DATA

■ Dermatopathology

Proliferation of atypical keratinocytes with variable differentiation of the epidermis and variably sized nests and islands invading the dermis. Foci of keratinization are noted in well-differentiated variants. Perineural involvement may be observed.

COURSE

SCC tends to be more aggressive than BCC, with a reported 2% to 3% incidence of metastasis. Mucocutaneous SCC has a higher rate of metastasis, as high as 11%. More aggressive forms of SCC are observed in immunosuppressed patients or SCC that arises within previously irradiated sites, scars, burns, and areas of inflammation. There is a higher metastatic potential for SCC arising on the ear and the lip.

KEY CONSULTATIVE QUESTIONS

Evaluate for past history of blistering sunburns and chronic sun exposure. Determine if other predisposing factors are present such as personal and family history of skin cancer and immunosuppression, especially organ transplantation.

MANAGEMENT

Preventative measures, such as sun avoidance and daily sunscreen use, are critical for long-term prevention. Treatment selection should be based upon the age, health, and preferences of the patient after a full discussion of treatment options, risks, and benefits. Given the metastatic potential of SCC, histological confirmation of complete removal is always advised. Surgical excision and histological evaluation remain the treatment of choice in most cases. Tumors fixed to underlying bone, especially the scalp, merit radiological workup prior to surgical excision or Mohs micrographic surgery. Prior to treatment, lymph node palpation is appropriate for large SCC, SCC in immunosuppressed patients, and high-risk SCCs. Topical therapies require close follow-up for any evidence of treatment failure or recurrence.

■ First-Line Therapies

- Excisional surgery: 4-mm margins are generally recommended
- Mohs micrographic surgery is the treatment of choice for high-risk anatomical locations (ie, "mask" area of the face), locations where tissue conservation is crucial

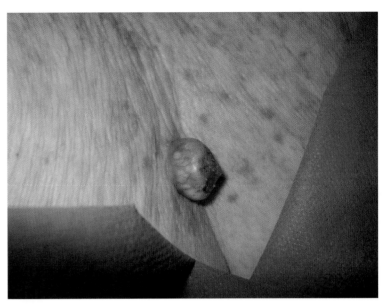

Figure 53.3 *Giant keratoacanthoma on the chest. Many authors regard keratoacanthomas as variants of well-differentiated squamous cell carcinoma*

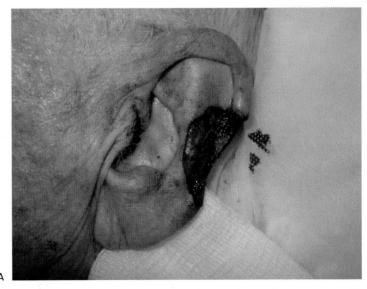

A

Figure 53.4 (A) *Defect on the ear after Mohs excision of a squamous cell carcinoma.*

for functional or cosmetic reasons, recurrent tumors, ill-defined clinical margins, histologically aggressive subtypes, tumors in immunosuppressed patients, tumors larger than 2 cm, irradiated skin, and perineural invasion on biopsy (Figs. 53.4 and 53.5). Cure rates of SCC depend on size, histological grade, perineural invasion, and immunosuppression. Larger lesions, less differentiated variants with perineural involvement, and lesions in immunocompromised patients demonstrate lower cure rates

- Electrodessication and curettage (usually not recommended due to lack of histologic confirmation of removal)
- Cryotherapy (usually not recommended due to lack of histological confirmation of removal)
- Radiotherapy (appropriate for poor surgical candidates)

■ Alternate Therapies

- Topical 5-fluorouraci is limited to SCC in situ
- Topical imiquimod is limited to SCC in situ
- Intralesional interferon
- Photodynamic therapy (PDT) using topical or systemic photosensitizers with lasers or noncoherent red light are most effective for SCC in situ. Clearance rates range from 72% to 94%. PDT can act as an alternative treatment for large lesions, especially for those patients who are poor surgical candidates. It can serve as an alternative treatment in patients with multiple SCCs. For these patients, PDT and close clinical follow-up may obviate the need for multiple surgeries. PDT is also effective for decreasing the number of actinic keratosis, thus acting as a preventative of future SCC development
- Carbon dioxide laser is highly effective for actinic cheilitis. It can also be used to treat SCC in situ

PITFALLS TO AVOID

Infection, bleeding, nerve damage, pain, hypertrophic scarring, poor cosmesis following surgical repair, and recurrence are all common pitfalls of SCC treatment and should be fully discussed with the patient prior to treatment. Nonsurgical therapies may provide better cosmesis but significantly higher rates of recurrence. Furthermore, nonsurgical interventions do not provide the opportunity for histological confirmation of complete removal. This is particularly crucial given the potential of metastatic spread with SCC. Thus, standard or Mohs micrographic surgical excision with histological confirmation of clear margins is always the treatment of choice for SCC.

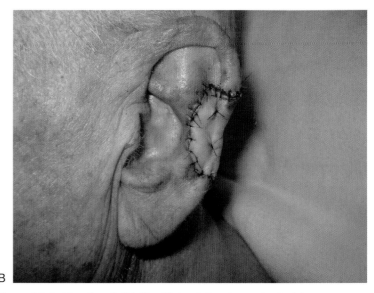

Figure 53.4 (*Continued*) (B) *The Mohs defect is repaired with a full-thickness skin graft*

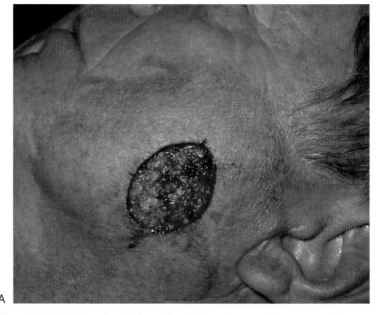

Figure 53.5 (A) *Surgical defect after Mohs micrographic surgery of an SCC on the left cheek.*

BIBLIOGRAPHY

Covadonga Martínez-González M, del Pozo J, Paradela S, Fernández-Jorge B, Fernández-Torres R, Fonseca E. Bowen's disease treated by carbon dioxide laser. A series of 44 patients. *J Dermatolog Treat.* 2008;19(5):293-299.

Morton CA, McKenna KE, Rhodes LE. British Association of Dermatologists Therapy Guidelines and Audit Subcommittee and the British Photodermatology Group. Guidelines for topical photodynamic therapy: *Update. Br J Dermatol.* 2008;159(6):1245-1246.

Preston DS, Stern RS. Nonmelanoma cancers of the skin. *N Engl J Med.* 1992;327:1649-1662.

Rowe DE, Carroll RJ, Day CL Jr. Prognostic factors for local recurrence, metastasis, and survival rates in squamous cell carcinoma of the skin, ear, and lip. Implications for treatment modality selection. *J Am Acad Dermatol.* 1992;26:976-990.

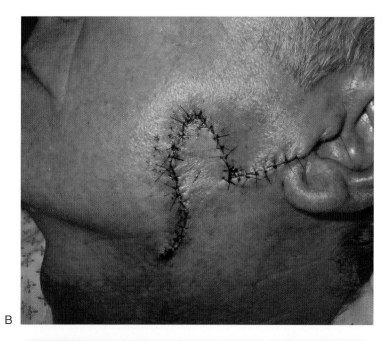

B

C

Figure 53.5 (*Continued*) (B) *The Mohs defect is repaired with a transposition flap.* **(C)** *After suture removal 1 week later*

SECTION NINE

Inflammatory Disorders

CHAPTER 54 Lichen Planus

Lichen planus (LP) is a common inflammatory disease involving the skin and mucous membranes. Many clinical variants exist that include atrophic, ulcerative, bullous, annular, linear, inverse, hypertrophic, lichen planopilaris, actinic LP and LP pigmentosus.

EPIDEMIOLOGY

Incidence: About 0.5%

Age: 30 to 60 years

Race: All races are affected equally in most variants

Sex: Higher incidence in females

Precipitating Factors: Most commonly idiopathic medications may induce a LP-like eruption

PATHOGENESIS

Primarily, a T-helper cell-mediated reaction

PHYSICAL EXAMINATION

Most commonly, primary lesions consist of multiple violaceous, polygonal, flat-topped, grouped papules, and plaques that are usually pruritic. Their surface is shiny or transparent and may exhibit small gray-white punctae or reticular fine white lines known as Wickham's striae. The lesions favor the oropharynx, flexural wrists, dorsal hands, medial thighs, shins, trunk, and genitalia. Postinflammatory hyperpigmentation is common. Actinic LP and LP pigmentosus can present with melasma-like hyperpigmented patches on the forehead and the face (Figs. 54.1–54.3).

DIFFERENTIAL DIAGNOSIS

Psoriasis, lichen simplex, lichenoid graft-versus-host disease, chronic cutaneous lupus erythematosus, lichenoid drug eruption, melasma.

LABORATORY DATA

Given the association with hepatitis B and C, hepatitis serologies can be investigated.

■ Dermatopathology

Pathology reveals lichenoid interface dermatitis, hyperkeratosis, hypergranulosis, saw-tooth acanthosis, associated with colloid or civatte bodies.

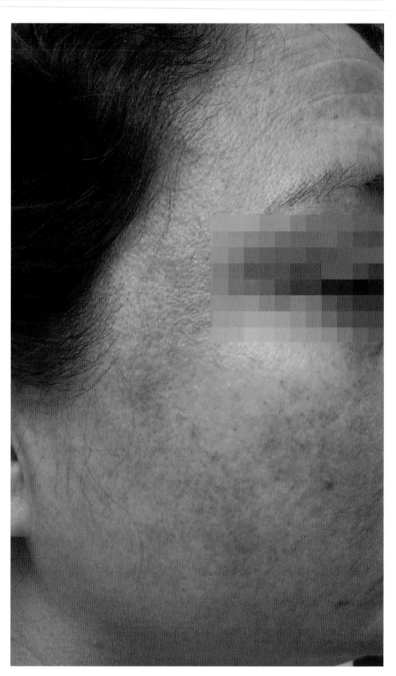

Figure 54.1 *Actinic LP on the forehead, temples, and lateral cheek, mimicking melasma*

COURSE

Spontaneous remission of cutaneous LP occurs within 1 year of onset in the majority of patients. Oral LP persists for many years. Squamous cell carcinoma may arise from these lesions, predominantly from the oral variant (Fig. 54.4).

MANAGEMENT

■ Topical Treatment

• Corticosteroids, topical, intralesional
• Immunomodulators, such as tacrolimus
• Cyclosporine retention mouthwash for oral LP

■ Systemic Treatment

• Corticosteroids
• Retinoids: isotretinoin and acitretin. Acitretin is the only systemic treatment that has been evaluated in a double-blind, placebo-controlled study
• Griseofulvin, metronidazole, antimalarials, methotrexate, cyclosporine, and mycophenolate mofetil

■ Light Treatment

• Narrow Band UVB
• PUVA
• 308-nm UVB excimer laser for oral LP
• CO_2 laser for oral LP: variable results with increased risks of side effects
• Extracorporeal photophoresis

BIBLIOGRAPHY

Dammak A, Masmoudi A, Boudaya S, Bouassida S, Marrekchi S, Turki H. Childhood actinic lichen planus (6 cases) [published online ahead of print January 18, 2008]. *Arch Pediatr.* 2008;15(2):111-114.

Laurberg G, Geiger JM, Hjorth N, et al. Treatment of lichen planus with acitretin. A double-blind, placebo-controlled study in 65 patients. *J Am Acad Dermatol* 1991;24(3):434-437.

Trehan M, Taylor CR. Low-dose excimer 308-nm laser for the treatment of oral lichen planus. *Arch Dermatol* 2004;140(4):415-420.

van der Hem PS, Egges M, van der Wal JE, Roodenburg JL. CO₂ laser evaporation of oral lichen planus. *Int J Oral Maxillofac Surg.* 2008;37(7):630-633.

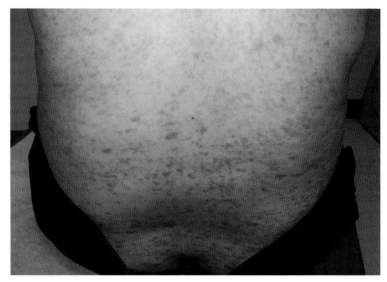

Figure 54.2 *Generalized lichen planus in a patient with skin type 1V–V involving the trunk and buttocks with postinflammatory hyperpigmentation*

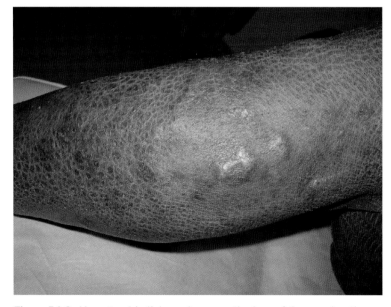

Figure 54.3 *Hypertrophic lichen planus on the legs of 4 years duration resistant to topical and intralesional steroid therapy. The patient improved markedly after 1 month treatment with acetretin*

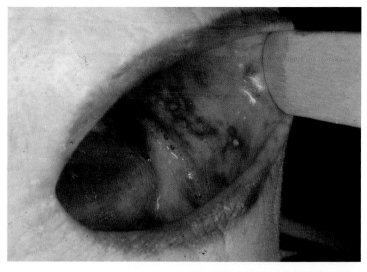

A

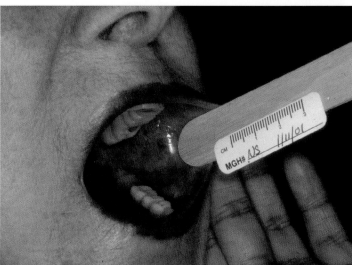

B

Figure 54.4 **(A)** *Oral lichen planus at baseline.* **(B)** *Two month follow-up after 18 treatments with excimer laser administered weekly (Courtesy of Charles Taylor, MD)*

CHAPTER 55 | Morphea

Morphea is localized scleroderma confined to the skin. It most commonly affects the trunk but also occurs on the face and extremities. The four clinical variants include plaque-type morphea, generalized morphea, linear morphea (en coup de sabre), and pansclerotic morphea of children (morphea profunda).

EPIDEMIOLOGY

Incidence: rare

Age: most commonly occurs in the second to fifth decade. Linear scleroderma and morphea profunda are more common in children

Race: slightly more common in Caucasians

Sex: females more than males (2–3:1)

Precipitating factors: Borrelia can trigger morphea in some cases, predominantly in Europe

PATHOGENESIS

Overproduction of collagen (types I, II, III) and glycosaminoglycans by skin fibroblasts and vascular damage. Probable T-cell mediated phenomenon.

PHYSICAL EXAMINATION

Ill-defined pink to violaceous, indurated 2- to 15-cm plaques that transform to smooth sclerotic ivory-colored plaques with a light violaceous border and a shiny surface. Postinflammatory hyperpigmentation is prevalent (Fig. 55.1). Linear morphea presents with a linear erythematous inflammatory streak that may progress to form a scar-like band involving underlying fascia, muscle, and tendons.

DIFFERENTIAL DIAGNOSES

Acrodermatitis chronica atrophicans, eosinophilic fasciitis, lichen sclerosus et atrophicus, scleredema, scleromyxedema, and nephrogenic systemic fibrosis.

LABORATORY DATA

■ Serology

Check for Borrelia antibodies.

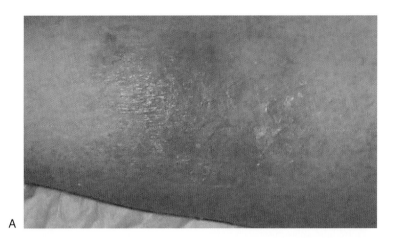

A

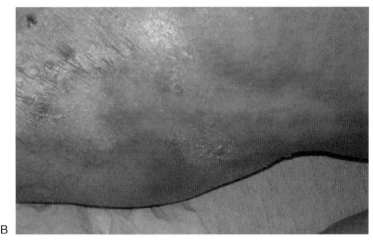

B

Figure 55.1 (A) *Early morphea on the left leg presenting as an erythematous plaque.* **(B)** *Same patient with late stage morphea on the right leg presenting as linear depressed yellowish to white hard plaques with erythematous margins*

■ Dermatopathology

Homogenization and thickening of dermal collagen bundles, trapped and atrophic eccrine glands, perivascular mononuclear infiltrate of lymphocytes and plasma cells with normal or atrophic overlying epidermis. Underlying subcutaneous fat may also be involved with sclerosis in advanced cases.

COURSE

Course is variable. Many patients remit spontaneously but others have a progressive course.

MANAGEMENT

Treatment for this condition can be frustrating due to frequent treatment failure. Patients should be counseled that therapy may not be effective.

- Topical treatment
  - Corticosteroids
  - Calcipotriene
- Systemic treatment
  - Corticosteroids, D-penicillamine, vitamin D_3, methotrexate
- Light treatment
  - Ultraviolet A1 phototherapy
  - Pulsed dye laser (585 nm, 5 J/cm^2 twice monthly), reported to be effective in single case report
- Subcision: subcision with a Nokor 18G needle may help to elevate the bound-down skin. It is most effective for linear morphea and facial hemiatrophy. Subcision is performed under local infiltrative anesthesia to the affected site with 1% lidocaine with 1:100,000 epinephrine. The Nokor needle is introduced at a 45-degree angle into the skin utilizing a sweeping motion to release any tethered areas. Multiple entrance sites should be performed for optimal benefit. Firm pressure is applied to the treatment sites for hemostasis
- Soft tissue augmentation: various fillers have been employed with variable success to augment the sclerotic sites. They are most commonly utilized for linear morphea and facial hemiatrophy. Temporary fillers currently recommended given the unpredictable course of morphea. Autologous fat transfer can provide significant augmentation of the affected sites (Fig. 55.2). Repeat injections generally required. En bloc autologous dermal fat graft reported to be effective in one case report.

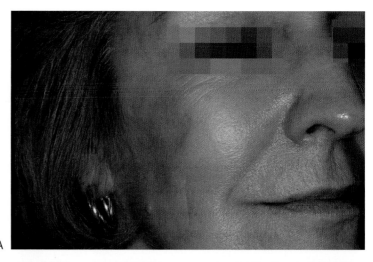
A

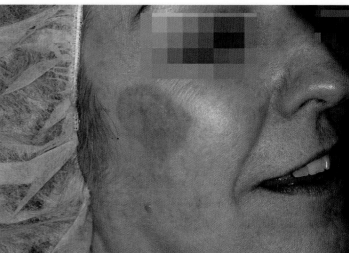
B

Figure 55.2 (A) *Morphea with significant epidermal, dermal, and subcutaneous atrophy.* **(B)** *Elevation of the atrophic plaque of morphea after a single autologous fat transfer. The associated telangiectasias were subsequently treated with the pulsed dye laser with substantial improvement*

PITFALL TO AVOID

Patients must be aware of the unpredictable nature of morphea, therefore the unpredictable nature of the treatment.

BIBLIOGRAPHY

Eisen D, Alster TS. Use of 585 nm pulsed dye laser for the treatment of morphea. *Dermatol Surg*. 2002;28(7): 615-616.

Lapiere JC, Aasi S, Cook B, Montalvo A. Successful correction of depressed scars of the forehead secondary to trauma and morphea en coup de sabre by en bloc autologous dermal fat graft. *Dermatol Surg*. 2000;26(8):793-797.

Nisticò SP, Saraceno R, Schipani C, Costanzo A, Chimenti S. Different applications of monochromatic excimer light in skin diseases. *Photomed Laser Surg*. 2009;27(4):647-654.

CHAPTER 56 | Psoriasis

Psoriasis is a common chronic inflammatory disease of the skin. They are symmetric in distribution and favor elbows, knees, scalp, retroauricular skin, and intertriginous areas. Many clinical variants exist and include plaque psoriasis, pustular psoriasis, guttate psoriasis, inverse psoriasis, and erythrodermic psoriasis, with the plaque variant being the most common type (Figs. 56.1 and 56.2). Nails and mucous membranes can be affected. Psoriasis is associated with psoriatic arthritis in at least 5% of patients.

EPIDEMIOLOGY

Incidence: About 1.5% to 2% of the world's population

Age: can occur at any age. Two peaks of onset, the second and sixth decades. Onset is earlier in women. Uncommonly affects children

Race: lower incidence in African Americans, Native Americans, and Asians

Sex: equal

Precipitating factors: bacterial infections, especially streptococcal infection (guttate psoriasis), trauma (Koebner phenomenon), stress, genetic predisposition, and medication use (most commonly lithium, beta blockers, antimalarials). Rapid corticosteroid tapers may induce pustular psoriasis

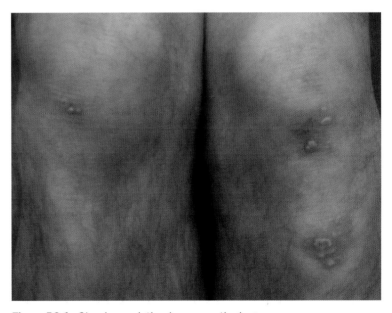

Figure 56.1 *Classic psoriatic plaques on the knees*

PATHOGENESIS

Polygenic disease with a 41% risk for a child to develop psoriasis if both the parents are affected. The primary pathophysiology involves hyperproliferation and abnormal differentiation of epidermal keratinocytes as well as abnormal cellular immune response.

PHYSICAL EXAMINATION

Plaque variant with well-demarcated, pink to erythematous papules and plaques with overlying silvery-white scale. Pinpoint bleeding observed with scale removal (Auspitz sign). Guttate variant with tear drop-shaped lesions. Erythematous generalized pustules are seen with pustular psoriasis.

DIFFERENTIAL DIAGNOSES

Tinea corporis, seborrheic dermatitis, eczematous dermatitis, mycosis fungoides, parapsoriasis, lichen simplex chronicus, pityriasis rubra pilaris, Reiter's disease, Bowen's disease.

LABORATORY DATA

■ Serology

Antistreptolysin O(ASO) titer for guttate psoriasis.

■ Dermatopathology

Regular psoriasiform epidermal hyperplasia with absent granular cell layer and thinning above the dermal papillae. Other characteristic features include collections of neutrophils in epidermis as well as tortuous blood vessels in the papillary dermis.

COURSE

This disease demonstrates a chronic course with multiple exacerbations and remissions, which can be seasonal or related to stress.

MANAGEMENT

There are multiple therapeutic options for treatment of psoriasis. Choosing an appropriate therapy depends on the age, health, and preferences of the patient. It also depends on the extent of the psoriasis. The costs of therapy vary dramatically as well. Alternative therapies are most appropriate in refractory cases. Assessing the side-effect profile of treatments is another crucial component

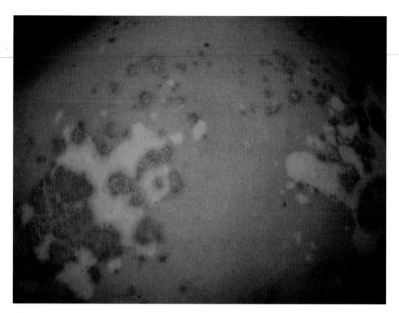

Figure 56.2 *Psoriatic plaques koebnerizing vitiligo patches*

of therapy. Combination therapies are generally most effective to decrease inflammation and reduce scale production.

- Topical Treatment
  - Corticosteroids, topical and intralesional
  - Calcipotriene
  - Tazarotene
  - Coal tar
  - Anthralin
  - Salicylic acid
- Systemic Treatment
  - Methorexate
  - Retinoids, predominanetly acitretin
  - Cyclosporine
  - Biologics such as alefacept, etanercept, efaluzimab, and infliximab
- Laser and Light Treatments
  - Psoralen with Ultraviolet A (PUVA)
  - Ultraviolet B (UVB), 311-nm narrowband-UVB (NB-UVB)
  - 308-nm UVB excimer laser
    - An alternative for treatment of mild-to-moderate psoriasis, where more conventional therapies have failed. It is especially helpful for localized refractory plaque psoriasis
    - Studies have demonstrated that this localized UVB treatment provides much lower cumulative doses of UVB to induce clearance of psoriatic plaques compared to NB-UVB therapy
    - The excimer laser might also produce longer remission periods, with minimization of UVB exposure to healthy surrounding skin
    - Excimer laser has proved to be effective and safe in treating refractory scalp psoriasis
    - Drawbacks of excimer laser in psoriasis treatment include limited availability, treatment expense and extensive treatment time needed per session
- Photodynamic therapy has been shown to improve psoriasis in multiple studies. The major side effects included pain and burning sensation associated with PDT
- Pulsed dye laser (0.45–1.5 ms, 7-mm spot, 7–9 J/cm^2, DCD 30–40/20) has been employed to target the vascularity associated with psoriatic lesions with noted benefit. In a recent study, PDL proved to be effective in the treatment of nail psoriasis (Fig. 56.3)
- In a recent study, Nd:YAG laser (1,064 nm) failed to improve localized plaque type psoriasis

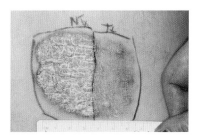
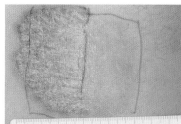
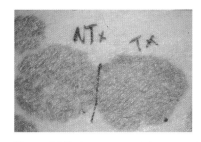
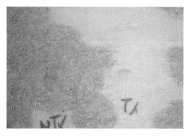

Figure 56.3 *Improvement in treated psoriatic plaque 3 months after pulsed dye laser treatment (585 nm, 10-mm spot size, 5 J/cm^2, no cooling, 0.45-ms pulse duration), as compared to the control site (Reproduced, with permission, from Brian Zelickson, MD)*

PITFALLS

- Patients should be counseled that psoriasis is a chronic condition with flares and remissions. Laser therapy, such as the excimer laser, is an alternative treatment that should only be considered after a patient has failed multiple other treatment regimens.

- Patients should be aware that any treatment administered, it may result in spread of the psoriasis (Koebner phenomenon). They should also be aware that surgical treatments performed for any reason may also result in similar spread.

BIBLIOGRAPHY

Fernández-Guarino M, Harto A, Sánchez-Ronco M, García-Morales I, Jaén P. Pulsed dye laser vs. photodynamic therapy in the treatment of refractory nail psoriasis: A comparative pilot study. *J Eur Acad Dermatol Venereol.* 2009;23(8):891-895.

Gattu S, Rashid RM, Wu JJ. 308-nm excimer laser in psoriasis vulgaris, scalp psoriasis, and palmoplantar psoriasis. *J Eur Acad Dermatol Venereol.* 2009;23(1):36-41.

Noborio R, Kurokawa M, Kobayashi K, Morita A. Evaluation of the clinical and immunohistological efficacy of the 585-nm pulsed dye laser in the treatment of psoriasis. *J Eur Acad Dermatol Venereol.* 2009;23(4):420-424.

Smits T, Kleinpenning MM, van Erp PE, van de Kerkhof PC, Gerritsen MJ. A placebo-controlled randomized study on the clinical effectiveness, immunohistochemical changes and protoporphyrin IX accumulation in fractionated 5-aminolaevulinic acid-photodynamic therapy in patients with psoriasis. *Br J Dermatol.* 2006;155(2):429-436

Taylor CR, Racette AL. A 308-nm excimer laser for the treatment of scalp psoriasis. *Lasers Surg Med.* 2004;34(2):136-140.

Van Lingen RG, de Jong EM, van Erp PE, van Meeteren WS, van De Kerkhof PC, Seyger MM. Nd: YAG laser (1,064 nm) fails to improve localized plaque type psoriasis: A clinical and immunohistochemical pilot study [published online ahead of print October 27, 2008]. *Eur J Dermatol.* 2008;18(6):671-676.

SECTION
TEN

Adipose Tissue Alterations

CHAPTER 57 | Gynecomastia

Gynecomastia is the increased presence of benign glandular tissue, in the form of a firm mass, around the nipple in males (Fig. 57.1). It is accompanied by increased fat deposition. In contrast, increased fat deposition alone, in the absence of glandular proliferation, is known as pseudogynecomastia. It can be bilateral or unilateral. It is common at birth, puberty, middle age, and in elderly adults. Many cases are idiopathic. Multiple precipitating factors exist including hormonal abnormalities, medication, cirrhosis, hypogonadism, testicular tumors, hyperthyroidism, and chronic renal insufficiency. For this reason, in the appropriate clinical setting, the appearance of gynecomastia demands a medical workup.

EPIDEMIOLOGY

Incidence: most common in newborns but also common in puberty and older males

Age: birth (0–3 weeks), puberty (10–17 years), middle-aged and elderly age groups (50–80 years)

Race: none

Sex: males

Precipitating factors: hormonal imbalances, hormonal therapy for prostate cancer, drugs such as, finasteride, cirrhosis, hypogonadism, testicular tumors, hyperthyroidism, chronic renal insufficiency. About one-quarter of cases are idiopathic

PATHOGENESIS

In cases of hormonal imbalances, the fundamental defect is a decrease in androgen levels with a concomitant increase in estrogen levels.

PHYSICAL LESIONS

A firm subcutaneous nodule extends concentrically from the nipple. It may be unilateral or bilateral. In pseudogynecomastia, the examined area is less firm as there is no excess glandular tissue.

DIFFERENTIAL DIAGNOSIS

Breast cancer, pseudogynecomastia, breast hypertrophy.

LABORATORY EXAMINATION

Serum hCG, LH, testosterone, estradiol levels should be investigated in the setting of pain, tenderness, or recent

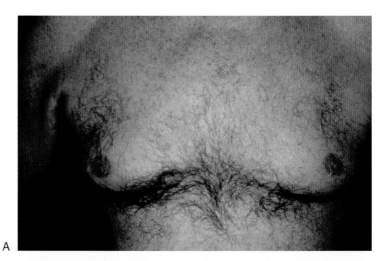

A

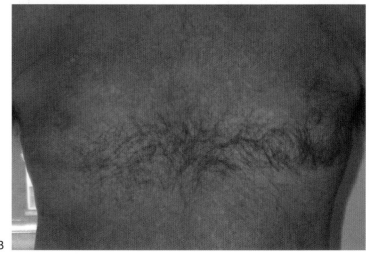

B

Figure 57.1 *Characteristic appearance of gynecomastia in a middle-aged male*

onset or clinical suspicion of endocrine abnormalities. Further workup is indicated in the event of unilateral breast enlargement.

COURSE

This depends on the etiology. Newborn gynecomastia persists for a few weeks. In teenagers, it may last a few years. Discontinuance of medication will ameliorate symptoms in drug-induced cases. In cases of hormonal imbalance, kidney disease, and hyperthyroidism, correction of the underlying illness will produce improvement.

KEY CONSULTATIVE QUESTIONS

- Medication history
- Hormonal changes
- Renal or thyroid disease
- Hormonal therapy for prostate cancer
- Associated symptoms
- Unilateral or bilateral

MANAGEMENT

Most gynecomastia is temporary and will resolve without therapy. If it is related to puberty, clinical observation and follow-up will likely be all that is needed. Discontinuation of an offending medication is typically all that is required to treat drug-induced gynecomastia. Unilateral gynecomastia requires a mammogram with appropriate follow-up as needed. Medical and surgical options are available for patients who have persistent gynecomastia into late puberty producing emotional distress, pain, or tenderness. Benign psuedogynecomastia is the most common cause of male breast enlargement.

TREATMENT

■ Oral Medications

Medical therapy for gynecomastia is beyond the scope of this textbook. It is best performed by a physician who is trained in internal medicine or endocrinology. Medications include androgens, antiestrogens, and aromatase inhibitors.

■ Prophylaxis in Prostate Cancer

Breast radiation can be performed prophylactically in patients undergoing antiandrogen therapy or orchiectomy for prostate cancer. Concomitant tamoxifen administration with finasteride/flutamide therapy can also be prophylactic for gynecomastia.

■ Surgery

In the event of medical treatment failure, surgical therapy is the next option. It is reserved for patients with refractory gynecomastia that has failed medical therapy. The treatments depend on the extent of gynecomastia. A few options are described below.

- Surgical excision including standard elliptical excision as well as subcutaneous mastectomy.

- Conventional and ultrasound-assisted liposuction, that is, localized removal of glandular tissue and/or excess fat. This is particularly successful in early stage and limited gynecomastia.

  - Liposuction is performed through small incisions in the axilla and sternum to minimize scarring

  - Liposuction is less effective in longstanding and substantial gynecomastia

  - In prostate cancer patients, earlier intervention is more efficacious

  - Residual periareolar fat may be noted postliposuction that can be improved with localized dissection of fat via a small periareolar incision

  - Postprocedure skin laxity may be noted

- Combination of surgical excision and tumescent liposuction. This involves liposuction, open excision, and skin reduction for laxity. Liposuction has also been combined with subcutaneous mastectomy.

- Surgical excision with plastic surgical repair, particularly in the event of breast tissue sagging. Excessive fat, glandular tissue, and loose skin are excised via elliptical excision, including the nipple and areola. The nipple/areola complex is then placed in the appropriate anatomic position as a full thickness skin graft after the excess glandular tissue is removed.

- Psuedogynecomastia can be treated with liposuction. Male breast fat tends to be relatively fibrous, and thus more difficult to treat. Further, care must be taken to avoid injury to the pectoralis muscle. In true gynecosmastia, excess glandular tissue renders the procedure even more challenging.

- While traditional liposuction and tumescent liposuction have dominated liposuction treatment of gynecomastia and pseudogynecomastia, laser-assisted liposuction is a recent addition to this field. There is no evidence to show that laser-assisted liposuction is superior to either of these forms of liposuction.

PITFALLS TO AVOID/COMPLICATIONS/ MANAGEMENT/OUTCOME EXPECTATIONS

- It is important to recognize that gynecomastia has multiple etiologies before attempting to treat it.

- In most cases, watchful waiting is the best therapy.

- In cases of an underlying systemic cause, referral to the appropriate specialist is mandated.

- In cases of drug-induced gynecomastia, discontinuation of the medication is the best management.

- In cases of refractory to medical management, there are several surgical options. Complications from these procedures include a poor cosmetic result, postoperative scarring, incomplete removal, postprocedure skin laxity, permanent numbness in the area, and hematoma formation.

BIBLIOGRAPHY

Aslan G, Tuncali D, Terzioglu A, Bingul F. Periareolar-transareolar-perithelial incision for the surgical treatment of gynecomastia. *Ann Plast Surg.* 2005;54(2):130-134.

Bembo SA, Carlson HE. Gynecomastia: Its features, and when and how to treat it. *Cleve Clin J Med.* 2004;71(6): 511-517.

Gabra HO, Morabito A, Bianchi A, Bowen J. Gynaecomastia in the adolescent: A surgically relevant condition. *Eur J Pediatr Surg.* 2004;14(1):3-6.

Gasperoni C, Salgarello M, Gasperoni P. Technical refinements in the surgical treatment of gynecomastia. *Ann Plast Surg.* 2000;44(4):455-458

Iwuagwu OC, Calvey TA, Ilsley D, Drew PJ. Ultrasound guided minimally invasive breast surgery (UMIBS): A superior technique for gynecomastia. *Ann Plast Surg.* 2004;52(2):131-133.

Rohrich RJ, Ha RY, Kenkel JM, Adams WP Jr. Classification and management of gynecomastia: Defining the role of ultrasound-assisted liposuction. *Plast Reconstr Surg.* 2003;111(2):909-923.

Graf R, Auersvald A, Damasio RC, Rippel R, de Araújo LR, Bigarelli LH, Franck CL. Ultrasound-assisted liposuction: An analysis of 348 cases. *Aesthetic Plast Surg.* 2003;27(2):146-153.

Zelickson BD, Dressel TD. Discussion of laser-assisted liposuction. *Lasers Surg Med.* 2009;41(10):709-913.

CHAPTER 58 | Cellulite

Cellulite describes an orange peel type dimpling of skin in the upper posterior thighs and buttocks (Fig. 58.1). Although there is no associated morbidity or mortality, it is among the most common cosmetic complaints among female patients. It is present in nearly all postpubertal females, regardless of weight. It is best thought of as a female secondary sexual characteristic. Importantly, treatments for fat removal and cellulite should be considered distinct. Effective treatments for fat removal typically have no benefit for cellulite.

EPIDEMIOLOGY

Incidence: 85% to 98% of postpubertal females, far less common in males

Age: begins in females after puberty

Race: more common in Caucasians

Sex: far more common in females, rare in males

Precipitating factors: female gender, androgen deficiency in males (rare)

PATHOGENESIS

Unknown.

PHYSICAL LESIONS

There is an orange peel or cottage cheese type dimpling of the upper and outer thighs and buttocks. Other common locations include the breasts, lower abdomen, upper arms, and nape of neck.

DIFFERENTIAL DIAGNOSIS

None.

LABORATORY EXAMINATION

None indicated as the clinical appearance is classic.

COURSE

Begins in puberty in females and persists throughout life. In males with androgen deficiencies, the clinical appearance worsens as the androgen deficiency becomes more severe. It may present de novo in males undergoing hormonal therapy for prostate cancer.

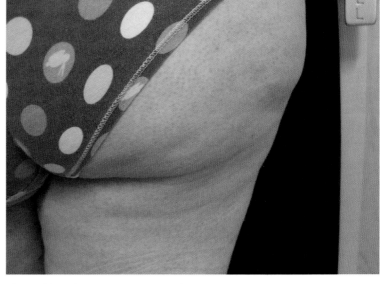

Figure 58.1 *Classic appearance of cellulite*

KEY CONSULTATIVE QUESTIONS

In males, inquire as to any possibility of endocrine abnormalities. This is a very rare association of cellulite in males.

MANAGEMENT

There is no medical indication to treat cellulite. Still, many patients request therapy. Currently, there are numerous purported therapies, none of which have proven to be very effective. Interestingly, despite the lack of scientific evidence of improvement, many patients report subjective improvement and satisfaction with therapy.

TREATMENTS

◼ Diet

- Weight has only a minor association with cellulite
- It is common in thin females and rare in obese males
- There is no data to show that diet and exercise are effective treatments

◼ Topical Treatments

- Aminophylline, retinoids, lactic acid, xanthines, and many others have all been used with little evidence of efficacy
- Some creams may produce more harm than benefit
- In fact, one study indicated 25% of cellulite creams examined contained known contact allergens

◼ Interventional Treatments

Liposuction

- There are a few published reports of improvement; however, typically it does not improve cellulite
- In some cases, it accentuates the appearance of cellulite
- Prior to performing a liposuction procedure, it is useful to inform patients that their cellulite will not resolve. This will protect against postprocedure disappointment

Endermologie

- Endermologie is an FDA cleared device to improve the appearance of cellulite
- Skin is kneaded by a handheld machine
- It is rolled over affected areas of the body that are covered by a nylon suit
- It purports to improve blood and lymphatic flow as well as skin architecture

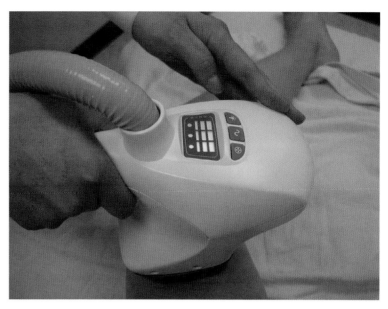

Figure 58.2 *VelaSmooth laser treatment of thigh of young female*

- Twice weekly treatments of 10 to 45 minutes each are recommended
- There is a little evidence to support its efficacy

Subcision

- Requires local anesthesia
- Using a scalpel or special 16-gauge needle, the fat septae are cut in the deep subcutaneous fat
- Side effects include pain, bruising, scar, and puckering
- Little data to support temporary efficacy

Mesotherapy

Phosphatidylcholine injections: not a recommended therapy.

- Injection of combinations of ingredients directly into subcutaneous fat
- Phosphatidylcholine and deoxycholate preparations are most commonly used
  - Deoxycholate is the active ingredient
- No published data to show efficacy

Laser

- VelaSmooth system (Syneron Inc., Richmond Hill, Ontario, Canada) combines near-infrared light at a wavelength of 700 to 2,000 nm, continuous-wave radio frequency, and mechanical suction (Fig. 58.2)
  - Twice weekly treatments for a total of eight to ten sessions have been recommended
  - There are no long-term data to support its efficacy in patients
- The TriActive Laserdermology (Cynosure, Inc, Chelmsford, Massachusetts) combines six near-infrared diode lasers at a wavelength of 810 nm, localized cooling, and mechanical massage
  - Three weekly treatments for 2 weeks and then biweekly treatments for 5 weeks are suggested
  - There are no long-term data to support its efficacy in patients
- Other FDA cleared devices include a unipolar radiofrequency device (Alma Accent, Alma, Inc., Buffalo Grove, Ill.) and a dual wavelength laser system (SmoothShapes, Eleme Medical, Inc., Merrimack, New Hampshire)

PITFALLS TO AVOID/COMPLICATIONS/ MANAGEMENT/OUTCOME EXPECTATIONS

Patients should be informed that there are no truly effective treatments for cellulite. It is also important to distinguish treatments for body contouring and fat removal from those of cellulite. Most of the positive results relating to cellulite treatment are anecdotal or reported in small, unscientific studies. Many of the therapies are expensive, especially given their lack of efficacy. Some may even produce more harm than benefit. There may be a more promising future for laser and light source treatments.

BIBLIOGRAPHY

Avram MM. Cellulite; A review of its physiology and treatment. *J Cosmet Laser Ther.* 2005;7:1-5.

Goldberg DJ, Fazeli A, Berlin AL. Clinical, laboratory, and MRI analysis of cellulite treatment with a unipolar radiofrequency device. *Dermatol Surg.* 2008;34(2):204-209.

Kinney BM. Cellulite treatment: A myth or reality: a prospective randomized, controlled trial of two therapies, endermologie and aminophylline cream. *Plast Reconstr Surg.* 1999;104:1115-1117.

Lis-Balchin M. Parallel-placebo-controlled clinical study of a mixture of herbs sold as a remedy for cellulite. *Phytother Res.* 1999;13:627-629.

Pierard-Franchimont C, Pierard GE, Henry F, Vroome V, Cauwenbergh G. A randomized, placebo-controlled trial of topical retinal in the treatment of cellulite. *Am J Clin Dermatol.* 2000;1:369-374.

Rao J, Gold MH, Goldman MP. A two-center, double-blinded, randomized trial testing the tolerability and efficacy of a novel therapeutic agent for cellulite reduction. *J Cosmet Dermatol.* 2005;4(2):93-102

Rossi AR, Vergnanini AL. Cellulite: A review. *J Eur Acad Dermatol Venereol.* 2000;14:251-262.

van Vliet M, Ortiz A, Avram MM, Yamauchi PS. An assessment of traditional and novel therapies for cellulite. *J Cosmet Laser Ther.* 2005;7(1):7-10.

Wanner M, Avram MM. An evidence-based assessment of treatments for cellulite. *J Drugs Dermatol.* 2008;7(4):341-345

CHAPTER 59 | HIV Lipodystrophy/Facial Lipoatrophy

HIV lipodystrophy describes a constellation of changes in subcutaneous and visceral fat distribution in patients on antiretroviral therapy. In distinction to "lipoatrophy" (which describes local fat loss), lipodystrophy refers to both the accumulation of fat as well as the loss of fat in other areas. In HIV lipostrophy, the findings include sub-cutaneous fat loss in the malar and buccal fat pads, ie, facial lipoatrophy, as well as on the extremities. It also features fat accumulation on the dorsocervical fat pad, (Fig 59.1) ie, buffalo hump, breasts, and intra-abdominal cavity. Its characteristic appearance is significant, in that it reduces patient compliance with antiretroviral therapy and deprives patients of HIV status privacy, particularly in communities where HIV rates are high. This disorder is also associated with a host of metabolic disorders with long-term impact on health including hyperglycemia, hyperlipidemia, and hypertriglyceridemia. Treatments vary according to the clinical findings.

EPIDEMIOLOGY

Incidence: 25% to 83% of patients treated with antiretro-virals depending on criteria used

Age: All ages, but older age is predictive of severity

Race: None

Sex: Equal, severe findings more frequent in females

PRECIPITATING FACTORS

Antiretroviral therapies are the precipitating factor. It also presents infrequently in HIV patients naïve to HIV ther-apy. Typically, patients are on combination therapies.

PATHOGENESIS

Pathogenesis remains unknown. It is a multifactorial dis-order that varies according to the medications taken.

DERMATOPATHOLOGY

Complete or near complete loss of fat. Juxtaposition of the dermis and fascia may be seen. Adipocytes are markedly reduced in number and size.

PHYSICAL LESIONS

Fat accumulation and fat loss are displayed.

• Fat accumulation

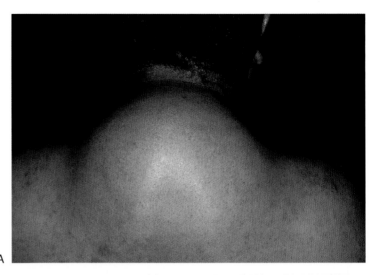

A

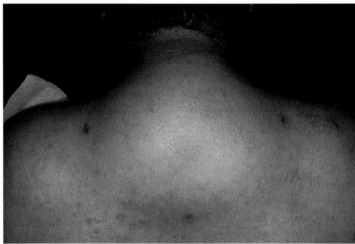

B

Figure 59.1 (A) *"Buffalo hump" in dorsocervical back of HIV-infected male.* **(B)** *Substantial reduction in size of buffalo hump after liposuction procedure*

- Dorsocervical fat pad, ie, buffalo hump
- Breasts
- Intra-abdominal cavity, ie, Crix belly
- Fat loss
  - Malar and buccal fat pads
  - Extremities and buttocks

DIFFERENTIAL DIAGNOSIS

Other lipodystrophies facial lipoatrophy from aging, HIV wasting syndrome, Cushing's disease, malnutrition states, anorexia nervosa, metabolic X syndrome, cachexia secondary to cancer, malabsorption syndromes, thyrotoxicosis, and multiple symmetric lipomatosis.

LABORATORY EXAMINATION

Biopsy is not useful. The clinical findings are sufficient to make a diagnosis. Laboratory workup should include assessment of blood glucose, lipids, and triglycerides. If Cushing's is clinically suspected, laboratory examination should be performed.

COURSE

HIV lipodystrophy does not spontaneously regress in the absence of treatment or medication change.

KEY CONSULTATIVE QUESTIONS

Medication use

Compliance

HIV status

Duration of lipodystoprhy

Associated hyperglycemia, hyperlipidemia, and hypertriglyceridemia

PREVENTION

Once a patient has been treated for the HIV virus, there is no prevention of HIV lipodystrophy.

MANAGEMENT

Cosmetic improvement can be essential to promoting a patient's adherence to their HIV medication regimen. There are several means by which the cosmetic appearance of HIV lipodystrophy can be improved. These include medication changes, filler substances, and liposuction. Diet and exercise can be helpful both for cosmesis and metabolic derangements. Treating the metabolic derangements is best referred to physicians skilled in treating hyperlipidemia, hypertriglyceridemia, and insulin resistance.

TREATMENTS

There are several treatments that can improve the cosmetic appearance of these disorders. They can be divided into two sections: treatment of lipoatrophy and treatment of fat accumulation. Additionally, changes in medications can be pursued. This is best entrusted to a physician who specializes in the care of patients with HIV.

■ Oral Medications

All changes to an antiretroviral regimen are best handled by physicians who specialize in HIV treatment. These changes can improve the appearance of HIV lipodystrophy. Medication changes include

• Discontinuance of antiretroviral therapy

  – Obvious risks of discontinuing medications for a life threatening illness

• Change HIV medications

  – Other HIV medications produce the same condition

  – Some antiretrovirals have a lower incidence of lipodystophy

■ Treatment of Facial Lipoatrophy

Temporary fillers

• Poly-L-lactic acid, Sculptra, is FDA cleared for the treatment of HIV facial lipoatrophy

  – Synthetic, biodegradable polymer

    ◦ The material used in Vicryl sutures

  – Several treatments are required, depending on severity of lipoatrophy

    ◦ Benefits are not seen until weeks after each treatment

  – 18 to 24 month duration of filler material

  – No need for allergy testing

• Calcium hydroxylapatite, Radiesee, is FDA cleared for the treatment of HIV facial lipoatrophy

  – Immediate correction

  – Duration up to 18 months

  – No need for allergy testing

Permanent fillers

• Silicone

  – Not FDA cleared

• A highly purified 1,000-cSt silicon oil has been examined in 77 patients

- The data showed that the number of treatments and amount of silicone required for full treatment was correlated to the initial severity of facial lipoatrophy
- The investigators noted no adverse events but cautioned that long-term efficacy and safety are yet to be determined

■ Treatment of Fat Accumulation

Liposuction/lipectomy

- Localized liposuction/lipectomy uses tumescent localized anesthesia rather than general anesthesia
- Ultrasound assisted liposuction has also been employed
- It is effective in removing excess fat in the dorsocervical region, that is, buffalo hump

PITFALLS TO AVOID/COMPLICATIONS/ MANAGEMENT/OUTCOME EXPECTATIONS

It is important to make certain that the multiple medical issues are being monitored appropriately in these patients. It is also important to emphasize the limited ability of these treatments in the face of extensive HIV lipodystrophy. Generally, however, patients are very eager to see improvement and grateful for the help they receive.

Fillers can be very effective for improving facial lipoatrophy. Temporary fillers, such as Sculptra or Radiesse, have the advantage of FDA clearance and studies documenting their efficacy. Further, their nonpermanent nature allows for temporary side effects in the event of poor results or granuloma formation. Unfortunately, temporary fillers require perpetual treatment sessions and expense.

Permanent fillers such as silicone are attractive in these patients because their disorder is permanent. Data are promising, but further long-term studies are needed to assess long-term efficacy and safety concerns. After a series of injections, further treatment and expense is not required. Unfortunately, poor technique and granuloma formation are hazards. While granulomas are infrequent side effects, they produce obvious cosmetic disfigurement. There is the potential of granuloma formation many years after initial treatment as well. These granulomas do not resolve with the relative rapidity of nonpermanent filler substances. Furthermore, silicone is not FDA cleared for the treatment of HIV lipodystrophy.

Liposuction can be very effective in patients with buffalo humps. Localized liposuction/lipectomy uses tumescent localized anesthesia rather than general anesthesia, which decreases the possibility of serious adverse events. Still, liposuction can be expensive and results vary according to the experience of the practitioner.

Facial plastic surgical procedures can be effective, but require major invasive surgery with its attendant risks of morbidity. There is also increased down time, pain, and the risk of general anesthesia.

BIBLIOGRAPHY

Boix V. Polylactic acid implants. A new smile for lipoatrophic faces? *AIDS*. 2003;17(17):2533-2535.

Carruthers A, Carruthers J. Evaluation of injectable calcium hydroxylapatite for the treatment of facial lipoatrophy associated with human immunodeficiency virus. *Dermatol Surg*. 2008;34(11):1486-1499.

Carruthers A, Liebeskind M, Carruthers J, Forster BB. Radiographic and computed tomographic studies of calcium hydroxylapatite for treatment of HIV-associated facial lipoatrophy and correction of nasolabial folds. *Dermatol Surg*. 2008;34(Suppl 1):S78-S84

Connolly N, Manders E, Riddler S. Short communication: Suction-assisted lipectomy for lipodystrophy. *AIDS Res Hum Retroviruses*. 2004;20(8):813-815.

Hadigan C, Yawetz S, Thomas A, Havers F, Sax PE, Grinspoon S. Metabolic effects of rosiglitazone in HIV lipodystrophy; A randomized, controlled trial. *Ann Intern Med*. 2004;786-794.

Jones DH, Carruthers A, Orentreich D, et al. Highly purified 1000 cst silicon oil for treatment of human immunodeficiency virus-associated facial lipoatrophy: An open pilot trial. *Dermatol Surg*. 2004;30(10):1279-1286.

Koutkia P, Canavan B, Breu J, Torriani M, Kissko J, Grinspoon S. Growth hormone-releasing hormonr in HIV-infected men with lipodystrophy: A randomized controlled trial. *JAMA*. 2004;292(2):210-218.

Levy RM, Redbord KP, Hanke CW. Treatment of HIV lipoatrophy and lipoatrophy of aging with poly-L-lactic acid: a prospective 3-year follow-up study. *J Am Acad Dermatol*. 2008;59(6):923-933.

Pilero PJ, Hubbard M, King J, Faragon JJ. Use of ultrasonography-assisted liposuction for the treatment of human immunodeficiency virus-associated enlargement of the dorsocervical fat pad. *Clin Infect Dis*. 2003;37:1374-1377.

Vleggaar D, Bauer U. Facial enhancement and the European experience with Sculptra (poly-L-lactic acid). *J Drugs Dermatol*. 2004;3(5):542-547.

CHAPTER 60 | Striae Distensae

Striae distensae, more commonly known as "stretch marks," are atrophic linear bands of skin that appear after certain precipitating factors such as pregnancy, steroid use, and dramatic changes in weight or muscle mass (Fig. 60.1). At presentation, they feature a purple or pink color (striae rubra) that fades to a paler white (striae alba) over time. They are most common in adult women.

EPIDEMIOLOGY

Incidence: common

Age: puberty, pregnancy

Race: more common in Caucasians

Sex: females > males (associated with puberty and pregnancy)

Precipitating factors: topical and oral steroid use, Cushing's syndrome, pregnancy, breast-feeding, puberty, genetic collagen defects, and dramatic changes in weight, height, or muscle mass

PATHOGENESIS

There are changes in the extracellular dermal matrix including fibrillin, elastin, and collagen, resulting from prolonged stretching of the skin.

PATHOLOGY

There are scar-like features. Typically, there is an atrophic epidermis with narrow collagen bundles arranged parallel to the skin surface. The rete ridges are effaced. In early striae, there is a superficial, deep, and interstitial lymphocytic perivascular infiltrate and occasional eosinophils. The infiltrate fades in older lesions.

PHYSICAL LESIONS

Multiple symmetric linear band-like plaques of atrophic skin that present most commonly in the outer thighs, breasts, and buttocks of women along the lines of cleavage. They present with a pink/purple hue (striae rubra) and become paler with fine wrinkling over time (striae alba). Striae are largest and most abundant in patients with Cushing's disease. In pregnancy, striae are most abundant on the abdomen. In weight lifters, they are most prominent on the shoulders. Topical corticosteroid use most commonly produces striae on the face, genitalia, flexural areas, and body folds.

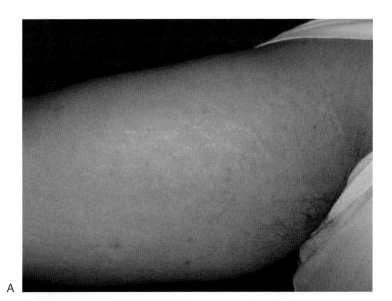

A

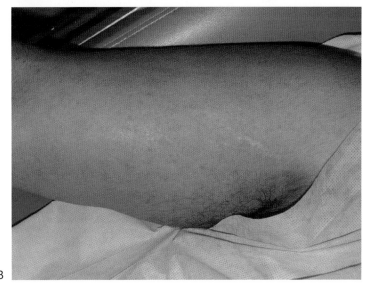

B

Figure 60.1 (A) *Striae alba at baseline.* **(B)** *Striae alba at 11 months follow-up after four treatments with a 1450-nm diode laser (Smoothbeam, Candela Corp., Wayland, MA) at energy settings of 13 to 14 J/cm², using a 6-mm spot size with a pulse duration of 30 ms. Treatment was performed at intervals of 2 to 3 months*

DIFFERENTIAL DIAGNOSIS

Linear focal elastosis.

LABORATORY EXAMINATION

The characteristic clinical appearance of striae negates any need for skin biopsy. Additional laboratory workup to rule out Cushing's disease is indicated in the appropriate clinical setting.

COURSE

Striae begin as pink or purple atrophic lesions that become paler and less obvious over time.

KEY CONSULTATIVE QUESTIONS

- Duration
- Skin phototype
- Pregnancy
- Assess for symptoms of Cushing's disease
- Use of corticosteroids
- History of weight change
- History of weight lifting

MANAGEMENT

There is no medical indication to treat striae. Still, many individuals are significantly bothered by their appearance and request treatment. There are numerous options to treat striae. Unfortunately, none of the treatments is completely successful. In fact, most treatments provide modest or no benefit. Thus, prior to treatment, patients' expectations need to be tempered. Combination treatment involving laser and topical regimens such as tretinoin is often a helpful method of treatment. More recently, nonablative and ablative fractional treatments have emerged. Fortunately, the appearance, particularly the color of striae, improves with time. Patients with skin phototypes I–III respond better than those with types IV–VI to laser therapy. Test sites prior to therapy are recommended. There is some data to show that treatments improve striae over nonintervention. The first priority is to establish whether stria rubra or stria alba are being treated, as their treatments differ significantly.

TREATMENT (Fig. 60.2)

- Stria rubra: the pulsed dye laser (585 nm) with a 7- or 10-mm spot size and 2 to 4 J/cm^2 fluence has been shown to improve the erythema of striae, but is associated with

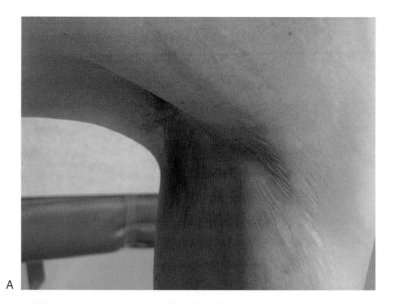

A

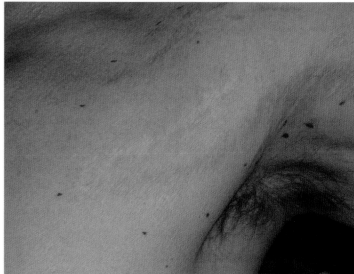

B

Figure 60.2 (A) *White striae, axilla. Prominent atrophy, textural changes, and depigmentation are observed.* **(B)** *White striae, axilla, following three fractional resurfacing laser treatments. Mild improvement of the atrophy and textural changes are noted. Mild post-inflammatory hyperpigmentation is observed, which resolved 3 weeks after the last laser treatment*

the risk of hyperpigmentation in darker skin phototypes. A clinical endpoint of deep erythema or light purpura is optimal. In our experience, lower fluences are more successful than higher fluences (Fig. 60.3).

- Pulsed dye laser treatments do little, if anything, to improve the texture and atrophy of striae.

- Improvement can be seen even in cases of poor initial response 6 months after treatment.

- Studies recommend against treating skin phototypes V–VI.

- Some data casts doubt on the effectiveness of pulsed dye laser.

• Stria alba: nonablative fractional resurfacing has been shown to provide some benefit for striae albae. Studies show a range of efficacy with these treatments.

There is little data to suggest whether deep depth, high coverage treatments are more effective than lower depth, lower coverage treatments. In our experience, most patients see a modest benefit from treatment. A minority sees more significant results.

• Short-pulsed erbium:YAG and CO_2 lasers can be modestly effective but are no longer commonly used due to such side effects as prolonged, difficult healing and pigmentary alteration. They are not recommended.

• The excimer laser (308 nm) has been examined for treatment of striae alba and scars in 31 adults. Treatments began at the Minimal Erythema Dose (MED) minus 50 mJ/cm² to affected areas and were performed biweekly for 10 weeks. An improvement in coloration, by visual inspection (60–70%) and colorimetric analysis (100%), was noted and correlated strongly with the number of treatments performed. The pigment correction, however, returned close to baseline after a 6-month follow-up. No blistering or pigmentary disturbances were noted.

TOPICAL TREATMENT

• Early striae

- Treninoin (0.1%) cream can improve the appearance of striae, particularly early striae, while decreasing their length and width.

• Mature striae

- Tretinoin (0.05%) and 20% glycolic acid can improve striae.

- Glycolic acid (20%) and 10% L-ascorbic acid can improve striae.

MICRODERMABRASION

Microdermabrasion can produce small improvement after six to ten treatments. Microdermabrasion can also

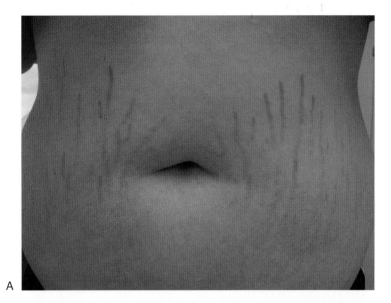

A

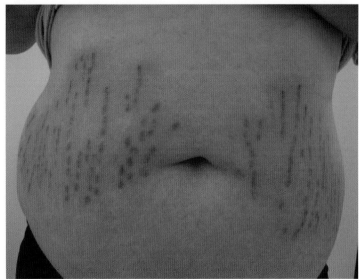

B

Figure 60.3 (A) *Numerous striae rubra and alba on the abdomen of a young woman.* **(B)** *Immediate endpoint of purpura following low energy, short pulse duration treatment with a pulsed dye laser*

be used in association with laser therapy given its fairly benign side-effect profile.

PITFALLS TO AVOID/OUTCOME EXPECTATIONS/COMPLICATIONS/ MANAGEMENT

- Patients should be informed that complete resolution is not realistic. Rather, mild-to-moderate benefit is most realistic. Thus, highly motivated patients with realistic expectations are the best candidates for treatment.
- Laser therapy must be used with caution in dark skin phototypes given the risk of hyperpigmentation.
- Topical tretinoin can produce skin irritation.

BIBLIOGRAPHY

Alexiades-Armenakas MR, Bernstein LJ, Friedman PM, Geronemus RG. The safety and efficacy of the 308-nm excimer laser for pigment correction of hypopigmented scars and striae alba. *Arch Dermatol.* 2004;140(8):955-960.

Ash K, Lord J, Zukowski M, McDaniel DH. Comparison of topical therapy for striae alba (20% glycolic acid/0.05% tretinoin versus 20% glycolic acid/10% L-ascorbic acid). *Dermatol Surg.* 1998;24(8):849-856.

Bak H, Kim BJ, Lee WJ, et al. Treatment of striae distensae with fractional photothermolysis. *Dermatol Surg.* 2009;35(5):826-832.

Goldberg DJ, Sarradet D, Hussain M. 308-nm Excimer laser treatment of mature hypopigmented striae. *Dermatol Surg.* 2003;29(6):596-598. Discussion 598–599.

Jimenez GP, Flores F, Berman B, Gunja-Smith Z. Treatment of striae rubra and striae alba with the 585-nm pulsed-dye laser. *Dermatol Surg.* 2003;29(4):362-365.

McDaniel DH, Ash K, Zukowski M. Treatment of stretch marks with the 585-nm flashlamp-pumped pulsed dye laser. *Dermatol Surg.* 1996;22(4):332-337.

Nehal KS, Lichtenstein DA, Kamino H, Levine VJ, Ashinoff R. Treatment of mature striae with the pulsed dye laser. *J Cutan Laser Ther.* 1999;1(1):41-44.

Nouri K, Romagosa R, Chartier T, Bowes L, Spencer JM. Comparison of the 585 nm pulse dye laser and the short pulsed CO_2 laser in the treatment of striae distensae in skin types IV and VI. *Dermatol Surg.* 1999;25(5):368-370.

Stotland M, Chapas AM, Brightman L, et al. The safety and efficacy of fractional photothermolysis for the correction of striae distensae. *J Drugs Dermatol.* 2008;7(9): 857-861.

SECTION ELEVEN

Wound Healing Alterations

CHAPTER 61 | Hypertrophic Scars, Keloids, and Acne Scars

INTRODUCTION

Hypertrophic scars and keloids are both characterized by excess fibrous tissue at a site of injury in the skin. Hypertrophic scars are confined to the original wound site, whereas keloids, by contrast, extend beyond the original wound site (Table 61.1). Both are common and frequently disturb patients greatly, both as an unsightly scar as well as a reminder of previous trauma or surgery. Acne scars result from the loss of underlying collagen and elastic tissue from dermal inflammation associated with acne, particularly cystic acne. Acne scars are also very common and a source of distress to the patient, both for their obvious appearance on the face as well as a reminder of previous acne.

HYPERTROPHIC SCARS AND KELOIDS: PHYSICAL EXAMINATION

Hypertrophic scars present as thick, firm linear plaques at the site of trauma. Initially, they may be erythematous but often become skin-colored with time. Keloids are firm, fibrous plaques that extend outside the site of injury with claw-like projections.

DIFFERENTIAL DIAGNOSIS

Dermatofibroma, scar sarcoid, dermatofibrosarcoma protuberans, granuloma.

LABORATORY EXAMINATION

None. If, however, a keloid is unresponsive to multiple therapies, skin biopsy to rule out dermatofibrosarcoma protuberans is indicated.

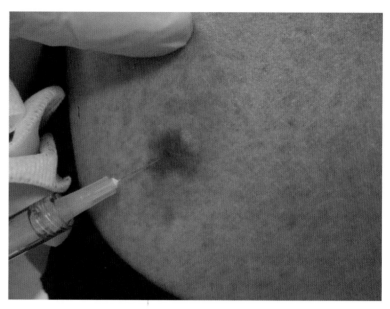

Figure 61.1 *Dermal injection of hypertrophic scar that resulted from a shave biopsy*

TABLE 61.1 ■ Hypertrophic Scars Versus Keloids

	Keloid	Hypertrophic scar
Definition	Excess fibrous tissue formation in a wound that extends beyond the original wound site	Excess fibrous tissue formation in a wound that remains within the original wound site
Course	Does not spontaneously regress	Often spontaneous regression months after the injury
	May arise weeks or months after injury	Usually arise within weeks of injury
Precipitating factors	Family history, surgery, trauma, burn, acne, earlobe piercing; most common in skin types IV–VI, but may arise in all skin types and all ages	Family history, surgery, trauma, burn, acne; may arise in any patient at all ages
Incidence	Common; Males = females	Common; Males = females
	Sternum: most common location	Sternum: most common location

MANAGEMENT

There are multiple therapies that are effective for decreasing the unsightly appearance of keloids and hypertrophic scars. None is completely satisfactory and none can be designated as a treatment of choice. Patients should be educated as to the refractory nature of keloids and hypertrophic scars and that multiple treatments over months are typically required for efficacy. Keloids tend to be more resistant to therapy than hypertrophic scars.

These treatment options include intralesional triamcinolone acetonide, intralesional 5-fluorouracil (5-FU), silicone sheeting, imiquimod, radiation, elliptical excision, fractional resurfacing, and pulsed dye laser (PDL) (595 nm). These treatments provide different benefits. Some reduce erythema, others flatten lesions, and some perform both the functions. Most often, intralesional steroids are a good initial therapy that can be combined with or followed by other therapies. Treatments can be broadly divided into laser and nonlaser therapies (Table 61.2).

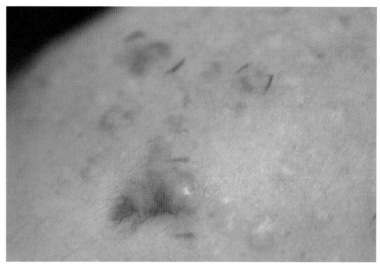

Figure 61.2 *Mild purpura after pulsed dye laser treatment of keloidal acne on back of a teenager. Intralesional kenalog was also used to produce eventual clinical improvement after a series of treatments*

TABLE 61.2 ■ Nonlaser Treatment Options

	Dose	Interval of time	Hypertrophic scar	Keloids	Comments
Intralesional 1 triamcinolone acetonide (Fig. 61.1)	5–40 mg/mL (site dependent)	Every 2–6 weeks	For most scars, moderate to dramatic improvement	Variable success; most successful with early intervention	Effective, safe, inexpensive; care to avoid atrophy
Intralesional 5-fluorouracil	50 mg/mL	1–3 times weekly for the first 1–2 weeks; then every 2–5 weeks	Can be effective; second-line therapy	Variable success	No clear advantage over triamcinolone acetonide
Silicone sheeting		12 hours per day for 12 weeks	Variable improvement	Variable improvement	Safe
Imiquimod	Induces tumor necrosis factor alpha and interferon alpha and gamma	Nightly application for 6–8 weeks starting the day of surgery	Not studied	Study showed no recurrences up to 6 months; risk hyperpigmentation in scar. Further study needed to confirm these results	No long-term studies for recurrence rates
Excision surgical			Mostly unsuccessful, not recommended without adjuvant therapy	Very high recurrence rate without adjunct therapy. All patients must be aware recurrent keloid may be worse than original	Immediate gratification but increased risk of recurrence

LASER

PDL (595 nm) has emerged as an important adjuvant for treatment of keloids and hypertrophic scars (Fig. 61.2). Given its selective targeting of superficial blood vessels, PDL can dramatically improve the erythema associated with hypertrophic scars and keloids (Table 61.3). Interestingly, lower fluence treatments at short pulse durations tend to be more successful than higher fluence treatments. It has also been shown help to flatten lesions as well.

Ablative and nonablative fractional resurfacing resurfacing has been shown to provide moderate improvement for acne, surgical, hypertrophic, and burn scars. It is still unknown whether high-density treatments are more effective than low-density treatments. Typically, scar remodeling with nonablative fractional resurfacing requires six to eight treatments to achieve about 50% benefit (Fig. 61.3). Significant improvement is seen with one to two treatments with ablative fractional resurfacing.

CO_2 laser treatment of these lesions, while reported successful in some of the literature, is not recommended due to a high rate of recurrence. Intralesional corticosteroids are a helpful adjuvant to laser therapy to help flatten lesions and reduce pruritus.

STUDIES

- One study examined the effect of a flashlamp pumped PDL at 585 nm or a flashlamp PDL at 510 nm on 15 patients with red hypertrophic scars. After an average of nearly two treatments, 77% improvement was noted. After three treatments, 7 of the 15 patients had complete resolution.

- Another study using the 585-nm PDL treated one half of median sternotomy hypertrophic scars/keloids in 16 patients and left the other side untreated. Patients received two treatments every 6 to 8 weeks and were examined after 6 months. Blinded observers and photography revealed "significant improvement" in redness, scar height, skin surface texture, and pruritis in laser-treated scar areas after 6 months.

TABLE 61.3 ■ **Pulsed Dye Laser for Hypertrophic Scars/Keloids**

Mechanism of action	Unknown
Expectation	Improves erythema, thickness, and pliability by up to 30–90%
PDL settings	3–7 J/cm², 7 or 10-mm spot, 0.45- or 1.5-ms pulse duration
Average number of treatments	4–6; but may require far more

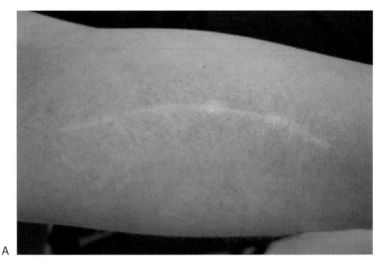

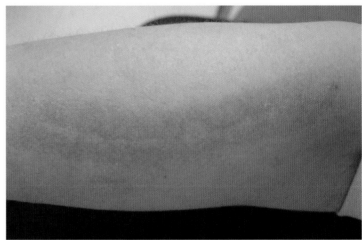

Figure 61.3 **(A)** *Pre- and* **(B)** *postappearance of a traumatic scar after a series of fractional resurfacing treatments. There is some mild residual PIH that faded within 1 to 2 weeks*

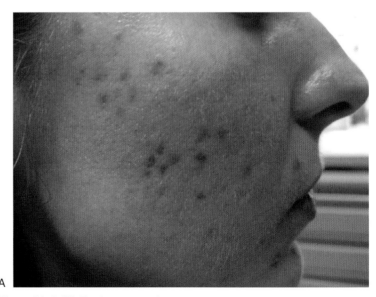

Figure 61.4 **(A)** *Erythematous deep acne scars.*

CLINICAL EXPERIENCE

- Avoid elective surgery in patients with a history of keloids/hypertrophic scarring.

- Consider beginning therapy at the time of surgery or at suture removal.

- Keloids are more difficult to treat and more unpredictable in their response than hypertrophic scars.

- Hypertrophic scars often improve with no treatment in 6 months.

  PDL and fractional resurfacing lasers are effective in improving hypertrophic scars,

  Fractional resurfacing can improve the texture and appearance of surgical and burn scars

ACNE SCARS

Acne scarring is a common sequela of severe inflammatory or cystic acne. It can present in a mild or cosmetically disfiguring form. The best prevention of acne scarring is aggressive treatment of acne vulgaris at the time of presentation, including, when appropriate, isotretinoin. Acne scars have several varieties including atrophic, ice-pick, rolling, and boxcar scars. Treatments vary according to the type of scar being treated. In fact, a combination of treatments is often merited, that is, PDL for scar erythema and subsequent nonablative fractional resurfacing for acne scars (Fig. 61.4) They also vary in terms of duration of efficacy and expense. Prior to surgical or ablative therapy, it is important to elicit any recent history of Accutane use within the previous 6 months as well as a history of hypertrophic or keloidal scarring to avoid poor wound healing and scarring after therapy.

■ Physical Lesions

- Atrophic scars are depressed from the skin surface and result from local loss of tissue from inflammation, intralesional steroids, skin surgery, weight loss, or rapid growth (Table 61.4).

- Ice-pick scars are narrow, deep, vertical, cylindrical depressions at the site of the infundibulum. Given their depth, they are more resistant to laser therapy. Punch excisions, followed by nonablative fractional resurfacing, can be helpful (Fig. 61.5).

- Rolling scars are shallow depressions that are best appreciated with a change in surface lighting. They can vary in size and often coalesce with neighboring rolling scars. They are wider than ice-pick scars. Their depressed appearance reflects an underlying fibrosis of the dermis and subcutaneous fat.

- Boxcar scars are wider than ice-pick scars but less deep. They have a well-defined circular or oval shape.

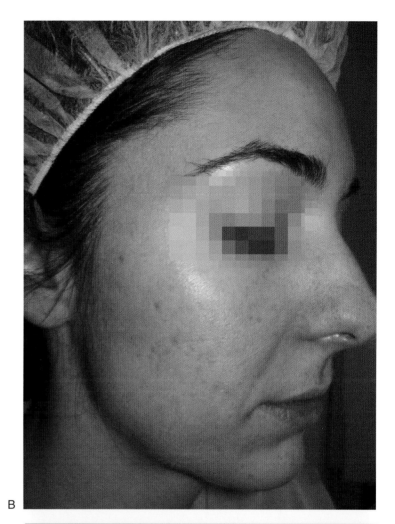

B

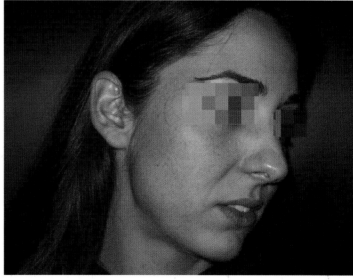

C

Figure 61.4 (*Continued*) **(B)** *Improvement in acne scar erythema after a series of pulsed dye laser treatments.* **(C)** *Further improvement with acne scars with subsequent nonablative fractional resurfacing*

TABLE 61.4 ■ **Treatment Options for Atrophic Scars**

Therapy	Type of therapy	Course	Comments
Topical	Tretinoin 0.05–1% nightly	Slight improvement after 6–12 months	Slight improvement as monotherapy. Most effective as an adjunct with other modalities. If initial irritation, apply every other night until better tolerated
Laser	1,450-nm diode: 12–13 J/cm^2, 6-mm spot size 30–40-ms cryogen cooling spray, three to four treatments over 4–6 months; treats active acne as well	10–30% improvement	Mild improvement Safe in all skin types Risk of transitory hyperpigmentation; postlaser erythema weeks to months; may cause acne flare
	Fractional resurfacing: five to six treatments; deeper depth of treatment is more effective, unclear if higher or lower density of treatment is more effective	Nonablative: moderate improvement after five to six treatments Ablative: moderate improvement after two treatments	Side effects include temporary erythema, edema, crusting, and mild pain Some may develop bronzing and mild flaking at 5–7 days Higher incidence of hyperpigmentation in darker skin phototypes Low risk for long-term adverse side effects; except that scarring may occur with ablative fractional devices
	Ultrapulsed pulse carbon dioxide laser	40–60% improvement; more effective than nonablative laser	More downtime and side effects than nonablative laser Postlaser erythema lasting weeks to months; risk of hyperpigmentation, infection, scar, and permanent hypopigmentation Best for shallow, wide scars such as boxcar scars Antivirals for patients with history of HSV
Fillers	Restylane (hyaluronic acid)	Dramatic improvement 6–8 months	Temporary Low-risk allergy, granuloma; do not overcorrect scars
Fillers	Autologous fat	Dramatic improvement and longer duration than other fillers	Longer duration No risk of allergy, granuloma More difficult to master effective technique
Fillers	Bovine collagen: Zyderm I, Zyderm II, Zyplast	Good, temporary improvement for 2–3 months	Requires test site for allergy Higher risk of allergy (ie, 1–3%) Technique: overcorrect scars Easier procedure for inexperienced practitioners than other fillers Adverse effects: shorter duration
Fillers	Human collagen	Good, temporary improvement for 2–3 months	

TABLE 61.4 ■ **Treatment Options for Atrophic Scars (*Continued*)**

Therapy	Type of therapy	Course	Comments
Mechanical/ chemical	Micodermabrasion, glycolic and salicylic acid peels (Fig. 61.4) TCA peels; dermabrasion	Mild improvement	Microdermabrasion/glycolic acid peels are safe; salicylic acid peels safe in skin types IV–VI; dermabrasion should not be performed except in extremely experienced hands
Surgical	Subcision (incision into dermis with mechanical trauma inducing fibrosis)	Mild improvement	Safe
Surgical	Punch excision Fig. 61.6), punch grafting, punch autografting, punch elevation	Good improvement	Time consuming. Multiple treatments. Better for ice-pick scars

■ Key Points in Treating Acne Scars

- Emphasize improvement rather than complete resolution as an obtainable result.

- Discuss all treatment options. All options have advantages and disadvantages.

- Many patients will benefit from a combination of therapy.

- Obtain complete medical history and medication use, that is, Accutane within 6 months of any surgical/ablative treatment.

- Make sure acne is being or has been treated to prevent future scars.

BIBLIOGRAPHY

Alster TS, Williams CM. Treatment of keloid sternotomy scars with 585 nm flashlamp-pumped pulsed-dye laser. *Lancet.* 1995;345(8959):1198-1200.

Avram MM, Tope WD, Yu T, Szacowicz E, Nelson JS. Hypertrophic scarring of the neck following ablative fractional carbon dioxide laser resurfacing. *Lasers Surg Med.* 2009;41(3):185-188.

Berman B, Kaufman J. Pilot study of the effect of postoperative imiquimod 5% cream on the recurrence rate of excised keloids. *J Am Acad Dermatol.* 2002;47(suppl 4):S209-S211.

Berman B, Viall A. Imiquimod 5% cream for keloid management. *Dermatol Surg.* 2003;29(10):1050-1051.

Chua SH, Ang P, Khoo LS, Goh CL. Nonablative 1450 nm diode laser in treatment of facial atrophic acne scars in type IV Asian skin. *Dermatol Surg.* 2004;(10):1287-1291.

Fitzpatrick RE. Treatment of inflamed hypertrophic scars using intralesional 5-FU. *Dermatol Surg.* 1999;25(3):224-232.

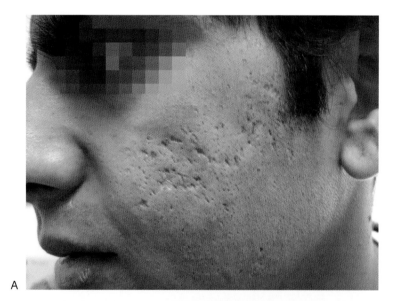

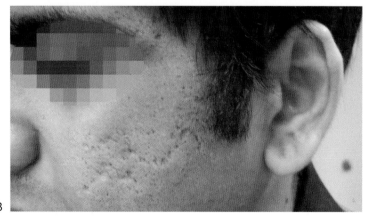

Figure 61.5 (A) *Ice pick scars prior to punch excisions.* **(B)** *Improvement of ice pick scars 1 week after suture removal. Further improvement was achieved with nonablative fractional resurfacing*

Glaich AS, Rahman Z, Goldberg LH, Friedman PM. Fractional resurfacing for the treatment of hypopigmented scars: A pilot study. *Dermatol Surg*. 2007;33(3): 289-294.

Haedersdal M, Moreau KE, Beyer DM, Nymann P, Alsbjorn B. Fractional nonablative 1540 nm laser resurfacing or thermal burn scars: A randomized controlled trial. *Lasers Surg Med*. 2009;41(3):189-195.

Jacob CI, Dover JS, Kaminer MS. Acne scarring: A classification system and review of treatment options. *J Am Acad Dermatol*. 2001;45(1):109-118.

Niwa AB, Mello AP, Torezan LA, Osorio N. Fractional photothermolysis for the treatment of hypertrophic scars: Clinical experience of eight cases. *Dermatol Surg*. 2009; 35(5):773-777.

Nouri K, Jimenez GP, Harrison-Balestra C, Elgart GW. 585 nm pulsed dye laser in treatment of surgical scars starting on suture removal day. *Dermatol Surg*. 2003; 29(1):65-73.

Waibel J, Beer K. Fractional laser resurfacing for thermal burns. *J Drugs Dermatol*. 2008;7(1):59-61.

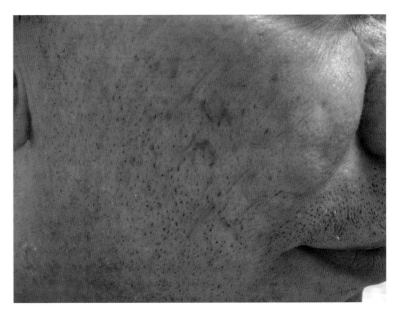

Figure 61.6 *Patient after numerous punch excisions. Sutures are removed 5 to 7 days after the procedure*

TABLE 61.5 ■ Ice-Pick/Boxcar Scar

	Advantage	Disdvantage
Punch harvesting and suture or punch harvest and implant full-thickness graft	Low cost, potential dramatic improvement; best for narrow, deep scars such as ice-pick scars or deep boxcar scars; punch excision can be followed by ablative or nonablative fractional resurfacing treatments	Unpredictable, risk of making cosmetic appearance worse; time consuming
Ablative CO_2/Erbium:YAG	Potential 40–60% long-term improvement; best for shallow boxcar scars	Postlaser erythema weeks to months; risk of hyperpigmentation, infection, scar, and permanent hypopigmentation
	Quick, significant improvement	Antivirals for patients with history of HSV
Fillers, ie, Restylane, collagen, etc. (see Table 61.4)		No permanent improvement
	Low risk	Need to repeat at least twice annually
	Lasts 4–8 months	
Nonablative laser ie,1,450-nm diode 12–13 J/cm² (one pass) lower fluencies (two passes) multiple monthly treatments	Low risk of serious side effects No downtime Treats any active acne	Improvement 10–30%

SECTION TWELVE

Exogenous Cutaneous Alterations

CHAPTER 62 | Ear Piercing

Ear piercing is performed to facilitate an individual's desire to wear earrings. By having the procedure performed in a medical facility by a physician, the patient is reassured that the procedure is being performed in a safe, controlled environment.

KEY CONSULTATIVE QUESTIONS

• Contact allergens to metals

• History of keloids or hypertrophic scarring

• Desired site of piercing

PHYSICAL EXAMINATION

Assess the thickness of earlobes.

MANAGEMENT

There are two common methods for ear piercing. It can be performed with a needle by hand or with the help of an automatic ear-piercing gun (Fig. 62.1). Before performing either procedure, it is important to make certain that the correct location for piercing has been selected. Symmetry with the contralateral ear is essential for a good cosmetic appearance. The patient should review the sites using a mirror prior to treatment.

TREATMENT

• Sterilize all instruments

• Sterilize and anesthetize both ear lobules

• Identify the exact sites to be pierced with a marking pen on the anterior and posterior portions of the ear lobule. Confirm proper placement with patient before proceeding

• Using slow pressure, advance a 14- to 18-gauge needle through the posterior lobule into the anterior lobule

• If an automatic ear-piercing gun is used, the gun is advanced from the anterior lobule toward the posterior lobule

• Use a sterilized earring with a stainless steel post

• A nickel-free post of the earring is advanced with the needle and the tip is pulled back through the ear

• The clasp is put on the posterior post

• Leave the earring in place for approximately 14 days until re-epithelialization of the track

• Clean the site with hydrogen peroxide and topical antibiotic ointment twice daily

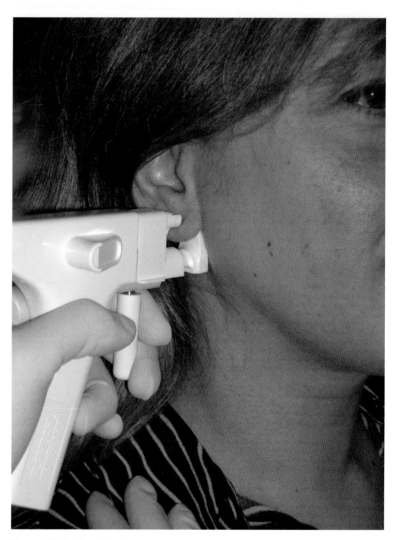

Figure 62.1 *Ear-piercing gun being used on earlobe of a young female*

PITFALLS TO AVOID/COMPLICATIONS/MANAGEMENT/OUTCOME EXPECTATIONS

- Thin earlobes may split, especially with heavier earrings

- Place earrings on the same level horizontally to assure symmetry

- A good clean sterile technique can avoid postprocedure infections

- It is important to elicit any history of hypertrophic scars or keloids in these patients (Fig. 62.2). Ear piercing should not be performed on these patients

- Any history of nickel or other metal allergens should be elicited prior to any procedure as well

- Educate patients as to wound care and the need to contact you in the event of infection

- In the event of contact dermatitis or allergy, topical steroids are the mainstay of treatment

BIBLIOGRAPHY

Atkin DH, Lask GP. Ear piercing and surgical repair of the earlobe. In: Lask GP, Moy RL, eds. *Principles and Techniques of Cutaneous Surgery*. New York: McGraw-Hill, Inc; 1996.

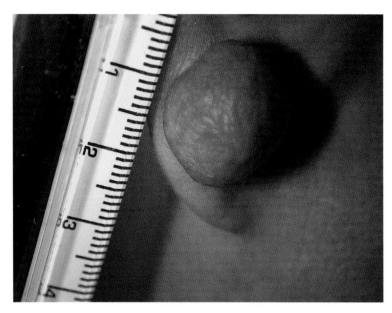

Figure 62.2 *Keloid on posterior earlobe secondary to ear piercing (Courtesy of Tomi Pandolfino, MD)*

CHAPTER 63 | Tattoo Removal

Tens of millions of Americans have tattoos. Over time, many decide that they want the tattoo to be removed. Quality-switched (Q-switched) lasers are effective in removing most tattoo pigments safely (Figs. 63.1–63.3). The appropriate laser wavelength is determined by the tattoo ink's absorption spectrum. It is believed that laser pulses in the nanosecond range target tattoo pigments and break them into smaller particles, thereby facilitating removal of the pigment transepidermally or via macrophages and local scavenger cells. In order to treat multicolored tattoos, several Q-switched laser wavelengths must be employed.

KEY CONSULTATIVE QUESTIONS

- Was the tattoo placed by an amateur or a professional tattoo artist?
- Was the tattoo placed for the purpose of radiation therapy?
- Is the tattoo the result of trauma or injury?
- What colors are contained within the tattoo? (Table 63.1)
- Previous treatments
- Use of isotretinoin within 6 months
- History of keloids/hypertrophic scars
- Duration of tattoo
- Skin phototype
- History of HSV at site of treatment
- History of allergic or granulomatous reaction to tattoo pigment

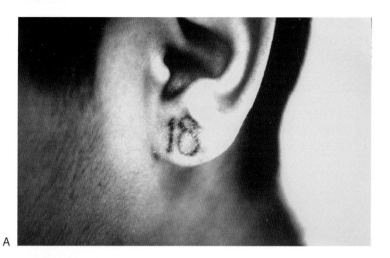

A

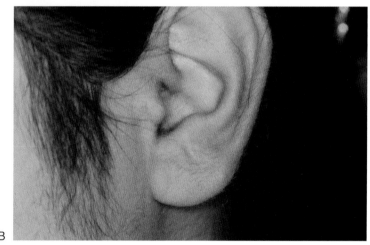

B

Figure 63.1 (A) *Tattoo on left earlobe prior to therapy.* **(B)** *Resolution after six treatments with 1,064-nm Q-switched Nd:YAG laser*

TABLE 63.1 ▪ Laser Therapy by Tattoo Color

Tattoo pigment	Light spectrum	Most effective lasers	Comment
Red	Green	Frequency-doubled Q-switched Nd:YAG (532 nm)	May cause pigment alteration in darker skin Least painful of Q-switched lasers
Yellow	Green	Frequency-doubled Q-switched Nd:YAG (532 nm)	Not very effective
Green	Red/near infrared	Q-switched ruby (694 nm) Q-switched alexandrite (755 nm)	May cause hypopigmentation in darker skin
Light blue	Red/near infrared	Q-switched ruby (694 nm) Q-switched alexandrite (755 nm)	May cause hypopigmentation in darker skin
Dark blue	Red/near infrared	Q-switched ruby (694 nm): light skin types only	
Black		Q-switched alexandrite (755 nm): light skin types only Q-switched Nd:YAG (1,064 nm): all skin types	Q-switched Nd:YAG (1,064 nm) safe in all skin types. Less pigment loss

- Is the tattoo placed over or covering another tattoo?
- History of gold ingestion
- Does the tattoo contain rust-colored or white pigment?

MANAGEMENT

It is important to ask the patient who placed the tattoo. Professional tattoo pigments are denser and placed deeper in the dermis than most amateur tattoos. This renders these tattoos more refractory to treatment, particularly those that are multicolored and contain metallic pigments. It is important to inform the patient prior to treatment that complete resolution is not always feasible. It is also important to counsel that multiple treatments over 1 to 2 years may be required for maximal improvement. There is no fixed answer as to the number of treatments for tattoo removal.

PRETREATMENT ASSESSMENT

- Patients with darker skin types are more likely to suffer pigmentary changes
- Professional tattoos require more treatments than amateur tattoos
- Older tattoos respond more favorably than new tattoos
- Black and dark blue tattoos respond more effectively than yellow tattoos
- Assess for suntan. If patient is tanned, delay treatment until tan resolves
- Multicolored tattoos are more difficult to successfully clear than single-color tattoos. During treatment, some patients may be frustrated at the nonuniform improvement of these tattoos
- Assess for scarring within the tattoo. If present, show the patient and document prior to treating

NUMBER OF TREATMENTS

- Professional tattoos require about 6 to 20 treatments prior to removal; not infrequently, more than 20 treatments are needed for maximal improvement
- Amateur tattoos contain less dense pigment particles and usually require about four to six treatments
- Radiation tattoos and traumatic tattoos are more superficial and less dense than professional tattoos, requiring only a few treatments for resolution (Fig. 63.4)
- In general, radiation tattoos can be removed in one to three treatments. Sometimes, they require additional treatments
- Lower fluences and larger spot sizes can be as effective as smaller spot sizes and increased fluences

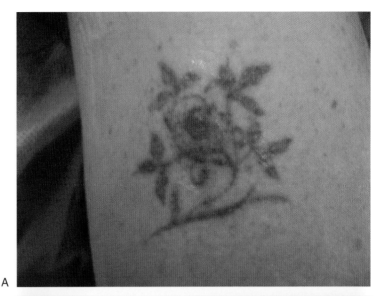

A

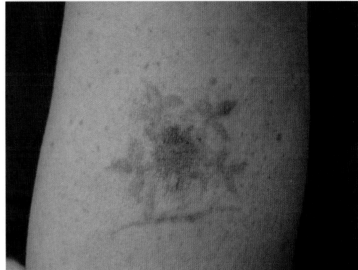

B

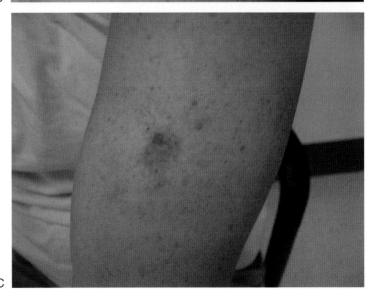

C

Figure 63.2 (A) *Tattoo on arm with underlying port-wine stain.* **(B)** *Note the selective removal of the tattoo, while the port-wine stain persists.* **(C)** *Tattoo clearance*

- Test spot may be appropriate in darker skin phototypes if concerning
- Test spots are clearly indicated for cosmetic tattoos, rust-colored tattoos, and white tattoos

TATTOO TREATMENT

- Photograph of tattoo prior to treatment
- Topical anesthesia or 1% lidocaine, in the form of local injection or nerve block, will make the treatment more comfortable for the patient
- Treat the affected areas with the appropriate Q-switched laser allowing for up to a 10% overlap (Table 63.2)
- The clinical endpoint is immediate tissue whitening. For the 1,064-nm Q-switched Nd:YAG, in addition to tissue whitening there may be a small amount of pinpoint bleeding at the site of treatment (Figs. 63.5 and 63.6)
- Tissue "splatter" (ie, epidermal/dermal disruption and bleeding) may produce scarring. If this occurs, decrease the fluence
- If the tattoo is multicolored, treat the red pigment first. Erythema and inflammation from other treated sites may obscure visualization of red tattoo pigment
- Apply topical hydrated petrolatum and a nonadherent dressing after completing the treatment
- Counsel sunscreen and sun avoidance to the treatment area

POSTTREATMENT CARE

- Sun avoidance, sunscreens
- Telfa dressing and hydrated petrolatum ointment with paper tape
- If tattoo is located in belt-line area or above ankles, caution patients from wearing tight belts or boots that may produce friction against the treated area
- Return for treatment in 6 to 8 weeks

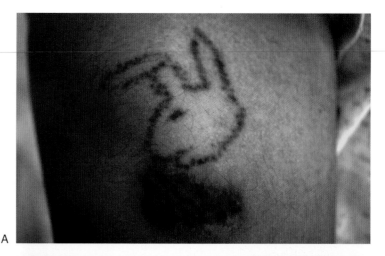

A

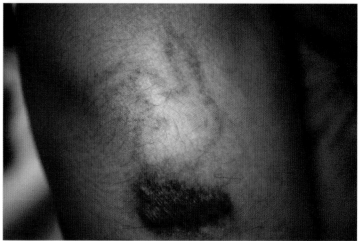

B

Figure 63.3 (A) *Left shoulder tattoo with inferior scar resulting from prior treatment with dermabrasion.* **(B)** *Improvement after six treatments with 1,064-nm Q-switched Nd:YAG laser. While improvement is not complete, the cosmetic result is far superior to that of dermabrasion*

TABLE 63.2 ■ Laser Therapy by Quality-Switched Lasers

Laser	Initial settings	Effective against these tattoo inks
Frequency doubled Q-switched Nd:YAG (532 nm)	1.5–5.0 J, 4.0–8.0 mm spot size	Red, orange, yellow
Q-switched ruby (694 nm)	3.0–8.0 J, 6.5 mm spot size	Green, blue, black
Q-switched alexandrite (755 nm)	5.0–6.5 J, 2.0–4.0 mm spot size	Green, blue, black
Q-switched Nd:YAG (1,064 nm)	3.0–12.0 J, 2.0–8.0 mm spot size	Blue, black (safest in dark skin types)

ADVERSE EFFECTS/PRECAUTIONS

- Pigmentary alteration

- Blistering (especially, Q-switched alexandrite and ruby) (Fig. 63.7)

- Scarring (Fig. 63.8)

- In a patient with an allergic reaction to tattoo ink in the past (Fig. 63.9), there is the possibility of a recurrence secondary to the release of tattoo ink following laser therapy. Allergic precautions should be taken. Systemic allergic reactions can occur with Q-switched lasers (unlike destructive modalities—dermabrasion, etc.)

- Rust-colored and white tattoos should be treated carefully as well as red and flesh-colored cosmetic tattoos, for example, lip liner. Sometimes white ink is mixed with other pigments (Fig. 63.10)

  - The tattoo may darken as a result of oxidation of iron or titanium oxide pigment within the tattoo

  - A test site can be performed 4 to 8 weeks prior to treatment for possible darkening

  - This darkening can sometimes be treated with lasers or may require excision

  - They respond slowly to laser therapy

- Perform a test spot prior to treating patients with history of gold salt ingestion. Chrysiasis, manifested as dark-blue pigmentation, can result from treatment with Q-switched lasers

- Rarely, patients will experience a transient immune response following a laser tattoo treatment. Such responses include flu-like symptoms and enlarged lymph nodes

PITFALLS TO AVOID/COMPLICATIONS/ MANAGEMENT/OUTCOME EXPECTATIONS

- Response to tattoo treatment is dependent upon the depth of pigment, the color of pigment, and the size of pigment particles. It can vary dramatically from one to tattoo to another

- Effective treatment for a professional tattoo may require up to a 20 or more treatment sessions over a period of 1 to 2 years. Furthermore, complete removal is often not feasible

- A successful treatment often leaves some residual tattoo pigment. This can be improved with nonablative fractional resurfacing

- Physicians should counsel patients that significant lightening may be the best feasible clinical result

- Tattoo treatment can produce hyper- and hypopigmentation in any patient, especially those with darker skin types

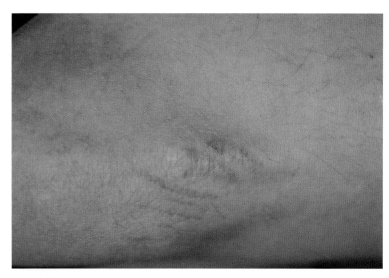

Figure 63.4 *Traumatic tattoo on knee of a female that has persisted 30 years after childhood bicycle fall. Q-switched 1,064-nm Nd:YAG cleared the tattoo in three treatments*

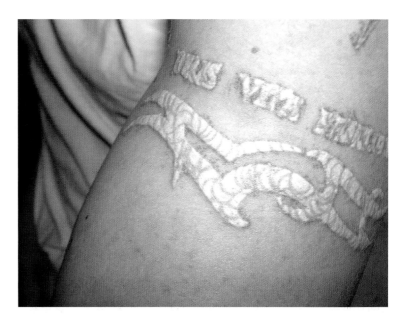

Figure 63.5 *Tissue whitening after treatment with the 532-nm frequency-doubled Q-switched Nd:YAG and 694-nm Q-switched ruby laser. Tissue whitening is the appropriate endpoint when treating tattoos with Q-switched lasers. Pinpoint bleeding resulted from injection of lidocaine with epinephrine prior to treatment*

- Treatment of tattoos in areas of hair growth (ie, eyebrows) may produce temporary hair removal

- The frequency-doubled Q-switched Nd:YAG, Q switched ruby, and Q-switched alexandrite lasers are more likely to cause durable pigmentary changes than the Q-switched Nd:YAG (1,064 nm)

- Most frequently, pigment alteration is temporary. Hyperpigmentation typically resolves more quickly

- Lower fluences and additional time between treatments should be employed in darker skin phototypes

BIBLIOGRAPHY

Alster T. Q-switched alexandrite laser (755 nm) treatment of professional and amateur tattoos. *J Am Acad Dermatol.* 1995;33:69-73.

Ferguson JE, August PJ. Evaluation of the Nd/YAG laser for treatment of amateur and professional tattoos. *Br J Dermatol.* 1996;135(4):586-591.

Fitzpatrick RE, Goldman MP. Tattoo removal using the alexandrite laser. *Arch Dermatol.* 1994;130:1508-1514.

Grevelink JM, Mulas MW, Hata TR, Goldman MP, Fitzpatrick RE, Grevelink JM. Laser treatment of tattoos in darkly pigmented patients: Efficacy and side effects. *J Am Acad Dermatol.* 1996;34:653-656.

Izikson L, Avram MM, Anderson RR. Transient immunoreactivity after laser tattoo removal: Report of two cases. *Lasers Surg Med.* 2008;40(4):231-232.

Kilmer SL, Anderson RR. Clinical use of the Q-switched ruby and the Q-switched Nd:YAG (1064 nm and 532 nm) lasers for treatment of tattoos. *J Dermatol Surg Oncol.* 1993;19(4):330-338.

Levine VJ, Geronemus RG. Tattoo removal with the Q-switched ruby laser and the Q-switched Nd: YAG laser: A comparative study. *Cutis.* 1995;55:291-296.

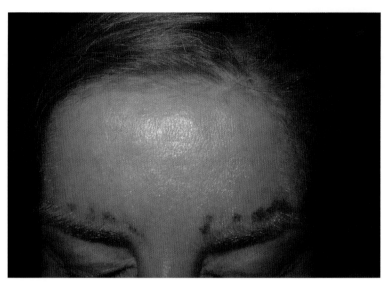

Figure 63.6 *Purpura immediately after treatment of an eyebrow tattoo with a Q-switched Nd:YAG laser*

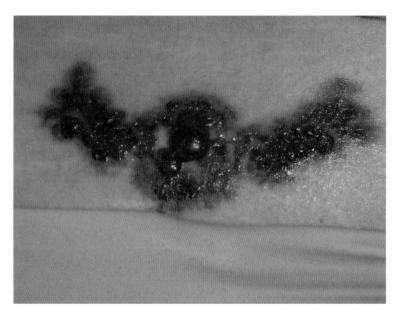

Figure 63.7 *Blistering after tattoo treatment. This reaction is common and usually resolves completely within a week with routine topical skin care*

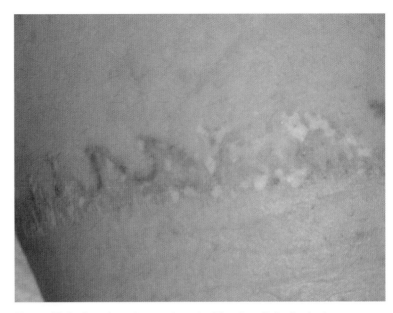

Figure 63.8 *Scarring after treatment with a Q-switched ruby laser (Courtesy of Teresa Soriano, MD)*

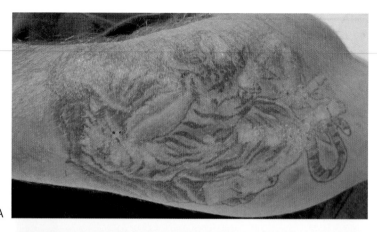

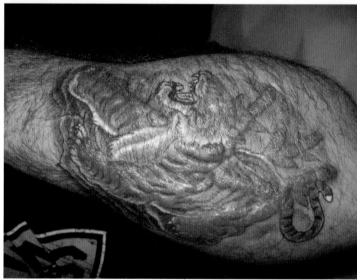

Figure 63.9 **(A)** *Allergic hypersensitivity reaction to tattoo (see elevated portions of tattoo).* **(B)** *To avoid systemic allergic reaction with traditional Q-switched laser treatment of the entire tattoo, focal treatment with an ablative fractional erbium laser was performed. Note focal improvement after several treatments*

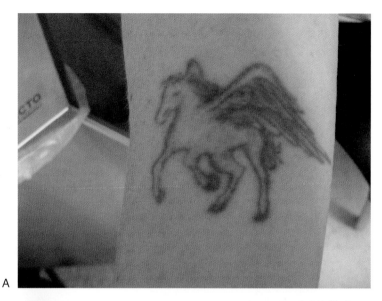

A

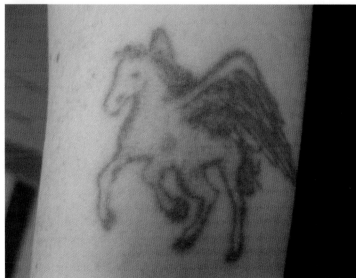

B

Figure 63.10 **(A)** *Tattoo prior to test spot treatment.* **(B)** *Test spot treatment of tattoo with a 694-nm Q-switched ruby laser produces discoloration. Tattoo ink combined blue and white inks*

CHAPTER 64 | Torn Earlobe

Torn earlobe and enlarged pierced earlobe canals are a common consequence of wearing heavy earrings for a prolonged period of time (Fig. 64.1) as well as other factors such as trauma, heavy earrings, infection, low placement of piercing, pressure necrosis, etc. It occurs most easily in thin ear lobules. Drooping or easily torn earlobes may also be secondary to a congenital defect or trauma.

KEY CONSULTATIVE QUESTIONS

• Precipitating event of earlobe tear

• History of keloids or hypertrophic scarring

• Does patient desire to wear earrings again after the repair?

MANAGEMENT

There are numerous surgical methods to repair completely and partially torn earlobes. Different techniques are suited for different tears. Partial tears are more easily treated and can be corrected via side-to-side closure as well as punch excision and repair.

TREATMENTS (Figs. 64.1–64.3)

Complete tears are more difficult to treat than partial tears. There are numerous different techniques that can be successful. Most commonly, the Z-plasty repair or interlocking Ls repair produce the best result.

• Sterile preparation and technique

• Local anesthesia should be injected into the repair site

• The epidermis of the opposing edges of the tear wound should be excised

  – Scalpel

  – Scissors

• Interrupted 6-0 epidermal sutures approximate and evert the wound edges of the anterior and posterior lobe

  – Be certain to approximate the wound edges of the inferior rim of the ear carefully to avoid distortion or misalignment

  – The wound edges should be under minimal tension

• No subcutaneous sutures are used

• Z-plasty repair (Fig. 64.2) or interlocking Ls repair on the rim will produce tissue approximation while preventing the dimpling of the inferior rim of the earlobe

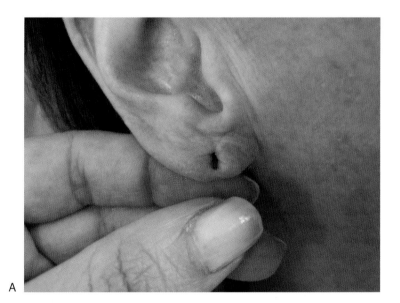

A

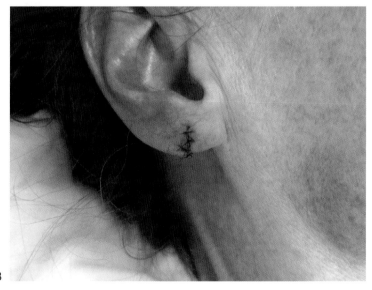

B

Figure 64.1 **(A)** *Female with large tear defect of earlobe at the site of heavy earring.* **(B)** *Torn earlobe reconstructed by primary repair*

- Patients should be counseled to refrain from wearing earrings for 3 months following the repair

PITFALLS TO AVOID/COMPLICATIONS/ MANAGEMENT/OUTCOME EXPECTATIONS

- Meticulous attention to approximating the wound edges and the inferior rim of the ear are essential for a satisfactory result. Notching of the inferior rim of the earlobe can occur easily, significantly compromising aesthetic appearance
- Caution in a patient with a history of keloids or hypertrophic scars
- Patient should not wear earrings for 2 to 3 months after surgery
- Wound strength is less than the original strength of the lobe. Avoid wearing heavy earrings to prevent recurrence

BIBLIOGRAPHY

Tipton JB. A simple technique for reduction of the earlobe. *Plast Reconstr Surg.* 1980;66:630-632.

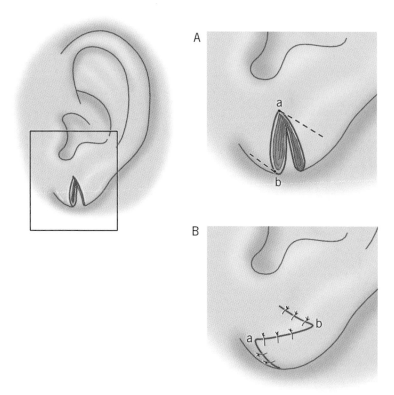

Figure 64.2 *Repair of complete earlobe tear utilizing a Z-plasty to prevent dimpling of the inferior aspect of earlobe*

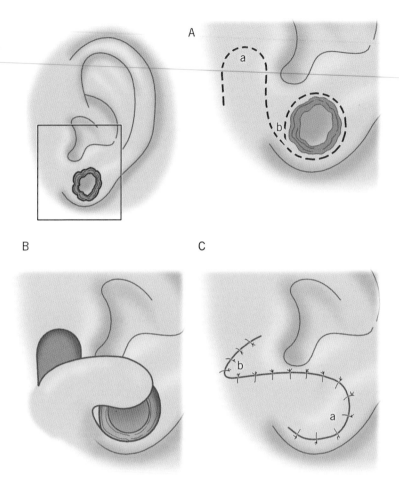

Figure 64.3 *One stage preauricular flap to repair earlobe deformities*

INDEX

Note: In this index, the letters "f" and "t" denote figures and tables, respectively.

1, 450-nm diode laser, 82, 82f, 83f
5-aminolevulinic acid (5-ALA), 75, 254
5-fluorouracil, 207, 224, 229
1320-nm Nd:YAG laser, 41
1450-nm diode laser, 41, 74

A

Ablative fractional laser resurfacing, 39, 57
  advantages of, 57
  indications, 58
  laser safety, 59
    adverse side effects, 60, 60f
    follow-up, 59–60, 59f
    infection, 60, 61f
    nonfacial skin, 60–61
    postoperative care, 57f, 58f, 59
  preoperative evaluation, 58
  prophylaxis/anesthesia, 58–59
Ablative laser resurfacing, 151t, 152
  absolute contraindications, 45
  anesthesia, 46–47
  for Becker's nevus, 218
  for epidermal nevus, 224
  ideal laser candidate, 45
  indications, 44
  less than ideal laser candidate, 45
  mechanism of action, 43
    carbon dioxide laser, 43, 43f, 44f
    Er:YAG, 43, 45f
  medications, 46
  for milia, 230
  postoperative care, 49, 50f, 51f
  preoperative evaluation, 44–45
  procedure, 48–49, 49f
  relative contraindications, 45–46
  safety measures, 47–48
  for seborrheic keratosis, 236
  treatment pearls, 50
ACE inhibitors. See Angiotensin-converting enzyme (ACE) inhibitors
Acetaminophen, 58
Acetone, 48
Acne scars, 290, 293
  physical lesions, 293–295
  treatment, 295
Acne vulgaris, 72, 76, 100
  vs. angiofibroma, 212
  course, 73
  differential diagnosis, 72
  epidemiology, 72
  laboratory data
    dermatopathology, 73
    endocrine studies, 72–73
  management, 73
    light treatment, 72f, 73f, 74–75, 75f
    surgical treatment, 74
    systemic treatment, 73–74
    topical treatment, 73

  pathogenesis, 72
  physical examination, 72
Acquired capillary hemangioma, 170–173
Acral amelanotic melanoma, 206
Actinic cheilitis, 248
Actinic keratosis (AK), 248
  consultative questions, 249
  course, 249
  dermatopathology, 248
  differential diagnosis, 248
  epidemiology, 248
  management, 249
  pathogenesis, 248
  physical examination, 248
  pitfalls, 250–251
  treatment, 249–250
Actinic kerotoses
  vs. warts, 206
Acyclovir, 32, 46, 54
Adapalene, 9, 73
Adatosil 5000, 14t, 15t
Adenoma sebaceum, 212
Affirm 1, 440 nm Nd:YAG laser, 56, 56t
Age-related textural changes, 2t
Aging, 2
Aging face and non-facial regions, analysis of
  anatomic considerations, 2–3, 2t
  preoperative evaluation, 3
    cartilage, bony structures, and supportive structures, changes in, 5
    facial musculature changes, 5
    Glogau Photoaging Classification, 2f, 3–4, 3f, 4f, 5f
    pigmentary changes, 4, 6f
    subcutaneous fat atrophy, 5
AK. See Actinic keratosis
ALA. See 5-aminolevulinic acid
Alcaine. See Topical proparacaine
Alcon, 28
Alcon Labs, 15t
Allergan, 14t, 15t, 21t
Allergic reactions
  to sclerotherapy, 201
Alloderm, 14t
Aloe vera, 10
Aloesin, 9t, 10
α-hydroxy acid, 32
  lotions, 182
  for postinflammatory hyperpigmentation, 160
  peels, 141
Aluminum chloride hexahydrate, 87
Ambulatory phlebectomy, 202
American Academy of Dermatology, 8
Amoxicillin, 73
Amyotrophic lateral sclerosis, 22
Anesthesia, 88
  for ablative fractional laser resurfacing, 58–59
  for ablative laser resurfacing, 46–47

for angiofibroma, 213
for lipoma treatment, 227
for neurofibroma, 236
for nonablative fractional laser resurfacing, 54
for nonablative laser resurfacing, 40
    mid-infrared lasers, 40f, 41
for soft tissue augmentation, 16f, 17
for wart removal, 207t, 208
Angiofibroma, 212–215
    consultative questions, 213
    course, 213, 213f
    dermatopathology, 212
    differential diagnosis, 212
    epidemiology, 212
    laboratory data, 213
    management, 213–214, 214f, 215f
    pathogenesis, 212
    physical examination, 212, 212f
    pitfalls, 214
Angiokeratoma, 168
    vs. angiomas, 171
    course management, 168–169, 169f
    dermatopathology, 168
    differential diagnoses, 168
    epidemiology, 168
    physical examination, 168
    pitfalls to avoid, 169
Angiolipoma, 226
Angiomas, cherry and spider, 170
    course, 171
    differential diagnoses, 171
    epidemiology, 170
    management, 171–172
    pathogenesis, 170
    pathology, 171
    physical examination, 171
    pitfalls to avoid, 172
Angiotensin-converting enzyme (ACE)
    inhibitors, 89
Anthralin, 224
Antibacterial agents, 73
Antibacterial therapy, 46, 53
Antibiotics, 73
Antimalarials, 175
Antioxidants, 8
Antiperspirant, 89
Antiviral medications, 49
Antiviral therapy, 46, 54
Apraclonidine hydrochloride, 28
Aquamid, 14t
Aquaphor Healing Ointment, 49
Arbutin, 9t, 10
Artefill, 14t
Arterial spider, 170–173
Ascorbic acid, 9t, 11
Ash leaf macule, 212, 213f
Aspergillus, 10
AstraZeneca, 17
Ataxiatelangiectasia, 67
Ativan, 58
Atrophic scars, 294–295
Atrophoderma vermiculatum (AV), 181
Avita, 9
Avobenzone, 7t
Azelaic acid, 9t, 10, 73, 77, 141, 151, 160
Azithromycin, 46, 73

B
B lupus miliaris disseminatus faciei, 76
B-HCG. *See* β-Human chorionic gonadotropin
Bannayan-Zonana syndrome, 226
Basal cell carcinoma (BCC), 81, 252–254
    epidermal nevus and, 222, 223
    consultative questions, 253
    course, 253
    dermatopathology, 252
    differential diagnoses, 252
    epidemiology, 252
    laboratory data, 253
    management, 253–254, 253f, 254f, 255f
    pathogenesis, 252
    physical examination, 252, 252f
    pitfalls, 254
Bearberry, 10
Becker's nevus, 216–218
    consultative questions, 217
    course, 217
    differential diagnosis, 216
    epidemiology, 216
    laboratory examination, 216
    management, 217–218, 217f
    pathogenesis, 216
    pathology, 216
    physical examination, 216, 216f
    pitfalls, 218
Belotero Basic, 14t
Belotero Soft, 14t
Benign growths
    angiofibroma, 212–215
    Becker's nevus, 216–218
    epidermal inclusion cyst, 219–221
    epidermal nevus, 222–225
Benzoyl peroxide, 73
β-Human chorionic gonadotropin (B-HCG)
Betacaine Enhanced Gel, 17
Betacaine Plus, 17
Bio-Alcamid, 14t
Bioform Medical, 15t
Biomatrix Inc., 15t
Biopsies
    epidermal inclusion cysts, 220
    epidermal nevus and, 223
    lipoma, 227
    neurofibroma, 232
    seborrheic keratosis, 235
Biotech Industry, 15t
Blaschko, lines of, 222
Bleaching creams, 46
Blepharochalasis, 64
Bloom's syndrome, 67, 136
Bornaprine, 87
Botox, 89. *See also* Botulinum toxin A
Botox Cosmetic, 21t
Botulinum toxin
    complications, 27
    contraindications
        absolute, 22
        relative, 22
    dilution, 22
    mechanism of action, 21
    muscle groups, 22f, 23
        forehead, 22f, 23–24, 23f

glabellar complex, 24, 24f
nasolabial fold, 25–26, 27f
neck, 26–27, 28f
perioral region, 26, 27f, 28f
periorbital region, 24–25, 25f
upper nasal root, 25, 26f
pharmacology, 21, 21t
postoperative considerations, 27
preoperative evaluation, 22
lower eyelid snap back test, 22–23
preparations, 21t
procedure, 23
treatment benefits, 27
treatment pearls, 28
Botulinum toxin A (BTX-A), 21, *22*, 87, 88, 88f
anesthesia, 88
antiperspirant, 89
Botox, 89
hyperhidrosis, mechanism of action in, 88f
injection sites of, 88f, 89f
medications, 89
surgery, 89
treatment, 88–89, 88f, 89f
Botulinum toxin B (BTX-B), 21
Botulinum toxin E (BTX-E), 21
Brindis, 14t
Broussonetia papyrifera, 10
Buccinator, 26, 27f, 28f

C

Café au lait macules (CALMs), 136
vs. Becker's nevus, 216
consultative questions, 137
course, 137
differential diagnosis, 136
epidemiology, 136
laboratory examination, 136
laser treatment, 137–138
management, 137
vs. neurofibromas, 232
pathogenesis, 136
pathology, 136
physical lesions, 136
pitfalls, 138
topical treatment, 138
Calcipotriol, 224
Campbell de Morgan spots, 170–173
Candela Corp., 41
Canderm, 17
Canderm Pharma, Inc., 14t
Caninus, 26, 27f, 28f
Cantharone, 207
Capillary, 177
Captique™, 14t
Carbon dioxide (CO_2) laser, 43, 43f, 48, 49, 57, 172, 239
Carbon dioxide laser resurfacing
for angiofibroma, 213, 214–215f
for angiomas, 172
for basal cell carcinoma, 254
for epidermal nevus, 224
for neurofibroma, 232
for seborrheic keratosis, 236
for squamous cell carcinoma, 258
for venous lakes, 208
for warts, 207t, 208

Cavernous hemangioma, 177–180
Cellulite, 276–279, 276f
consultative questions, 277
course, 276
epidemiology, 276
laboratory examination, 276
management, 277
physical lesions, 276
pitfalls, 278–279
treatments, 277–278, 277f
Centrofacial telangiectasias, 194f
Chemical peels, 30, 74, 141
complications, 34, 38f
contraindications, 31–32
ideal candidate, 31
less ideal candidate, 31
medications, 32
peel types, 33
postoperative care, 34
procedure, 33–34, 36f, 37f
treatment pearls, 34–35
wound depth, 32
Chemical sunscreen, 7–8, 7t
Cherry angiomas, 170–173, 172f
Cinoxate, 7t
Ciprofloxacin, 46
Clindamycin, 73
Clofazimine, 175
Clostridium botulinum, 21
CO_2 laser ablation, 82
CO_2 resurfacing. *See* Carbon dioxide (CO_2) laser
Coenzyme Q10, 8
Colchicine, 175
Collagen, in angiofibroma, 212
Collagenase, 9
Comedone extraction, 74
Common warts, 206–209
Complete tears, 308
Compression stockings, 200
Congenital adrenal hyperplasia, 92
Congenital hemangiomas, 177
Congenital nevus, 216
Contura International, 14t
Cooltouch Inc., 41
Corrective hair transplant surgery, 110, 110t
Corrugator supercilii, 24, 24f
Corticosteroids, 164, 175
for epidermal nevi, 224
for epidermal inclusion cysts, 221
for milia, 229
Cosmoderm™, 14t
Cosmoplast™, 14t
Cross-hatching, 18
Cryogen spray cooling (CSC), 185
Cryosurgery, 175
Cryotherapy
for dermatosis papulosa nigra, 242
for ephelides, 142
for epidermal nevus, 224
for lentigines, 146
for sebaceous hyperplasia, 83
for seborrheic keratosis, 236
for squamous cell carcinoma, 258
for venous lakes, 204
for wart removal, 209
for seborrheic keratosis, 236, 237, 237f

Curettage
for epidermal nevus, 224
for wart removal, 209
Cushing's disease, 92, 285
Cutting tool, 44
Cymetra Life Cell Corp., 14t
Cynosure, 56, 56t
Cyproterone acetate, 128
Cysts
epidermal inclusion cysts, 219–221
horn, 235
milia, 229–230
pilar cysts, 220

D

DAO. *See* Depressor anguli oris
Dapsone, 175
Deep-depth strength peels, 30t, 33
Deep hemangioma (DH), 177
Deep vein thrombosis, 198
Demodex folliculorum, 77
Depilation, 94
Depressor anguli oris (DAO), 26, 27f, 28f
Dercum's disease, 226
Dermabrasion, 175
for epidermal nevus, 224
for angiofibroma, 214
Dermal melasma, 149
Dermatochalasis, 64
consultative questions, 65
course, 65
dermatopathology, 65
differential diagnosis, 64
epidemiology, 64
management, 65
pathogenesis, 64
physical examination, 64
pitfalls, 65–66
treatment, 65
Dermatosis papulosa nigra (DPNs),
241, 241f
consultative questions, 242
course, 241
differential diagnosis, 241
epidemiology, 241
laboratory examination, 241
laser treatments, 242–243
management, 242
pathogenesis, 241
pathology, 241
physical lesions, 241
pitfalls, 243
Dermik, 15t
Destructive modalities, 83
of sebaceous hyperplasia
Diazepam, 17
Dicloxacillin, 46
Diode laser treatments
for Becker's nevus, 218
for venous lakes, 204
Dioxybenzone, 7t
Dow-Corning, 14t
Doxycycline, 73, 77
DPNs. *See* Dermatosis papulosa nigra

Dyschromia
from wart removal, 207t, 208, 209
Dysport, 21t

E

Ear piercing, 298
consultative questions, 298
management, 298, 298f
physical examination, 298
pitfalls, 299, 299f
treatment, 298
Ectopic adrenocorticotropic hormone production, 92
Electrocautery, 239
for epidermal nevus, 224
Electrodesiccation, 83
for angiofibromas, 213
for seborrheic keratoses, 236
Electrolysis, 94, 217
Electrosection, 77
Electrosurgery, 76f, 77, 77f, 82, 175
for venous lakes, 204
Elliptical excision, 213, 219f, 227, 2132
Elliptical strip harvesting, 106
vs. follicular unit extraction (FUE), 107, 107t
Ellman Surgitron, 78
Embolization, 180
Endermologie
for cellulite, 277–278
Endocrine studies, of acne vulgaris, 72–73
Endocrinology, consultation with, 93
Endoscopic/classic sympathectomy, 88
Eosinophilic granuloma, 174
Ephelides, 139
consultative questions, 140
course, 140
differential diagnosis, 140
epidemiology, 139
laboratory examination, 140
management, 140
pathogenesis, 139
pathology, 140
physical lesions, 140
vs. solar lentigo, 145t
treatments
chemical peels, 141–142
cryotherapy, 142
laser therapy, 142–143
pitfalls to avoid/complications/management, 143
topical treatment, 140–141
Epidermal acanthosis, 65, 67
Epidermal inclusion cysts (EIC), 219–221
consultative questions, 220
course, 220
differential diagnosis, 220
epidemiology, 219
laboratory data, 220
management, 220
pathogenesis, 219
pathology, 219
physical examination, 219, 219f
pitfalls, 221
treatment, 220–221, 219f, 220f
Epidermal melasma, 32f, 149
Epidermal nevus (EN), 222
vs. Becker's nevus, 216

consultative questions, 223
course, 223
differential diagnosis, 223
epidemiology, 222
laboratory data, 223
pathogenesis, 222
pathology, 222
physical examination, 223
pitfalls, 225
vs. seborrheic keratosis, 223, 235
treatment, 224–225
Epidermis
and epidermal inclusion cysts, 219
in lipoma, 226
Epidermoid cyst, 219
Epiluminescence microscopy (ELM), 203
Epinephrine, 59
Er:YAG. *See* Erbium:Yttrium-Aluminum Garnet Laser
Erbium ablative resurfacing lasers, 57
Erbium:Yttrium-Aluminum Garnet (Er:YAG) laser
and ablative laser resurfacing, 43, 45f, 48, 49
and epidermal nevus, 224
and seborrheic keratosis, 236
Erythematotelangiectatic rosacea. *See* Vascular rosacea
Erythromycin, 73
Eutectic mixture of local anesthetic (EMLA), 17, 40
Excimer laser, 165, 287
Excision surgical, 253, 257, 291, 291t
Eye injuries
and lasers, 98f

F

Facial age-related contour changes, 2t
Facial musculature changes, 5
Facial telangiectasias, 192, 192f
course, 192
dermatopathology, 192
epidemiology, 192
management, 192–194
physical examination, 192
pitfalls to avoid, 194
prior to long pulse-duration pulsed dye laser
treatment, 195f
prior to pulsed dye laser treatment, 193f
Fanning, 18
Fascia Biomaterials, 15t
Fascian, 15t
Fat accumulation
treatment of, 283
FDA-approved medications, for male pattern hair loss, 104, 104t
Female pattern hair loss, 126, 126f. *See also* Male pattern hair loss
chief complaint, 131
consult, 131–132
consultative questions, 126
course, 126
differential diagnosis, 127
epidemiology, 126
female hair transplantation, 131
to correct altered temporal hairline, from lifting procedure, 131
female surgical planning, 129
postoperative instructions, 130
postoperative period, 130–131
preoperative instructions, 130
vs. male pattern hair loss, 129, 129t, 131f

medical therapy, 127–128
non-FDA approved medications, 128
pathogenesis, 126
physical examination, 126, 128–129
surgery, 128
Female surgical planning, 129
postoperative instructions, 130
postoperative period, 130–131
preoperative instructions, 130
Ferndale Labs, 17
Fibrous papules, 212
Filiform warts, 206
Fillers
permanent, 282–283
temporary, 282
Finasteride, 104, 104t, 128, 133
Fitzpatrick skin phototype, 31
Fitzpatrick's classification, of skin types, 4t
Flashlamp, 78f, 79, 79f, 80f
treatment, 193
Flavonoids, 9t
Foam sclerotherapy, 199–200
Follicular infundibulum, 219
Follicular unit extraction (FUE), 106t, 107, 108t
vs. elliptical strip harvesting, 107t
Folliculitis, 100
Forehead, 22f, 23–24, 24f
milia, 229–230
Fractional photothermolysis (FP)
Fractional resurfacing, 151t, 152, 153f
Fraxel Restore, 56, 56t
Freckles. *See* Ephelides
Frontalis muscle, 22f, 23–24, 23f
Frontalis muscles, 24, 24f
FUE. *See* Follicular unit extraction

G

Gelatinase, 9
Genital warts, 206–209
Gentisic acid, 9t
Glabellar complex, 24, 24f
Glabridin, 10
Glogau Photoaging Classification, 2f, 3–4, 3f, 4f, 5f
Glycolic acid, 9t, 30t
Glycolic acid peel, 32, 33f, 74, 160
and ephilides, 141
and melasma, 151, 151t
Glycopyrronium bromide, 87
Glycyrrhiza glabra linneva, 10
Gold injections, 175
Grafts, skin, 225f
Granuloma faciale, 174, 174f, 176f
course, 174
dermatopathology, 174
differential diagnoses, 174
epidemiology, 174
light treatment, 175
management, 175
multiple lesions of, 175f
pathogenesis, 174
physical examination, 174
pitfalls to avoid, 175
systemic treatment, 175
topical treatment, 175

Granuloma gravidarum, 188–191
Granuloma telangiectaticum, 188–191
Granulomatous rosacea, 76
Gynecomastia, 272–275, 272f
  consultative questions, 273
  course, 273
  differential diagnosis, 272
  epidemiology, 272
  laboratory examination, 272–273
  management, 273
  pathogenesis, 272
  physical lesions, 272
  pitfalls/complications/outcome expectations, 274–275
  treatment, 273–274

H
Hair loss. *See* Female pattern hair loss; Male pattern hair loss
Hair removal, 217
Hair transplantation, 104–105
Hairline design, 108
Hamartoma, 216, 222
Hemangioma, segmental, 180f
Hemangioma, ulcerated, 179f
Hemangiomas, 177
Hibernoma, 226
Hibiclens, 48
Hirsutism, 92
  consultative questions, 93
  course, 93
  differential diagnosis, 92–93
  epidemiology, 92
  laboratory tests, 93
  management, 93
    electrolysis, 94
    endocrinology, consultation with, 93
    just prior to treatment, 96
    laser hair removal technique, 95, 96–98
    nonlaser therapies, 93–94
    patient consultation, 95–96
    posttreatment instructions to patient, 98
  physical examination, 92
  pitfalls, 94f, 98–99
HIV lipodystrophy/facial lipoatrophy, 280–284
  consultative questions, 281
  course, 281
  dermatopathology, 280
  differential diagnosis, 281
  epidemiology, 280
  laboratory examination, 281
  management, 281–282
  pathogenesis, 280
  physical lesions, 280–281
  pitfalls, 283–284
  precipitating factors, 280
  prevention, 281
  treatments, 282–283
Homosalate, 7t
Hormones, 73
Human papillomavirus (HPV), 206–209
Hyaluronidase, 47
Hydroquinone, 9, 9t, 13, 140, 146, 151t, 160,
Hydroxy acid, 73
Hydroxycoumarins, 9t
Hylaform®, 15t
Hyperhidrosis, 86

botulinum toxin A, 88, 88f
  anesthesia, 88
  antiperspirant, 89
  botox, 89
  medications, 89
  surgery, 89
  treatment, 88–89, 88f, 89f
consultative questions, 87
course, 86
dermatopathology, 86
differential diagnosis, 86
epidemiology, 86
laboratory examination, 86, 86f
management, 87, 87f
oral medications, 87
pathogenesis, 86
physical findings, 86
pitfalls, 89–90
surgery, 88
topical medications, 87
Hyperhidrosis
  sites of, 90f
  treatment diagram, 87f
Hyperpigmentation
  and cryotherapy, 209
  and post-sclerotherapy, 200
Hypersensitive reactions, of soft tissue augmentation, 18
Hypertonic saline, 199, 200t, 201t
Hypertrichosis, 216, 217
Hypertrophic scars, 290
  clinical experience, 293
  differential diagnosis, 290
  vs. keloids, 290t
  laboratory examination, 290
  laser, 291f, 292, 292f
  management, 291
  physical examination, 290
  pulsed dye laser, 292t
  studies, 292
Hypopigmentation, 67, 187f
  and cryotherapy, 209, 236
  and laser treatments, 218

I
Ice-Pick/Boxcar Scar
Icodin, 58
Idebenone, 8
Imiquimod, 179, 207, 291, 291T
Inamed Corp, 14t
Inamed Corp., 15t
Infantile hemangioma (IH), 177, 177f, 178f
  ancillary tests, 178
  complications, 178
  course, 178
  dermatopathology, 177
  differential diagnoses, 177
  epidemiology, 177
  laboratory tests, 177
  management, 178–180
  physical examination, 177
  pitfalls to avoid, 180
Intense pulsed light lasers
  for pseudofolliculitis, 101
  for Becker's nevus, 218
  for cherry and spider angiomas, 172

for port-wine stains, 185
for postsclerotherapy hyperpigmentation, 201–202, 201f, 202f
for venous lakes, 204
Interferon-α, 179
Interlocking Ls repair, 308
Intralesional 5-fluorouracil (5-FU), 291, 291t
Intralesional steroid injection, 74
Intralesional triamcinolone acetonides, 291, 291t
Iopidine, 28
IPL. *See* Intense pulsed light
Ipsen Limited, 21t
Isolagen, 15t
Isopropyl alcohol, 48
Isotretinoin, 40, 58, 74, 77

J

Jessner, 30t, 35f
Jessner peels, 141, 160
Juvederm™, 15t

K

Keflex, 17, 46
Keloids
    differential diagnosis, 290
    vs. hypertrophic scars, 290t
    vs. keloids, 290t
    laboratory examination, 290
    laser, 291f, 292, 292f
    management, 291
    physical examination, 290
    pulsed dye laser, 292t
    studies, 292
Keratinocytes, 140, 222
Keratolytic agents, 73
Keratoses
    seborrheic, 223
Keratosis follicularis spinulosa decalvans (KFSD), 181
Keratosis pilaris atrophicans (KPA), 181, 181f, 182f
    course, 181
    dermatopathology, 181
    differential diagnosis, 181
    epidemiology, 181
    management, 182
    pathogenesis, 181
    physical examination, 181
    pitfalls to avoid, 182
Keratosis pilaris atrophicans faciei (KPAF), 181
Kerotoses
    actinic, 206
    seborrheic, 206, 234–237
Kindler syndrome, 67
Koenen's tumor, 212
Kojic acid, 9t, 10, 141
KTP laser. *See* Potassium-titanyl-phosphate laser

L

L-M-X-4 and 5, 17
Lactic acid, 182
Lactic acid, 9t
LAMB syndrome, 144
Lanzhou Institute of Biological Products, 21t
Laser hair removal

and hirsutism, 95
and pseudofolliculitis, 100f, 101, 101f
technique, 96–98
Laser light firing, 93f
Laser safety, 97f
    nonablative laser resurfacing, 41
    for ablative fractional laser resurfacing, 59
        adverse side effects, 60, 60f
        follow-up, 59–60, 59f
        infection, 60, 61f
        nonfacial skin, 60–61
        postoperative care, 57f, 58f, 59
Laser therapy
    for dermatochalasis, 65
    for granuloma faciale, 175
    for Poikiloderma of Civatte, 68, 68f
    for sebaceous hyperplasia, 82–83, 82f, 83f
Laser-assisted photodynamic therapy, 82
Lasers, 74
Lecithins, 9t
Lentigines, 144
    chemical peels, 146
    consultative questions, 145–146
    course, 145
    cryotherapy, 146
    differential diagnosis, 145
    epidemiology, 144
    laboratory examination, 145
    laser and light source treatment, 146–147
    management, 145
    pathogenesis, 144
    pathology, 144
    physical lesions, 144
    pitfalls to avoid/complications/management/outcome expectations,
        147–148
    vs. seborrheic keratosis, 235
    topical medications, 145–146
Lentigo simplex, 144
LEOPARD syndrome, 144
Lichen planus (LP), 262–264
    course, 263, 264f
    dermatopathology, 262
    differential diagnosis, 262
    epidemiology, 262
    laboratory data, 262
    management, 263
    pathogenesis, 262
    physical examination, 262, 262f, 263f
Lichen striatus, 223
Licorice extract, 9t, 10
Lidocaine, 47, 59, 107
    for wart removal, 208
Life Cell Corp., 14t
Light treatment, of acne vulgaris, 72f, 73f, 74–75, 75f
Light cryotherapy, 82
Linear focal elastosis.
Linear threading, 18
Linoleic acid, 9t
Lipectomy, 283
Lipoma, 226–228
    consultative questions, 227
    course, 227
    differential diagnosis, 226
    epidemiology, 226
    laboratory data, 227
    pathology, 226

physical examination, 226, 226f, 227f, 228f
    pitfalls, 228
    treatment, 227–228, 227f, 228f
Liposarcoma, 226
Liposuction, 88
    for cellulite, 277
    for gynecomastia, 274
    for HIV lipodystrophy/facial lipoatrophy, 283
    for lipoma, 227
Liver spots. *See* Solar lentigos
LLLT. *See* Low level light laser therapy
Lobular capillary hemangioma, 188–191
Long-pulsed alexandrite laser, 101
Long-pulsed Nd:YAG laser, 101
Low level light laser therapy (LLLT), 133, 133f, 134f
    mechanism of action, 133
    pearls of wisdom, 133
    use of, 133
Lower extremity telangiectasias, 198–202
Lower eyelid snap back test, 22–23
Lower face, 3
Lower lid horizontal laxity, 64
LP. *See* Lichen planus
Lux 1, 540 nm laser, 56, 56t

M
Macules, 216, 223
Madelung's disease, 226
Male pattern hair loss, 103. *See also* Female
    pattern hair loss
    consult, 105
    differential diagnosis, 103
    epidemiology, 103
    vs. female pattern hair loss, 129, 129t, 131f
    hair transplantation, 104–105
    laboratory examination, 104
    medical therapy, 104, 104t
    natural progression, 103
    pathogenesis, 103
    physical examination, 103, 103f, 105f
    surgical procedure
        corrective hair transplant surgery, 110, 110t
        day of procedure, 106
        donor harvesting techniques, 106, 106f, 106t, 107t
        donor region, anesthesia in, 106
        follicular unit extraction (FUE), 107, 107t
        graft creation, 107
        graft placement, 108–109, 113f
        hairline design, 108
        post hair transplant side effects, 109
        postoperative period, 109
        postsurgical period after sutures/staples
          removed, 109–110
        preoperative instructions, 106
        rare side effects, 109
        recipient region, anesthesia in, 108
        recipient site creation, 108, 112f
McCune–Albright syndrome, 136
McGhan Medical, 15t
MED. *See* Minimal erythema dose
Medial orbicularis oculi, 24, 24f
Medicis, 15t
Medicis Esthetics, 21t
Medium-depth peel, 30t, 33, 34f, 35f
Medy-Tox, Inc, 21t

Melanin
    in post-sclerotherapy hyperpigmentation, 200
    in seborrheic keratosis, 236
Melanocyte cytotoxic agents, 9t
Melanocyte transfer inhibition, 9t
Melanoma
    vs. seborrheic keratosis, 235
    venous lakes and, 203
    warts and, 206
Melanophages, 144
Melasma, 149, 149f
    ablative laser, 152
    chemical peels, 151–152
    consultative questions, 150
    course, 150
    dermatopathology, 149
    differential diagnosis, 150
    epidemiology, 149
    fractional resurfacing, 152, 153f
    laboratory examination, 150
    management, 150, 150f, 151f, 152f
    pathogenesis, 149
    physical lesions, 149
    pitfalls, 152–153
    Q-switched laser, 152
    topical treatment, 151, 151t
MEND. *See* Microscopic epidermal necrotic debris
Mentalis muscle, 26, 27f, 28f
Mentor Corporation, 15t
Mequinol, 9t
Merz Pharma, 14t, 21t
Mesotherapy
    for cellulite, 278
Methanthelium bromide, 87
Methyl aminolevulinic acid (MAL), 254
Methyl anthranilate, 7t
Metronidazole, 77
Mexoryl SX, 7t
Mexoryl XL, 7t
Microdermabrasion, 74, 229, 287
Microscopic epidermal necrotic debris (MEND), 52
Microthermal treatment zones (MTZs), 52
Midface, 3
Mid-infrared lasers, 40f, 41
Mild atrophy, 67
Milia, 229–230
    consultative questions, 230
    course, 230
    epidemiology, 229
    pathogenesis, 229
    pathology, 229
    physical examination, 229, 229f, 230f
    pitfalls, 230
    treatment, 230, 230f
Minimal erythema dose (MED), 8
Minocycline, 73, 77
Minoxidil, 104, 104t, 127–128, 127t, 131, 133
Mixed dermal melasma, 149
Mixed superficial and deep hemangioma (MH), 177
Mohs micrographic surgery, 254, 257–258
Monobenzone, 9t
Morphea, 265–267
    course, 266
    dermatopathology, 266
    differential diagnosis, 265
    epidemiology, 265

laboratory data, 265–266
management, 266, 266f
pathogenesis, 265
physical examination, 265, 265f
pitfall, 267
MTZs. *See* Microthermal treatment zones
Mulberry extract, 9t
Muscle groups, 23
  forehead, 23–24
  glabellar complex, 24, 24f
  nasolabial fold, 25–26, 27f
  neck, 26–27, 28f
  perioral region, 26, 27f, 28f
  periorbital region, 24–25, 25f
  upper nasal root, 25, 26f
Myasthenia gravis, 22
Myobloc, 21t

N

NAFR. *See* Nonablative fractional laser resurfacing
Nasal sebaceous hyperplasia. *See* Rhinophyma
Nasolabial fold, 25–26, 27f
Nd:YAG laser, 99, 193
  for seborrheic keratosis, 236
Neck, 26–27, 28f
Neurofibromas (NF), 231–234
  consultative questions, 232
  course, 232
  differential diagnosis, 231
  epidemiology, 231
  laboratory data, 232
  management, 232
  pathogenesis, 231
  pathology, 231
  physical examination, 231, 231f
  pitfalls, 223–224
  treatment, 232–233, 232f
Neurofibromatosis, 136
Neuronox, 21t
Nevus araneus, 170–173
Nevus, Becker's, 216–218
Nevus, epidermal, 222–225, 235
Nevus fuscoceruleus ophthalmomaxillaris, 154
Nevus of Ota, 154
  consultative questions, 155
  course, 155
  differential diagnosis, 154
  epidemiology, 154
  laboratory examination, 155
  management, 155
  pathogenesis, 154
  pathology, 154
  physical lesions, 154
  pitfalls, 157
  topical treatment, 155
  treatment, 155–156
Nevus sebaceous, 223
Niacinamide, 9t, 10
Nonablative fractional laser resurfacing (NAFR)
  anesthesia, 54
  contraindications, 53
  dermatopathology, 52, 52f
  devices, 56, 56t
  indications, 52
  mechanism of action, 52, 52f

  medications, 53–54
  postoperative care, 55
  preoperative evaluation, 52–53, 53f, 54f
  preoperative preparation, 54
  procedural tips, 54–55
  treatment pearls, 55–56
Nonablative fractional lasers, 57
Nonablative fractional resurfacing, 39, 60
Nonablative laser resurfacing, 39, 39f
  adverse side effects, 4, 41f1
    postoperative care, 41–42
  indications, 40
  laser safety, 41
  preoperative evaluation, 40
  prophylaxis/anesthesia, 40
    mid-infrared lasers, 40f, 41
Nonfacial skin, 60–61
Non-FDA approved medications, for female pattern hair loss, 128
Non-hypersensitive reactions, of soft tissue augmentation, 18–19
Nonlaser therapy, 93
  depilation, 94
  topical eflornithine, 94
Norwood classification, 103f

O

Octocrylene, 7t
Octyl methoxycinnamate, 7t
Octyl salicylate, 7t
Ocular rosacea, 76
Oral medications
  in hyperhidrosis, 87
Oral therapy, 165
Orbicularis oculi, 24–25, 25f
Orbicularis oculi tone, 64
Orbicularis oris, 26, 27f, 28f
Oxybenzone, 7t

P

p^{53} tumor suppressor gene, 252
PABA. *See* Para-aminobenzoic acid
Padimate O, 7t
Palmoplantar warts, 206–209
Palomar Medical Technologies, 56, 56t, 79
Paper mulberry, 10
Papules
  in angiofibromas, 212
  in epidermal nevus, 223
  in warts, 206
Papulopustular rosacea, 76
Para-aminobenzoic acid (PABA), 7t
Partial tears, 308
Patient consultation, 95
  prior to treatment, 95–96
PDL. *See* Pulsed dye laser
PDT. *See* Photodynamic therapy
Pearly penile papules, 212
Peel types, 33
  and clinical indications, 30t
Peeling agent characteristics, 30t
Penicillium, 10
Perifollicular erythema, characteristic posttreatment, 93f
Perioral dermatitis, 76
Periorbital region, 24–25, 25f, 26, 27f, 28f
Periorbital rhytides, 55f

Periungual fibromas, 212
Perlane, 15t
Perlane I ™, 15t
Peutz–Jeghers syndrome, 144
PHACE syndrome, 178
Phenol, 30t
Phenyl benzimidazole sulfonic acid, 7t
Photodynamic therapy (PDT), 75
Photodynamic therapy, 254, 258, 269
Phototherapy, 75, 165
Phymatous rosacea. *See* Sebaceous hyperplasia
Physical screen, 8, 8t
Pigmentary changes, in face, 4, 6f
PIH. *See* Postinflammatory hyperpigmentation; Pregnancy-induced
    hypertension
Pilar cysts, 220, 226
Pimecrolimus, 164
Pityrosporum ovale, 10
Plane warts, 206–209
Plantar warts, 206
Plaques
    in angiofibroma, 212
    in Becker's nevus, 216
    in seborrheic keratosis, 235
Platysma muscle complex, 26–27, 28f
POC. *See* Poikiloderma of Civatte
Podophyllin, 224
Podophyllotoxin, 207
Poikiloderma of Civatte (POC), 67
    consultative questions, 68
    course, 68
    dermatopathology, 67
    differential diagnosis, 67
    epidemiology, 67
    management, 68
    pathogenesis, 67
    physical examination, 67, 67f, 68f
    pitfalls, 68–69, 69f
    pretreatment, 68f
    treatment, 68, 68f
Polidocanol, 199, 200, 200t
Poly-L-lactic acid, 18
Pontocaine. *See* Topical tetracaine
Port-wine stains (PWS), 183, 184f, 185f, 186f
    ancillary tests, 183
    course, 183
    dermatopathology, 183
    differential diagnosis, 183
    epidemiology, 183
    management, 183
    physical examination, 183
    pitfalls to avoid, 183
Post hair transplant side effects, 109
Postinflammatory erythema
    and curettage, 237f
Postinflammatory hyperpigmentation (PIH), 158, 158f
    chemical peels, 160–161
    consultative questions, 159
    course, 159
    dermatopathology, 158
    differential diagnosis, 158
    epidemiology, 158
    laboratory examination, 158
    lasers, 161
        treatment, 218, 233
    management, 159

pathogenesis, 158
physical lesions, 158
pitfalls to avoid/complications/management/outcome
    expectations, 161
sunprotection, 159
topical treatment, 160
Postsclerotherapy hyperpigmentation (PSH), 200
Potassium-titanyl-phosphate laser, 79, 193
Prednisone, 130, 179
Pregnancy
    and telangiectasias, 198, 201
Pregnancy-induced hypertension (PIH), 60
Prevelle silk, 15t
Primary androgen-producing neoplasms, 92
Procerus, 24, 24f
Propantheline, 87
Prophylactic antibiotics, 49, 53
Propranolol, 179
Prosigne, 21t
Prostate cancer
    prophylaxis in, 273
Proteus syndrome, 226
Pseudofolliculitis, 99
    course, 100
    dermatopathology, 100
    differential diagnosis, 100
    epidemiology, 99
    laboratory examination, 100
    management, 100
    pathogenesis, 99
    physical lesions, 100
    pitfalls, 101–102, 101f, 102f
    treatment
        laser hair removal, 100f, 101, 101f
        shaving cessation, 100
        shaving technique, modification of, 100–101
        topical treatment, 101
Pseudofolliculitis, and etrology, 101f
Pseudogynecomastia, 272
Pseudo-ochronosis, 34, 159f
Psoralen and ultraviolet A (PUVA), 165, 175
Psoriasis, 267–270, 267f, 268f
    course, 268
    differential diagnosis, 268
    epidemiology, 267
    laboratory data, 268
    management, 268–269, 269f
    pathogenesis, 268
    physical examination, 268
    pitfalls, 270
Psuedogynecomastia, 274
Pulsed carbon dioxide laser, 250
Pulsed dye laser (PDL)
    for acne vulgaris, 75
    for angiofibroma, 213
    for angiokeratomas, 169
    for cherry and spider angiomas, 171
    for facial telangiectasia, 203, 203f, 205f
    for facial telangiectasias, 192
    for hypertrophic scars/keloids, 292t
    for infantile hemangiomas, 179
    for keratosis pilaris atrophicans, 182
    for morphea, 266
    for Poikiloderma of Civatte, 68
    for port-wine stains, 185
    for psorias, 269

for pyogenic granuloma, 189
for rosacea, 78
for sebacious hyperplasia, 82
for striae distensae, 287
for telangiectasias, 201
for venous lakes, 203, 205f
for warts, 206f, 208, 208f, 209f
for warts, 208
Punch excision, 213
Purpura, 204, 208
PUVA. *See* Psoralen and ultraviolet A
Pyogenic granuloma (PG), 188, 188f, 189f
    biopsy-proven, 191f
    course, 188
    dermatopathology, 188
    differential diagnoses, 188
    epidemiology, 188
    laser treatment, 189
    management, 189
    pathogenesis, 188
    physical examination, 188
    pitfalls to avoid, 189
    surgical treatment, 189
    vs. venous lakes, 203

Q
Q-Med AB, 15t
Q-switched lasers, 152
    alexandrite
        for Becker's nevus, 217, 218f
        for café au lait macules, 137, 138
        for dermatosis papulosa nigra, 242
        for epidermal nevus, 225
        for nevus of Ota, 155, 156
        for seborrheic keratosis, 236
    argon
        and granuloma faciale, 175
    Nd:YAG
        for Becker's nevus, 217, 218f
        for café au lait macules, 137, 138
        and ephilides, 142
        and lentigines, 146
        for nevus of Ota, 155
        for tattoo removal, 300t, 302
    ruby
        for Becker's nevus, 217, 218f
        for dermatosis papulosa nigra, 242
        for ephilides, 142
        for lentigines, 146, 147
        for nevus of Ota, 155
        for seborrheic keratosis, 236
        for tattoo removal, 300t, 302t

R
Radiation dermatitis, 67
Radiation therapy, 254
Radiesse™, 15t
Radiofrequency (RF) technology, 62
Radiotherapy, 258
Re-epithelialization, 49
Reloxin, 21t
Renova, 9
Restylane, 15t
Restylane-L, 15t

Rete ridges
    in epidermal nevus, 222
Reticular veins, 198–202
Reticulated hyperpigmentation, 67
Retin-A, 182
Retinaldehyde, 8, 9
Retinoic acid, 8–9, 9t, 10, 12
    chemical structures of, 8f
Retinoids, 73, 141, 151, 151t, 160, 182
Retinol, 8
Retinyl esters, 8
RF technology. *See* Radiofrequency (RF) technology
Rhinophyma, 76, 76f, 77–78
Rhytides, 58
Rosacea, 76
    course, 77
    dermatopathology, 77
    differential diagnosis, 76
    epidemiology, 76
    management, 77
        surgical therapy, 77–79
        systemic therapy, 77
        topical therapy, 77
    pathogenesis, 76
    physical examination, 76
Rothmund–Thomson syndrome, 67
Ruby spot, 170–173. *See also* Cherry angiomas
Russell–Silver syndrome, 136

S
Salicylic acid, 73, 207
Saline
    and warts, 207, 208
    and telangiectasias, 201
Scarring
    from angiofibroma treatment, 214
    from surgical incision, 224, 228
    from wart removal, 207t, 208, 209
SCC. *See* Squamous cell carcinoma
Sclerotherapy, 199–201, 198f, 199f, 200f, 200t, 201t, 204
Scoliosis, 232
Sculptra™, 15t
Sebaceous cyst, 219
Sebaceous hyperplasia, 76, 77, 81, 81f
    consultative questions, 81
    course, 81
    differential diagnosis, 81
    epidemiology, 81
    for seborrheic keratosis, 236f
    laboratory examination, 81
    management, 82
    pathogenesis, 81
    pathology, 81
    physical lesions, 81
    pitfalls, 83
    treatments, 82
        destructive modalities, 82
        laser therapy, 82–83, 82f, 83f
Seborrheic dermatitis, 76
Seborrheic keratosis, 234–237. *See also* Dermatosis papulosa nigra
    consultative questions, 235
    course, 235
    differential diagnosis, 235
    epidemiology, 234
    vs. epidermal nevus, 223, 235

management, 235–236
pathology, 235
physical examination, 235
pitfalls, 237
treatment, 236
vs. warts, 206
Segmental hemangioma, 180f
Senile hemangiomas, 170–173
Serial puncture, 18
Serial salicylic acid peels, 74
Sharplan FeatherTouch, 169
Shave biopsies and excisions
for angiofibromas, 213
for epidermal nevus, 224
for lipoma, 227, 227f
for neurofibromas, 236
for seborrheic keratosis, 236
Shaving cessation, 100
Shaving technique, modification of, 100–101
Short-pulsed erbium, 287
Silicone, 18
Silicone sheeting, 291, 291t
Silikone-1000, 15t
Skin grafts, 225f
Skin lightening agents, 9–11
Skin testing, 16
Skin turnover acceleration, 9t
Skin types
and Becker's nevus, 218
Smoothbeam, 41
SNAP-25, 21
Sodium morrhuate, 199
Sodium sulfacetamide, 73, 77
Sodium tetradecyl sulfate, 199, 200t, 201t
Soft tissue augmentation
adverse reactions
hypersensitive, 18
non-hypersensitive, 18–19
technique complications, 19
anesthesia, 16f, 17
degree of correction, 18
duration of correction, 18
ideal filler, 14, 14t–15t
injection technique, 18, 18f, 19f
level of injection, 17–18, 17f, 18f
mechanism of action, 14
preoperative evaluation, 15–16
procedural medications, 17
skin testing, 16
treatment pearls, 19
Softform, 15t
Solar lentigo *vs.* ephelid, 145t
Solar lentigos, 144
Solta Medical, Inc., 56, 56t
Soltice Neurosciences, 21t
Sotradechol, 200
Soy, 10
Soybean/milk extracts, 9t
SPF. *See* Sun protective factor
Spider angiomas, 170–173, 171f
Spider telangiectasia, 170–173
Spinal dysraphism, 227
Spironolactone, 73, 128
Squamous cell carcinoma (SCC), 256–258
consultative questions, 257
course, 257

dermatopathology, 257
differential diagnosis, 256, 257f
epidemiology, 256
vs. epidermal nevus, 223
laboratory data, 257
management, 257–258, 258f, 259f
pathogenesis, 256
physical examination, 256, 256f
pitfalls, 258
vs. seborrheic keratosis, 235
vs. warts, 206, 207
Starch-iodine test, 88
Starlux Lux G handpiece, 79
Steroid rosacea, 76
Stockings, elastic compression, 200
Strawberry, 177–180
Stretch marks. *See* Striae distensae
Stria alba, 287
Stria rubra, 286–287, 287f
Striae distensae, 285, 285f
consultative questions, 286
course, 286
differential diagnosis, 286
epidemiology, 285
laboratory examination, 286
management, 286
microdermabrasion, 287
pathogenesis, 285
pathology, 285
physical lesions, 285
pitfalls, 288
topical treatment, 287
treatment, 286–287
Stromelysin, 9
Sturge–Weber syndrome (SWS), 184
Subcision, 278
Subcutaneous fat, in lipoma, 226
Subcutaneous fat, 15t
Subcutaneous fat atrophy, 5
Sulfur, 73
Sulisobenzone, 7t
Sun exposure
and sclerotherapy, 200
and venous lakes, 203
Sun protective factor (SPF), 8
Sunscreen, 7–8, 7f, 7t
Superficial hemangioma (SH), 177, 179
Superficial peel, 30t, 32f, 33, 33f
Surgery
in hyperhidrosis, 88
Surgical excision, 175
Surgical procedure, for hair transplantation
corrective hair transplant surgery, 110, 110t
day of procedure, 106
donor harvesting techniques, 106, 106f, 106t, 107t
donor region, anesthesia in, 106
follicular unit extraction (FUE), 107, 107t
graft creation, 107
graft placement, 108–109, 113f
hairline design, 108
post hair transplant side effects, 109
postoperative period, 109
postsurgical period after sutures/staples
removed, 109–110
preoperative instructions, 106
rare side effects, 109

recipient region, anesthesia in, 108
recipient site creation, 108, 112f
Surgical therapy
  of acne vulgaris, 74
  for angiofibroma, 213
  for Becker's nevus, 217
   for Dermatochalasis, 64f, 65
  for epidermal inclusion cysts, 220
  for epidermal nevus, 224
  for lipoma, 227, 227f, 228f
  for neurofibroma, 232–233, 232f
  of Rosacea, 76f, 77–79, 79f, 80f
  for venous lakes, 204
  for wart removal, 207–209
Syringoma, 238, 238f
  consultative questions, 239
  course, 239
  differential diagnosis, 238
  epidemiology, 238
  laboratory examination, 238
  management, 239
  pathogenesis, 238
  pathology, 238
  physical lesions, 238, 238f
  pitfalls, 239f, 240, 240f
  treatment, 239–240
Systemic lupus erythematosus, 76
Systemic therapy
  of acne vulgaris, 73–74
  of Rosacea, 77

T
Tacrolimus, 164
Tacrolimus ointment, 175
Talkesthesia, 17
Tap water iontophoresis, 87
Tattoo removal, 300, 300f
  adverse effects/precautions, 303, 304f, 305f, 306, 307f
  consultative questions, 300–301
  laser therapy, 300t
  management, 301
  pitfalls, 303–304
  posttreatment care, 302
  pretreatment assessment, 301
  tattoo treatment, 302, 302t, 303f, 304f
  treatment, 301–302, 303f
Tazarotene, 9, 73, 182
TCA peels. *See* Trichloroacetic acid peels
Telangiectases, 67
Telangiectasias, 78–79, 78f, 79f, 80f
  lower extremity, 198–202
    epidemiology, 198
    laboratory data, 198
    management, 199–202, 198f, 199f, 200f
    pathophysiology, 198
    physical examination, 198
Telangiectatic matting ™, 201
Telogen effluvium, 129, 130–131
Tetracycline, 73, 77
Thrombophlebitis, 198
Thyroid-stimulating hormone (TSH), 163
Tissue tightening, 62
  candidate selection, 62
  clinical pearls, 63
  mechanism of action, 62

procedure, 62
  checklist, 62–63
  side effects, 63
Topical 5-fluorouracil, 254
Topical eflornithine, 94
Topical imiquimod, 254
Topical medications, in hyperhidrosis, 87
Topical proparacaine, 47, 59
Topical retinoic acid, 32
Topical tetracaine, 47, 59
Topical therapy
  of acne vulgaris, 73
  for dermatochalasis, 65
  for Poikiloderma of Civatte, 68
  of pseudofolliculitis, 101
  of Rosacea, 77
Topical treatment options
  application techniques, 11–12
  complications, 12
  contraindications, 11
  ideal candidate, 11
  indications, 11
  less than ideal candidate, 11
  mechanism of action, 7–11
  posttreatment care, 12
  pretreatment evaluation, 11
  treatment pearls, 12–13
Topical tretinoin, 46, 146
Torn earlobe, 308
  key consultative questions, 308
  management, 308
  pitfalls to avoid/complications/management/outcome expectations, 309
  treatments, 308–309, 308f, 309f, 310f
Traditional PDL, 78
Traditional resurfacing, 39
Tretinoin, 9, 46, 54, 73
  and epidermal nevus, 224
  and milium, 230
TriActive Laserdermology, 278
Triamcinolone acetonide, 179
Triangularis muscles, 26, 27f, 28f
Trichloracetic acid (TCA) peels, 30t, 74
  for wart removal, 207
Triluma, 146
Trolamine salicylate, 7t
TSH. *See* Thyroid-stimulating hormone
Tuberous sclerosis, 136
Tuberous sclerosis, 213, 213f
Tumors, 220
Tylenol, 109
Tyrosinase, 9
Tyrosinase inhibitors, 9t

U
Ulcerated hemangioma, 179f
Ultra, 15t
Ultra Plus, 15t
Ultra Plus XC, 15t
Ultra XC, 15t
Ultrasound, 198
Ultraviolet A (UVA), 67
Ultraviolet B (UVB), 67
Upper and midfacial musculature, anatomical illustration
  of, 22f
Upper face, 2–3

Upper nasal root, 25, 26f
U.S. Food and Drug Administration, 94
UVA. *See* Ultraviolet A
UVB exposure, 9
UVB. *See* Ultraviolet B

V

Valacyclovir, 46
Valacyclovir, 54
Valtrex, 17, 32
Vaniqa. *See* Topical eflornithine
Vaporizing tool, 44
Variable-pulse PDL, 78
Varicose veins, 198–202
Vascular alterations
　　lower extremity telangiectasias, 198–202
　　reticular and varicose veins, 198–202
　　venous lakes, 203–205
　　warts, 206–209
Vascular alterations
　　venous lakes, 203–205
　　warts, 206–209
Vascular ectasia, 77
Vascular lasers, 39
Vascular rosacea, 76
Vascular spider, 170–173
Vaseline, 34
Veins, reticular and varicose, 198–202
VelaSmooth system, 278
Venous lakes, 203–205
　　course, 203
　　dermatopathology, 203
　　differential diagnosis, 203
　　epidemiology, 203
　　epiluminescence microscopy (ELM), 203
　　management, 203–204, 203f, 204f, 205f
　　physical examination, 203
　　pitfalls, 204
Venous obstruction, 198
Venous valvular incompetence, 198
Verruca, 223, 235
Vincristine, 179
Vitamin C, 8
Vitamin E, 8
Vitiligo, 163
　　consultative questions, 164
　　course, 163–164
　　dermatopathology, 163
　　differential diagnosis, 163
　　epidemiology, 163

laboratory examination, 163
laser therapy
　　excimer laser, 165
management, 164
oral therapy, 165
pathogenesis, 163
phototherapy, 165
physical lesions, 163
pitfalls to avoid/complications/management/
　　outcome expectations, 166
prevention, 164
surgical treatments, 165
topical treatment, 164

W

Warts, 206–209
　　course, 207
　　dermatopathology, 206
　　differential diagnosis, 206
　　epidemiology, 206
　　pathogenesis, 206
　　physical examination, 206
　　pitfalls, 209
　　treatment, 207–209, 206f, 207f, 205f, 209f
Watson's syndrome, 136
Westerhof's syndrome, 136
Wickham's striae, 262
Wood's lamp evaluation, 31, 31f, 163
Wydase. *See* Hyaluronidase

X

Xanthelasma palpebrarum. *See* Xanthelasmas
Xanthelasmas, 243
　　course, 244
　　dermatopathology, 244
　　differential diagnosis, 244
　　epidemiology, 243
　　management, 244
　　pathogenesis, 243
　　physical examination, 244
　　pitfalls, 244
Xeomin, 21t

Z

Z-plasty repair, 308
Zyderm®, 15t
Zyplast®, 15t